Clinical Management of
VITILIGO

Clinical Management of
VITILIGO

Editors

Madhulika Mhatre
MBBS MD(Gold Medalist) FRGUHS(Aesthetic Dermatology)
Director and Consultant Dermatologist
Skin Saga Centre for Dermatology
Mumbai, Maharashtra, India
Founding Secretary – Vitiligo Foundation of India

Sqn Ldr (Dr) Aseem Sharma
MBBS MD DNB MBA
Director and Chief Dermatologist
Skin Saga Center for Dermatology
Director, ADMIRE Academy
Ex-Assistant Professor of Dermatology, LTMMC and GH
Mumbai, Maharashtra, India

Foreword

John E Harris

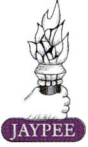

JAYPEE BROTHERS MEDICAL PUBLISHERS
The Health Sciences Publisher
New Delhi | London

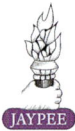 **Jaypee Brothers Medical Publishers (P) Ltd**

Headquarters
EMCA House
23/23-B, Ansari Road, Daryaganj
New Delhi 110 002, India
Landline: +91-11-23272143, +91-11-23272703
+91-11-23282021, +91-11-23245672
E-mail: jaypee@jaypeebrothers.com

Corporate Office
Jaypee Brothers Medical Publishers (P) Ltd.
4838/24, Ansari Road, Daryaganj
New Delhi 110 002, India
Phone: +91-11-43574357
Fax: +91-11-43574314
E-mail: jaypee@jaypeebrothers.com

Overseas Office
JP Medical Ltd.
83, Victoria Street, London
SW1H 0HW (UK)
Phone: +44-20 3170 8910
Fax: +44(0)20 3008 6180
E-mail: info@jpmedpub.com

Website: www.jaypeebrothers.com
Website: www.jaypeedigital.com

© 2025, Jaypee Brothers Medical Publishers

The views and opinions expressed in this book are solely those of the original contributor(s)/author(s) and do not necessarily represent those of editor(s) or publisher of the book.

All rights reserved. No part of this publication may be reproduced, stored or transmitted in any form or by any means, electronic, mechanical, photocopying, recording or otherwise, without the prior permission in writing of the publishers.

All brand names and product names used in this book are trade names, service marks, trademarks or registered trademarks of their respective owners. The publisher is not associated with any product or vendor mentioned in this book.

Medical knowledge and practice change constantly. This book is designed to provide accurate, authoritative information about the subject matter in question. However, readers are advised to check the most current information available on procedures included and check information from the manufacturer of each product to be administered, to verify the recommended dose, formula, method and duration of administration, adverse effects and contraindications. It is the responsibility of the practitioner to take all appropriate safety precautions. Neither the publisher nor the author(s)/editor(s) assume any liability for any injury and/or damage to persons or property arising from or related to use of material in this book.

This book is sold on the understanding that the publisher is not engaged in providing professional medical services. If such advice or services are required, the services of a competent medical professional should be sought.

Every effort has been made where necessary to contact holders of copyright to obtain permission to reproduce copyright material. If any have been inadvertently overlooked, the publisher will be pleased to make the necessary arrangements at the first opportunity.

Inquiries for bulk sales may be solicited at: jaypee@jaypeebrothers.com

Clinical Management of Vitiligo / **Madhulika Mhatre, Sqn Ldr (Dr) Aseem Sharma**

First Edition: **2025**

ISBN: 978-93-6616-883-8

Printed at: Samrat Offset Pvt. Ltd.

Dedication

To the late Dr Sanjeev Mulekar, whose unparalleled expertise in vitiligo has been a guiding light, and to the late Dr SC Sharma, my father, who taught us the true essence of life.

CONTRIBUTORS

Aaqib Aslam MBBS MD(Dermatology)
Consultant
Q-Derma Skin Clinic
Srinagar, Jammu and Kashmir, India

Abhijit Saha MBBS MD
Consultant Pediatric Dermatologist
Institute of Child Health
Kolkata, West Bengal, India

Sqn Ldr (Dr) Aseem Sharma MBBS MD DNB MBA
Director and Chief Dermatologist
Skin Saga Center for Dermatology
Director, ADMIRE Academy
Ex-Assistant Professor of Dermatology, LTMMC and GH
Mumbai, Maharashtra, India

Davinder Parsad MBBS MD
Professor
Department of Dermatology, Venereology and Leprology
Postgraduate Institute of Medical Education and Research
Chandigarh, India

Deepak Mohana MBBS MD(Skin and VD) PGDHA
Director
Dr Mohana's Skin Hair and Laser Center
Indore, Madhya Pradesh, India

Deepti Ghia MBBS MD DNB FCPS DDV
Consultant Dermatologist
South Mumbai Dermatology
Jaslok Hospital
Mumbai, Maharashtra, India

Iltefat H Hamzavi MBBS MD FAAD
Consultant Dermatologist, Henry Ford Hospital-Detroit, Michigan
Hamzavi Dermatology Specialists-SE Michigan
Founding Board Member Global Vitiligo Foundation
Clinical Associate Professor
Wayne State University SOM
Global Vitiligo Foundation –
Co-founder and Past President
Hidradenitis Suppurativa Foundation –
Past President

Imran Majid MBBS MD FRCP(Edinburgh)
Director
CUTIS Institute of Dermatology
Srinagar, Jammu and Kashmir, India

Kanika Sahni MBBS MD
Additional Professor
Department of Dermatology and Venereology
All India Institute of Medical Sciences
New Delhi, India

Koushik Lahiri MBBS DVD(Calcutta) FIAD FFAADV iFAAD FRCP(Glasgow) FRCP(Edinburgh) FRCP(London)
Adjunct Professor and Distinguished Academician of Apollo Hospitals Educational and Research Foundation (AHERF)
President, PsychoDermatology Association of India (PDAI), (2025–2027)
President, IADVL WB (2023–2024)
Director, International Society of Dermatology (2021–2025)

Madhulika Mhatre MBBS MD(Gold Medalist) FRGUHS(Aesthetic Dermatology)
Director and Consultant Dermatologist
Skin Saga Centre for Dermatology
Mumbai, Maharashtra, India
Founding Secretary – Vitiligo Foundation of India

Mansi M Bhatt MBBS MD
Consultant Dermatologist
Dermacare Clinic
Mumbai, Maharashtra, India

Maya Shriram Tulpule MBBS MS DA
Consultant, Sahawas Hospital
President and Founder
Shweta Association – Vitiligo Patient Support Group
Pune, Maharashtra, India

Mukesh D Shah MBBS MD DVD DDV FCPS
Senior Consultant Dermatologist and Director
Manek Skin Clinic
Kalyan, Maharashtra, India

Mukta Tulpule MBBS DDV
Consultant Dermatologist
Sahawas Hospital
Honorary Advisory Dermatologist
Shweta Association – Vitiligo Patient Support Group
Pune, Maharashtra, India

Munish Paul MBBS MD
Consultant – Dermatology
Manipal Hospitals, Dwarka
Consultant – Dermatology
Dr Paul's Skin Laser Centre,
Paschim Vihar
New Delhi, India

Muthu Sendhil Kumaran MBBS MD
Professor
Department of Dermatology, Venereology, and Leprology
Postgraduate Institute of Medical Education and Research
Chandigarh, India

Narayanan Baskaran MBBS MD
Senior Resident
Department of Dermatology, Venereology, and Leprology
Sree Balaji Medical College and Hospital
Chennai, Tamil Nadu, India

Neha Akhoon MBBS MD Pharmacology (AFMC)
Resident
Department of Dermatology, Venereology and Leprosy
Government Medical College
Jammu, Jammu and Kashmir, India

Nidhi Pugalia MBBS MD(Dermatology, Venereology and Leprosy)
Consultant Dermatologist
South Mumbai Dermatology Clinic
Mumbai, Maharashtra, India

Pradnya Prakash Manwatkar MBBS DDVL
Founder Consultant
Skin Matra Clinic
Mumbai, Maharashtra, India

Priyansh Gupta MBBS MD DNB
Senior Resident
Department of Dermatology, Venereology and Leprology
Postgraduate Institute of Medical Education and Research
Chandigarh, India

Ravina Surve MBBS MD DNB
Consultant Dermatologist
Manek Skin Clinic
Kalyan, Maharashtra, India

Salim Thurakkal MBBS MD DNB MNAMS
Senior Consultant and Clinical Head
Cutis Institute of Dermatology and Aesthetic Sciences
Kozhikode, Kerala, India

Samkit Shah MBBS MD(DVL)
Associate Professor
Vedanta Institute of Medical Sciences
Palghar, Maharashtra, India

Seerat Fatima MBBS MD(Dermatology)
Senior Resident
SKIMS Medical College
Srinagar, Jammu and Kashmir, India

Shivangi Garg MBBS MD
Senior Resident
Department of Dermatology and Venereology
All India Institute of Medical Sciences
New Delhi, India

Shreya K Gowda MBBS MD(Dermatology and Venereology)
Senior Resident
All India Institute of Medical Sciences
New Delhi, India

Somesh Gupta MBBS MD(Dermatology and Venereology)
Professor
All India Institute of Medical Sciences
New Delhi, India

Sonali Gupta MBBS MD(Dermatology and Venereology)
Senior Resident
All India Institute of Medical Sciences
New Delhi, India

S Prasannakumar MBBS MD
Senior Consultant in Dermatology
Cutis Institute of Dermatology and Aesthetic Sciences
Kozhikode, Kerala, India

Sumit Gupta MBBS MD(Dermatology, Venereology and Leprosy)
Consultant Dermatologist
EXCEL Hospital
Sir Ganga Ram Hospital
Skinnovation Clinics
New Delhi, India

FOREWORD

Vitiligo, a condition once shrouded in mystery and stigma that lasted for thousands of years, has seen remarkable advancements in understanding and management over recent years. This compendium, *"Clinical Management of Vitiligo"* stands as a testament to the resilience of those living with vitiligo and the dedication of clinicians and researchers who strive to transform their journeys.

In celebrating this landmark, I wish to honor the legacy of Dr Sanjeev Mulekar, a pioneer in vitiligo surgery, whose contributions have redefined the possibilities for patients. His innovative work continues to inspire me and practitioners worldwide, setting a benchmark for excellence and compassion in this evolving field.

I extend my heartfelt congratulations to Dr Madhulika Mhatre and Sqn Ldr (Dr) Aseem Sharma for their outstanding editorial leadership. They have brought together an eminent group of experts to produce a comprehensive and invaluable resource. This compendium will undoubtedly guide clinicians, inspire researchers, and provide hope to countless patients worldwide.

With immense gratitude for the effort and vision poured into this book, I am confident that it will leave a lasting impact on the field of dermatology and the lives of those it serves.

John E Harris MD PhD
Lambi and Sarah Adams Endowed Professor and Chair
Department of Dermatology
Founding Director, Vitiligo Clinic and Research Center
Department of Dermatology
UMass Chan Medical School
Founding Director, Autoimmune Therapeutics Institute

PREFACE

Vitiligo is more than just a condition; it is a complex interplay of science, art, and empathy that challenges clinicians to offer not just treatment but also hope to their patients. Over the years, advances in the understanding and management of vitiligo have transformed what was once deemed an enigma into a field rich with possibilities. It is with this spirit of progress and commitment to excellence that we present this *"Clinical Management of Vitiligo"*.

This book brings together the collective wisdom of leading researchers and experts who have dedicated their careers to unraveling the intricacies of this condition. Each chapter has been carefully curated to provide insights into cutting-edge treatments, innovative surgical techniques, and practical approaches to managing vitiligo in diverse clinical settings. Whether you are a budding dermatologist, an experienced practitioner, or a researcher, this compendium is designed to be the only resource you will need to master the art and science of treating vitiligo.

We owe immense gratitude to our authors for their timely contributions, which reflect not only their expertise but also their passion for advancing vitiligo care. To our publishers, we extend our heartfelt thanks for their support, persistence, and encouragement throughout this journey.

Lastly, we are deeply thankful for the partnership we share with each other—driven by constant motivation, mutual respect, and a shared vision to create a work that empowers and educates.

It is our hope that this compendium serves as a definitive resource, inspiring practitioners to approach vitiligo with both confidence and compassion.

Warm regards,
Madhulika Mhatre
Sqn Ldr (Dr) Aseem Sharma

CONTENTS

1. **Introduction: Overview of Vitiligo and Historical Perspective**   1
   Shreya K Gowda, Sonali Gupta, Somesh Gupta

2. **Etiology and Pathophysiology**   12
   Sumit Gupta

3. **Clinical Presentation and Diagnosis (Classifying Vitiligo: Types and Patterns; Diagnostic Tools and Criteria)**   26
   Madhulika Mhatre, Aseem Sharma

4. **Stability of Vitiligo: Recommendations and Controversies**   35
   Koushik Lahiri, Abhijit Saha

5. **Topical Treatments**   43
   Deepak Mohana

6A. **Systemic Treatments in Vitiligo: Immunosuppressants—Oral Mini Pulse, Methotrexate, Cyclosporine, and Others**   51
   Narayanan Baskaran, Muthu Sendhil Kumaran

6B. **Systemic Treatments in Vitiligo: Emerging Biologics and Systemic Janus Kinase Inhibitors**   63
   Priyansh Gupta, Davinder Parsad

7A. **Tissue Grafting Techniques in Vitiligo**   72
   Imran Majid, Seerat Fatima, Aaqib Aslam

7B. **Surgical and Adjunctive Therapies: Cellular Grafting in Vitiligo**   91
   Salim Thurakkal, S Prasannakumar

8. **Role of Lasers and Medication in Depigmentation in Vitiligo**   105
   Munish Paul

9. **Light-based Therapy in Vitiligo**   116
   Deepti Ghia, Nidhi Pugalia

10. **Vitiligo: Special Considerations** *Ravina Surve, Mukesh D Shah*	133
11. **Psychosocial Aspects of Vitiligo** *Pradnya Prakash Manwatkar*	145
12. **Camouflaging Techniques for Vitiligo** *Kanika Sahni, Shivangi Garg*	153
13. **Vitiligo Future Trends and Diet** *Samkit Shah, Mansi M Bhatt*	165
14A. **Resources: Guidelines for Practitioners—Algorithmic Approach** *Neha Akhoon*	176
14B. **Resources: Role of Patient Education and Support Groups in Vitiligo** *Maya Shriram Tulpule, Mukta Tulpule*	182
14C. **Resources: List of Phototherapy Chambers and Excimer Lamps in India** *Deepti Ghia*	186
15. **Remembering Dr Sanjeev Mulekar** *Madhulika Mhatre, Deepti Ghia, Iltefat H Hamzavi, Munish Paul*	205
Index	213

CHAPTER 1

Introduction: Overview of Vitiligo and Historical Perspective

Shreya K Gowda, Sonali Gupta, Somesh Gupta

INTRODUCTION

Vitiligo is a more prevalent depigmenting disorder characterized by the lack or near absence of functioning melanocytes in the afflicted areas histologically and clinically presents as white patches in layman's terms or depigmented macules in dermatological perspective. Segmental, generalized, and localized patterns are three distinct clinical forms of vitiligo. However, the most accepted classification includes two types: (1) segmental vitiligo (SV) and (2) nonsegmental vitiligo (NSV).[1] SV is characterized by early onset of depigmented macules arranged in a patterned distribution usually not crossing the mid-line. It can be unisegmental, bisegmental, or plurisegmental. On the other side, nonsegmental can be classified as acrofacial, mucosal (involving more than one mucosal site), generalized, universal, mixed (along with segmental), and few other variants.[2]

The condition creates a lot of social stigma and cosmetically concerning especially in skin of color. It progresses in different ways, and many lesions stabilize with or without therapy. Various theories describing the pathomechanisms of vitiligo have been described such as a complex interplay of immunologic, genetic, and environmental variables leading to the loss of melanocytes. Only 30–40% of the patients require surgical management.[3] Acral, bony, and nonhairy areas are resistant to medical therapies. Such refractory areas and persistent lesions can benefit from surgical therapy. However, most patients respond well to traditional medical treatments including immunomodulators, topical and systemic corticosteroids, and physical therapies such as lasers and phototherapy.

Our chapter focuses on the overview of the historical aspects of vitiligo, various medical therapies available, principles of management, and current updates in vitiligo.

HISTORICAL ASPECTS OF VITILIGO

Vitiligo was described in Indian and Egyptian texts 3,500 years ago. Even then, the social stigma associated with this disfiguring disease was evident. The Atharvaveda, an ancient text written in India between 1500 and 1000 BCE, records details of "white patches on the skin", as do the Egyptian Ebers Papyrus (1500 BCE) and the book of "Leviticus" in the Hebrew Bible from approximately the same time. Indian literature indicates that marriage of a son or daughter to one who has these white patches is "abhorred".[4] Early Buddhist literature states that men and women with vitiligo were not eligible for ordainment, and Hindu texts suggest that those who suffered from this disease may have stolen clothes in their former existence.[5]

Around 250 BC, Ptolemy II translated the Bible and in the Leviticus 13 (Old Testament), different skin conditions were referred to as "Zara'at," which was translated as "lepros" (scales) that was misinterpreted later on as leprosy and other hypopigmented disorders defined as unclean diseases.[6] Indian Manu Smriti, in 250 BC, described "Sweta Kushtha" meaning "white disease," that probably referred to vitiligo. Many centuries went by and vitiligo continued to be one of the most important depigmentation ailments worldwide provoking discrimination or segregation in certain cultures, where affected individuals were unable to get jobs or even get married most probably based upon ancient religious beliefs.

The name "vitiligo" was first used by the famous Roman physician Celsus in second century BC in his medical classic "De Medicina." The word "vitiligo" has often been said to have derived from "vitium" (defect or blemish) rather than "vitellus" meaning calf.[7]

In medieval Europe as well as the Islamic world, vitiligo continued to be misunderstood and frequently misdiagnosed as leprosy, exacerbating social ostracism. The stigma of vitiligo in the subcontinent is so ingrained that to this day, women with the disease would be considered unmarriageable. In certain Hindu texts, a person who is said to have committed a particular offense of insulting a religious teacher in a previous life, suffers vitiligo in the next life. The first Prime Minister of India, Jawaharlal Nehru, ranked vitiligo alongside malaria and leprosy as the three major medical "curses" afflicting his country.

Several studies in the late 19th century reported that there was a propensity for depigmentation in traumatized clinically normal skin of vitiligo subjects. There appeared to be a minimal threshold of injury, required for a depigmented patch to occur,[8] that came to be known later as "Koebner phenomenon."

In the late 20th century, the elusive nature of vitiligo has led to prudent definitions excluding disorders of established etiology. "*Vitiligo can be described as an acquired primary, usually progressive, melanocyte loss of still mysterious etiology, clinically characterized by circumscribed achromic macules often associated with leukotrichia, and progressive disappearance of melanocytes in the involved skin.*"[9]

Treatments listed for vitiligo in historical texts include cow dung or urine; elephant stool; cobra snake bones; topical acids; and heavy metals, including arsenic. While these have thankfully been abandoned, one ancient treatment is still used today. Photochemotherapy was practiced in the ancient world by physicians and herbalists who used boiled extracts of leaves, seeds, or the roots of "Ammi majus Linnaeus" in Egypt or *Psoralea corylifolia* in India, which contain psoralens and several furocoumarins. They are currently used in purified forms and combined with ultraviolet A (UVA) light to treat skin diseases, a therapy called "psoralen ultraviolet A therapy (PUVA)," for psoralen plus UVA light. Therefore, a version of this modern vitiligo therapy was used over three millennia ago, and this treatment was then rediscovered in the 20th century.[10-13]

Throughout history, vitiligo has been misunderstood and stigmatized, and in many cases, associated with curses, divine punishments or contagion. This continues till today with famous pop star late Michael Jackson being subject to stigma for his vitiligo. The disease was so poorly understood by the layman and there were rumors of him using skin bleaching creams to justify his altered appearance. This had an everlasting impact on his career and vitiligo continues to be a life-altering disease for millions worldwide.[14]

CLASSIFICATION OF VITILIGO[1]

Nonsegmental vitiligo:
- Focal
- Generalized
- Mucosal
- Acrofacial
- Universal

Segmental vitiligo:
- Unisegmental
- Bisegmental
- Plurisegmental

Mixed vitiligo: NSV + SV

Unclassified vitiligo:
- Focal
- Multifocal
- Asymmetrical nonsegmental
- Mucosal (involving one site)

PRINCIPLE OF MEDICAL MANAGEMENT OF VITILIGO

Vitiligo is a completely reversible disorder, in contrast to the most autoimmune conditions. The pigment-producing melanocytes, which are found in the interfollicular epidermis, are the main targets of vitiligo. While the melanocytes at the immune privilege sites such as hair follicles, brain, eye, and inner ear are spared. Additionally, hair follicles contain melanocytic stem cells that can produce new and functional melanocytes with the ability to restore normal pigmentation on the epidermis of a vitiligo patch. Areas of vitiligo patches without hair or leukotrichia do not respond well to medical management.[15] Whereas, hairy sites and photoexposed sites demonstrate predominantly punctate, or perifollicular and perilesional patterns of repigmentation. Successful management of vitiligo two therapeutic objectives must be met: suppression of vitiligo activity (appearance of new patches, or expansion of old patches) and melanocyte regeneration from the stem cell niche in the hair follicle. Immunosuppression is a crucial part of stabilizing the vitiligo. Repigmentation is documented by topical corticosteroids (TCS) and calcineurin inhibitors, whereas systemic corticosteroid therapy and Janus kinase (JAK) inhibitors also show some degree of repigmentation. However, the drugs used for repigmentation have some role in stabilizing and vice versa.[16,17]

DRUGS FOR STABILITY OF VITILIGO

Topical Corticosteroids

Due to its affordability and ease of use, TCS therapy is regarded as a first-line treatment for vitiligo. The possibility of local side effects, including atrophy, striae, and telangiectasias, as well as infrequent systemic side effects, outweigh its usefulness. Studies suggest using TCS with high potencies for localized vitiligo, but given their side effects, their usage should be restricted to 2–4 months periods.[18] A meta-analysis of nonsurgical treatments revealed that TCS was much more effective than tacrolimus, with a success rate of 33% compared to 0% in the placebo group.[19]

Topical Calcineurin Inhibitors

Topical calcineurin inhibitors are superior to topical steroids because neocollagenesis is not dependent on calcineurin, which eliminates the possibility of skin atrophy that TCS administration causes. By inhibiting proinflammatory cytokines and preventing the transcription of interleukin *(IL)-2* genes, which are critical for the growth of cytotoxic T cells, topical tacrolimus and pimecrolimus, calcineurin inhibitors, and regulate T-cell activity. Additionally, they work by preventing the transcription and synthesis of tumor necrosis factor-α (TNF-α), interferon-γ (IFN-γ), IL-10, IL-5, and IL-4. Compared to TCS, calcineurin inhibitors have shown comparable efficacy without the possibility of cutaneous atrophy over time.[20,21]

Vitamin D3 Analogs

Calcipotriol is a topical vitamin D3 analog that enhances melanocyte development, and melanogenesis and has immunomodulatory effects. It acts on vitamin D receptors in T cells and keratinocytes. Calcipotriol by itself does not seem to be as effective as corticosteroid monotherapy in causing repigmentation. According to one trial, calcitriol and betamethasone combination therapy induced noticeable repigmentation (50–75%) with improved tolerability and was superior to either treatment alone. Topical calcipotriene is safe; hypercalcemia may rarely occur.[22]

Oral Steroids

The first-line treatment for rapidly progressive vitiligo is systemic corticosteroids. In vitiligo, oral steroids inhibit T-cell function, and migration, and slow the disease's progression. It also promotes repigmentation from the melanocyte reservoir at the periphery of the lesions and perifollicular region. It takes a few weeks and months to achieve stability. After stability is attained, which is defined as the absence of new lesions and the extension of preexisting ones, the steroid dosage needs to be gradually reduced while further immunosuppressive techniques are added to promote repigmentation.[23] Every time there is a relapse, episodic treatment for 8–12 weeks at a time might be administered in addition to maintenance therapy. Phototherapy or photochemotherapy may also be used in conjunction with systemic corticosteroids in cases where disease activity temporarily changes or worsens. In 69% of cases, adverse symptoms included weight gain, sleeplessness, anxiety, acne, irregular menstruation, and hypertrichosis.[24]

Azathioprine

To compare the effectiveness of oral azathioprine and betamethasone oral minipulse (OMP) in treating rapidly progressive NSV. They found that both treatments were effective in stopping the disease's progression, but those patients in the OMP group responded to the treatment much sooner than those receiving azathioprine. Nevertheless, azathioprine was only slightly less effective than OMP after the 6-month research period (85% in the OMP group vs. 77.8% in the azathioprine group). After 6 months, 2 out of the 28 patients in the OMP group had >20% repigmentation, but none in the azathioprine group achieved repigmentation.[25]

Cyclosporine

Cyclosporine reduces the migration of activated T lymphocytes and antigen-presenting cells in the epidermis, inhibits calcineurin by creating a complex with cyclophilin, and lowers IL-2 production. It also influences the "trafficking" of different inflammatory cells and downregulates *ICAM-1* (intercellular adhesion molecule-1). There was no comprehensive data on the patients who were treated. Hypertension and renal impairment were the most common adverse outcomes. Sometimes cyclosporine is used in patients 6 weeks prior to surgery to optimize disease activity if the surgery is considered to vitiligo patch with regional stability.[26]

Minocycline

Minocycline involves inhibiting the synthesis of cytokines and free radicals. Both groups demonstrated a significant reduction in disease progression following 6 months of treatment in a trial by Singh et al. that compared OMP (2.5 mg dexamethasone on 2 consecutive days in a week) with minocycline (100 mg/day).[27]

Janus Kinase/Signal Transducer and Activator of Transcription Proteins Inhibitors

Ruxolitinib targets Janus kinase 1 (JAK1) and Janus kinase 2 (JAK2) specifically. Patients of vitiligo receiving oral (20 mg twice daily) or topical ruxolitinib (1.5% twice daily) showed rapid skin repigmentation. Following treatment, there was a noticeable drop in serum CXCL10 levels due to disruption of JAKs and IFN-γ signaling. Additionally, it suppressed the migration and development of human dendritic cells (DCs), which decreased the induction of CD8+ cytotoxic T-cell responses and the antigen-specific CD4+ and CD8+ T-cell responses generated by DCs.[28-30]

In addition, 16 individuals with vitiligo, including 11 with generalized vitiligo, received topical 2% tofacitinib cream. In patients with darker skin types and face lesions, repigmentation was more pronounced; concurrent phototherapy did not result in any better responses. After receiving tofacitinib therapy for an average of 9.9 months at a dosage of 5–10 mg daily or twice daily, only half of the patients experienced repigmentation in areas exposed to the sun or those that exclusively received phototherapy.[30,31]

DRUGS FOR REPIGMENTATION

Psoralen Ultraviolet A Therapy

Psoralen ultraviolet A therapy transforms psoralen molecules into oxidative, DNA-reactive chemicals that promote melanocyte proliferation and pigmentation while suppressing immunological function. The significant effectiveness of PUVA as a treatment for vitiligo may be explained by its combined immunosuppressive and pigment-stimulating qualities. However, narrowband-UVB (NBUVB) phototherapy offers better vitiligo lesion repigmentation with fewer negative side effects. Thus, NBUVB has largely replaced PUVA as first-line therapy for vitiligo, and conventional treatment strategies now incorporate NBUVB phototherapy in combination with TCS and/or topical calcineurin inhibitors. Current treatments for vitiligo remain far from ideal, as they are not universally effective in all patients, they do not repigment all anatomic locations, and they can be quite cumbersome for patients to use.[32-34]

Khellin-UVA

Vitiligo has been treated with khellin, a furochrome extract of the plant Ammi visnaga (5,8-dimethyl-2-methyl-4,5 furo-6,7-chromone) with UVA. However, there aren't many randomized controlled trials evaluating the effectiveness of this strategy, and oral khellin-UVA (KUVA) is not used in view of severe liver damage.[35]

Narrowband Ultraviolet B

Targeted phototherapy such as excimer lasers or lamps is especially well-suited for treating localized diseases because they emit light in the UVB spectrum, which peaks at 308 nm. Numerous investigations have been carried out to assess whether NBUVB phototherapy, either by itself or in conjunction with other modalities, can restore pigmentation to vitiligo lesions. In research comparing NBUVB with oral minocycline in individuals with unstable vitiligo, Siadat et al. found that stability was induced in 16 out of 21 patients (76.1%) in the NBUVB group and in 7 out of 21 (33.3%) in the minocycline group.[36]

NEWER THERAPY IN VITILIGO

Biologicals in Vitiligo

Biologicals and biosimilars target immunological and cytokine pathways. Numerous monoclonal antibodies, including pembrolizumab, nivolumab, infliximab, and adalimumab, have been implicated in vitiligo. Nevertheless, there have also been reports of TNF-α inhibitors and monoclonal anti-CD20 chimeric antibodies stabilizing vitiligo's increasing illness.[37-40]

Tables 1 and 2 summarize the other newer repigmenting agents and lasers utilized in vitiligo.[41-46]

TABLE 1: Summarizes the other newer repigmenting laser therapy utilized in vitiligo.[41-43]

Modality	Wavelength	Sittings	Repigmentation	Side effects	Comments
Bioskin	311 nm	Once a week	• 72%: G4 (monotherapy) • 90%: G4 (+betamethasone)	–	<30% BSA
UV-A1 laser	355 nm	Once/week for 6 months	• 17/21: G4 • 3/21: G3	Mild erythema, itching, and burning	
PDT (5-ALA) (case series)	633 nm	1.5% ALA + UVA 80 mW/cm² (once/week)	• All—chest, face, and neck • Begun after three sessions • Persists at 1 year follow-up	Mild pain, burning, and desquamation	Decreased pigment island on stoppage
Titanium sapphire laser	311 nm	• Twice a week • 13–47 session • + tacrolimus 0.1%	• G4 in 79% (21 sessions and 3 months) • Face and neck	Persistent erythema × 2 days in one-third	Comparable to excimer

(ALA: aminolevulinic acid; BSA: body surface area; PDT: photodynamic therapy; UVA: ultraviolet A)

TABLE 2: Summarizes the other newer repigmenting agents utilized in vitiligo.[41-43]

Target	Drugs	Study	Administration	Results				Side effects
				Site	Onset	NBUVB	Repigmentation	
MC1R agonist	Afamelanotide	• RCT (56) • Generalized vitiligo	Subcutaneous implant (16) monthly	• Face • Upper extremities	Earlier	• +(27) • Monotherapy +28 combined therapy	• 48.4% in combination group • NBUVB only—33%	• Nausea • Erythema • Hyperpigmentation (unacceptable)
β-FGF	Decapeptide	RCT (30)	Topical	Nonsegmental vitiligo	–	+	9/30–40% repigmentation	
Prostaglandin analogs	Latanoprost	Double blind trial (22)	• Topical 0.005% • BD	• Face (LT) • UL, LL, Trunk (LT + NB)	1 month	• + (LT + NBUVB-8) • + (only NBUVB-7)	• 43% excellent • Maintained in 75% in 6 months FU	• Mild irritation • Burning
	Bimatoprost	Open label	Topical 0.03% BD	• Face • Nonfacial (+mometasone)	–	–	• 4/8 >75% repigmentation • 3/8 had 50–75% repigmentation	"
PDE-4 inhibitors	Apremilast	Case series	oral	–	+	No significant improvement	–	Myalgia, diarrhea, mild elevation of creatine phosphokinase, and headache

(FGF: fibroblast growth factor; LL: lower limb; MC1R: melanocortin 1 receptor; NB: narrowband; NBUVB: narrowband ultraviolet B; PDE-4: phosphodiesterase 4; RCT: randomized controlled trial; UL: upper limb)

CONCLUSION

Managing vitiligo is challenging because stabilizing disease activity and achieving repigmentation in depigmented skin lesions may need long-term immunosuppression. However, medical management plays a major role in vitiligo.

REFERENCES

1. Taieb A, Alomar A, Böhm M, Dell'anna ML, De Pase A, Eleftheriadou V, et al. Guidelines for the management of vitiligo: the European Dermatology Forum consensus. Br J Dermatol. 2013;168:5-19.
2. Khaitan BK, Kathuria S, Ramam M. A descriptive study to characterize segmental vitiligo. Indian J Dermatol Venereol Leprol. 2012;78:715-21.
3. Rodrigues M, Ezzedine K, Hamzavi I, Pandya AG, Harris JE; Vitiligo Working Group. New discoveries in the pathogenesis and classification of vitiligo. J Am Acad Dermatol. 2017; 77(1):1-13.
4. Barman S. Switra and its treatment in Veda. Anc Sci Life. 1995;15:71-4
5. Singh G, Ansari Z, Dwivedi RN. Vitiligo in ancient Indian medicine. Arch Dermatol. 1974; 109(6):913.
6. Goldman L, Richard S, Moraites R. White spots in biblical times. Arch Derm. 1966;93:744-53.
7. Panda AK. The medico historical perspective of vitiligo (Switra). Bull Ind Hist Med. 2005; 35(1):41-6.
8. Sagi L, Trau H. The Koebner phenomenon. Clin Dermatol. 2011;29(2):231-6.
9. Prasad PV, Bhatnagar VK. Medico-historical study of "Kilasa" (vitiligo/leucoderma) a common skin disorder. Bull Ind Inst Hist Med. 2003;33:113-27.
10. Lerner AB. Vitiligo. J Invest Dermatol. 1959;32:285-310.
11. Pathak M, Daniels F, Fitzpatrick TB. The presently known distribution of furocoumarins (psoralens) in plants. J Invest Dermatol. 1962;39:225-39.
12. Pathak M, Fitzpatrick TB. The evolution of photochemotherapy with psoralens and UVA (PUVA) 2000 BC to 1992 AD. J Photochem Photobiol. 1992;14:3-22.
13. Sidi E, Bourgeois-Gavardin J. The treatment of vitiligo with Ammi Majus Linn. J Invest Dermatol. 1952;18:391-6.
14. Frisoli ML, Harris JE. Vitiligo: Mechanistic insights lead to novel treatments. J Allergy Clin Immunol. 2017;140(3):654-62.
15. Passeron T. Medical and maintenance treatments for vitiligo. Dermatol Clin. 2017;35(2):163-70.
16. Radakovic-Fijan S, Fürnsinn-Friedl AM, Hönigsmann H, Tanew A. Oral dexamethasone pulse treatment for vitiligo. J Am Acad Dermatol. 2001;44(5):814-7.
17. Kanwar AJ, Mahajan R, Parsad D. Low-dose oral mini-pulse dexamethasone therapy in progressive unstable vitiligo. J Cutan Med Surg. 2013;17(4):259-68.
18. Whitton ME, Pinart M, Batchelor J, Leonardi-Bee J, González U, Jiyad Z, et al. Interventions for vitiligo. Cochrane Database Syst Rev. 2015;2015(2):CD003263.
19. Njoo MD, Spuls PI, Bos JD, Westerhof W, Bossuyt PM. Nonsurgical repigmentation therapies in vitiligo: meta-analysis of the literature. Arch Dermatol. 1998;134:1532-40.
20. Kostovic K, Pasic A. New treatment modalities for vitiligo: focus on topical immunomodulators. Drugs. 2005;65:447-59.
21. Khandpur S, Sharma VK, Sumanth K. Topical immunomodulators in dermatology. J Postgrad Med. 2004;50:131-9.
22. Xing C, Xu A. The effect of combined calcipotriol and betamethasone dipropionate ointment in the treatment of vitiligo: an open, uncontrolled trial. J Drugs Dermatol. 2012; 11:e52-4.
23. Pasricha JS, Khaitan BK. Oral mini-pulse therapy with betamethasone in vitiligo patients having extensive or fast-spreading disease. Int J Dermatol. 1993;32:753-7.

24. Majid I, Masood Q, Hassan I, Khan D, Chisti M. Childhood vitiligo: response to methylprednisolone oral minipulse therapy and topical fluticasone combination. Indian J Dermatol. 2009;54:124-7.
25. Patra S, Khaitan BK, Sharma VK, Khanna N. A randomized comparative study of the effect of betamethasone oral mini-pulse therapy versus oral azathioprine in progressive nonsegmental vitiligo. J Am Acad Dermatol. 2021;85(3):728-9.
26. Gupta AK, Ellis CN, Nickoloff BJ, Goldfarb MT, Ho VC, Rocher LL, et al. Oral cyclosporine in the treatment of inflammatory and noninflammatory dermatoses. A clinical and immunopathologic analysis. Arch Dermatol. 1990;126(3):339-50.
27. Singh A, Kanwar AJ, Parsad D, Mahajan R. Randomized controlled study to evaluate the effectiveness of dexamethasone oral minipulse therapy versus oral minocycline in patients with active vitiligo vulgaris. Indian J Dermatol Venereol Leprol. 2014;80:29-35.
28. Kim SR, Heaton H, Liu LY, King BA. Rapid repigmentation of vitiligo using tofacitinib plus low-dose, narrowband UV-B phototherapy. JAMA Dermatol. 2018;154(3):370-1.
29. Liu LY, Strassner JP, Refat MA, Harris JE, King BA. Repigmentation in vitiligo using the Janus kinase inhibitor tofacitinib may require concomitant light exposure. J Am Acad Dermatol. 2017;77(4):675-82.e1.
30. Rothstein B, Joshipura D, Saraiya A, Abdat R, Ashkar H, Turkowski Y, et al. Treatment of vitiligo with the topical Janus kinase inhibitor ruxolitinib. J Am Acad Dermatol. 2017;76(6):1054-60.e1.
31. Mobasher P, Guerra R, Li SJ, Frangos J, Ganesan AK, Huang V. Open-label pilot study of tofacitinib 2% for the treatment of refractory vitiligo. Br J Dermatol. 2020;182(4):1047-9.
32. Pacifico A, Leone G. Photo(chemo)therapy for vitiligo. Photodermatol Photoimmunol Photomed. 2011;27(5):261-77.
33. Lotti T, Prignano F, Buggiani G. New and experimental treatments of vitiligo and other hypomelanoses. Dermatol Clin. 2007;25(3):393-400.
34. Shenoi SD, Prabhu S. Photochemotherapy (PUVA) in psoriasis and vitiligo. Indian Association of Dermatologists, Venereologists and Leprologists. Indian J Dermatol Venereol Leprol. 2014;80:497-504.
35. Orecchia G, Perfetti L. Photochemotherapy with topical khellin and sunlight in vitiligo. Dermatology. 1992;184:120-3.
36. Siadat AH, Zeinali N, Iraji F, Abtahi-Naeini B, Nilforoushzadeh MA, Jamshidi K, et al. Narrow-band ultraviolet B versus oral minocycline in treatment of unstable vitiligo: A prospective comparative trial. Dermatol Res Pract. 2014;2014:240856.
37. Hua C, Boussemart L, Mateus C, Routier E, Boutros C, Cazenave H, et al. Association of vitiligo with tumor response in patient with metastatic melanoma treated with pembrolizumab. JAMA Dermatol. 2016;152:45-51.
38. Uenami T, Hosono Y, Ishijima M, Kanazu M, Akazawa Y, Yano Y, et al. Vitiligo in a patient with lung adenocarcinoma treated with nivolumab: A case report. Lung Cancer. 2017;109:42-4.
39. Carvalho CLDB, Ortigosa LCM. Segmental vitiligo after infliximab use for rheumatoid arthritis: A case report. Anais Brasileiros de Dermatologia. 2014;89:154-6.
40. Toussirot E, Salard D, Algros MP, Aubin F. Occurrence of vitiligo in a patient with ankylosing spondylitis receiving adalimumab. Dermatol Venereol. 2013;140:801-2.
41. Lim HW, Grimes PE, Agbai O, Hamzavi I, Henderson M, Haddican M, et al. Afamelanotide and narrowband UV-B phototherapy for the treatment of vitiligo: a randomized multicenter trial. JAMA Dermatol. 2015;151(1):42-50.
42. Nayak CS, Kura MM, Banerjee G, Patil SP, Deshpande A, Sekar S, et al. Efficacy and safety comparison of basic fibroblast growth factor-related decapeptide 0.1% solution (bFGFrP) plus oral PUVA combination therapy with oral PUVA monotherapy in the treatment of vitiligo. J Cutan Aesthet Surg. 2023;16(1):28-33.
43. Pourriyahi H, Hosseini NS, Nooshabadi MP, Pourriahi H, Baradaran HR, Abtahi-Naeini B, et al. Utility of prostaglandin analogues and phosphodiesterase inhibitors as promising last resorts for the treatment of vitiligo: A systematic review, from mechanisms of action to mono-, combination and comparative therapies. J Cosmet Dermatol. 2024;23(11):3466-87.

44. Lotti T, Buggiani G, Troiano M, Assad GB, Delescluse J, De Giorgi V, et al. Targeted and combination treatments for vitiligo. Comparative evaluation of different current modalities in 458 subjects. Dermatol Ther. 2008;21(Suppl 1):S20-6.
45. Giorgio CM, Caccavale S, Fulgione E, Moscarella E, Babino G, Argenziano G. Efficacy of microneedling and photodynamic therapy in vitiligo. Dermatol Surg. 2019;45(11):1424-6.
46. Park MJ, Shon U, Seong GH, Kim MH, Park BC, Hong SP. A comparative clinical trial to evaluate efficacy and safety of the 308-nm excimer laser and the gain-switched 311-nm titanium: sapphire laser in the treatment of vitiligo. Photodermatol Photoimmunol Photomed. 2020; 36(2):97-104.

CHAPTER 2

Etiology and Pathophysiology

Sumit Gupta

INTRODUCTION

Vitiligo is a chronic skin condition characterized by the loss of melanocytes, leading to depigmented patches on the skin. This disorder can significantly impact the quality of life due to its visible nature and association with psychological distress. The etiology and pathogenesis of vitiligo are multifactorial, involving genetic predispositions, environmental triggers, autoimmune responses, and oxidative stress. A comprehensive understanding of the etiology and pathogenesis of vitiligo is essential for the development of targeted therapies and the enhancement of patient outcomes.

HISTORICAL CONTEXT OF VITILIGO RESEARCH

Vitiligo, a condition marked by the loss of skin pigmentation, has been recognized for thousands of years across various cultures. Exploring the historical context of vitiligo research is vital as it underscores the evolution of knowledge regarding this condition, societal attitudes, and advancements in medical treatment. Our understanding of vitiligo has evolved significantly over centuries. The following timeline outlines key milestones in our evolving understanding of vitiligo, highlighting significant research that has influenced its management and comprehension:

- *Ancient Egypt (~1500 BCE)*: Psoralen-containing plants (e.g., *Ammi majus*) were used in combination with sunlight to treat depigmentation, as documented in "the Ebers Papyrus". This early practice provided a foundation for light-based therapy.[1]
- *Ancient India (~600 BCE)*: The *Atharva Veda* described the use of Bakuchi (*Psoralea corylifolia*), a psoralen-rich herb, combined with sun exposure for repigmentation. This practice evolved into the precursor to modern psoralen and ultraviolet A (PUVA) therapy.[2]
- *Ancient China (~200 BCE)*: Traditional Chinese medicine (TCM) used herbs like Bai Zhi (*Angelica dahurica*) and Qing Dai (*Indigo naturalis*) alongside acupuncture and sun exposure to address skin disorders.[3]

- *Ancient Greece (~400 BCE)*: Hippocrates advocated heliotherapy (sunlight therapy) for skin conditions, reinforcing the connection between sunlight and skin healing.[4]
- *16th to 17th centuries*: After the middle ages, Andreas Vesalius (1533) highlighted that the skin has two layers. Later, Jean Riolan the Younger (1580–1657) described the skin of a Black individual as having an upper black layer (horny layer) and a lower white layer (dermis). In 1819, Giosué Sangiovanni first identified melanocytes in squids, calling them "chromatophores."[5]
- *19th century*: Austrian dermatologist Moritz Kaposi observed pigment granule absence in affected areas, shifting focus toward biological mechanisms of vitiligo.[6]
- *1974*: Parrish and Fitzpatrick introduced PUVA therapy, marking a significant milestone in modern vitiligo treatment.[7]
- *1980s*: Narrowband ultraviolet B (NB-UVB) phototherapy emerged as a safer and more effective alternative to PUVA.[8]
- *1990s*: Studies confirmed the role of T-cell-mediated cytotoxicity and oxidative stress in melanocyte destruction.[9,10]
- *2000s*: Genome-wide association studies (GWAS) identified susceptibility loci, linking vitiligo to other autoimmune diseases.[11]
- *2010s*: Studies on the cytokine interferon-γ (IFN-γ) and its downstream targets (e.g., CXCL10/CXCR3) identified actionable immune pathways. The introduction of Janus kinase (JAK) inhibitors, such as tofacitinib and ruxolitinib, demonstrated impressive repigmentation results in clinical trials.[12]

ETIOLOGY OF VITILIGO

Vitiligo is a complex disorder with a multifactorial etiology. The primary factors contributing to its development include genetic predisposition, autoimmune mechanisms, oxidative stress, neurogenic factors, and environmental triggers. Understanding these factors is crucial for developing targeted therapies and improving patient's outcomes.

Genetic Factors

Family History and Heritability
- *Incidence in first-degree relatives*: Vitiligo often clusters in families, suggesting a genetic component. Research indicates that approximately 20–30% of individuals with vitiligo have a first-degree relative affected by the condition, suggesting a notable hereditary component.[13]
- *Twin studies and concordance rates*: Twin studies have provided valuable insights into the heritability of vitiligo. Monozygotic (identical) twins have a higher concordance rate for vitiligo compared to dizygotic (fraternal) twins. However, the incomplete concordance among monozygotic twins indicates that environmental factors also play a crucial role in the disease's development.[14]

Genetic Susceptibility Loci
- *Overview of GWAS*:
  - Genome-wide association studies have identified numerous loci associated with vitiligo, with many of these loci overlapping with other autoimmune diseases. Some key loci include:[15]
    - *NOD-like receptor family pyrin domain containing 1 (NLRP1)*: This gene is involved in the regulation of the inflammasome, a multiprotein complex that activates inflammatory responses. Variants in *NLRP1* have been associated with an increased risk of vitiligo and other autoimmune diseases.
    - *Tyrosinase (TYR)*: Encodes the key enzyme for melanin biosynthesis. Mutations or polymorphisms enhance melanocyte vulnerability.
    - *Protein tyrosine phosphatase non-receptor type 22 (PTPN22)*: PTPN22 is a well-known risk gene for multiple autoimmune disorders. It encodes a phosphatase that negatively regulates T-cell activation, and mutations in this gene are associated with heightened immune responses against melanocytes.
    - *Human leukocyte antigen (HLA) genes*: The HLA region is highly polymorphic and plays a central role in immune system regulation. Specific HLA class I and II alleles (e.g., *HLA-A02:01, HLA-DRB104-DQB10301*) have been linked to an increased susceptibility to vitiligo.
    - *FOXP3*: Regulates Tregs (regulatory T cells), which dysfunction is critical in autoimmune diseases.
    - *PINK1 and NFE2L2*: These genes regulate antioxidant responses, and their impairment increases susceptibility to oxidative stress.
- *Recent advances*:
  - *Noncoding RNAs*: Recent research has explored the role of noncoding RNAs (e.g., microRNAs, long noncoding RNAs) in vitiligo. These RNAs do not code for proteins but regulate gene expression at the transcriptional and posttranscriptional levels. Dysregulation of specific microRNAs, such as miR-155 and miR-146a, has been implicated in the autoimmune response and melanocyte apoptosis.[16]
  - *Epigenetic modifications*: Epigenetic changes, including DNA methylation and histone modifications, can alter gene expression without changing the underlying DNA sequence. These modifications can be influenced by environmental factors and may play a role in the onset and progression of vitiligo.[17]

Autoimmune Hypothesis

Evidence of Autoimmunity
- *Association with other autoimmune diseases*: Vitiligo frequently coexists with other autoimmune conditions, such as autoimmune thyroid disease, type 1 diabetes mellitus, and pernicious anemia. The cooccurrence of these

autoimmune disorders implies shared genetic and immunological pathways contributing to their development.
- *Melanocyte-specific autoantibodies*: Patients with vitiligo often have circulating autoantibodies against melanocyte-specific antigens, such as tyrosinase and melanin-concentrating hormone receptor 1 (MCHR1). These autoantibodies can be detected in the serum and are thought to contribute to melanocyte destruction.[18]
- *Cytotoxic T-cell response*: CD8+ cytotoxic T-cells play a critical role in the immune-mediated destruction of melanocytes. These T-cells recognize melanocyte antigens presented by HLA class I molecules and induce apoptosis through the release of perforin and granzymes. The presence of activated CD8+ T-cells in vitiligo lesions supports the autoimmune nature of the disease.[19]

Autoimmune Pathways

- *Cytokines and chemokines*:
  - Cytokines such as IFN-γ and tumor necrosis factor-alpha (TNF-α) are upregulated in vitiligo and contribute to the inflammatory microenvironment that promotes melanocyte apoptosis. IFN-γ, in particular, plays a central role in the recruitment and activation of immune cells in vitiligo lesions.[20]
  - Chemokines such as *CXCL10* (C-X-C motif chemokine ligand-10) are crucial for the recruitment of CD8+ T-cells to the skin, where they exert their cytotoxic effects on melanocytes.[21]
- *Regulatory T-cells (Tregs)*: Regulatory T cells are essential for maintaining immune tolerance and preventing autoimmune responses. In vitiligo, there is evidence of Treg dysfunction, characterized by reduced numbers or impaired suppressive function, leading to an unchecked immune response against melanocytes.[22]

Recent Research

- *Checkpoint inhibitors*: Immune checkpoints are regulators of immune responses, preventing excessive activation that can lead to autoimmunity. Recent studies have shown that checkpoint inhibitors, such as those targeting the programmed cell death 1 (PD-1)/programmed cell death ligand 1 (PD-L1) axis, can exacerbate or induce vitiligo in patients undergoing cancer immunotherapy. This observation underscores the role of immune checkpoints in maintaining tolerance to melanocytes.[23]
- *Single-cell RNA sequencing (scRNA-seq)*: Single-cell RNA sequencing has provided new insights into the heterogeneity of immune cells in vitiligo lesions. This technology allows for the identification of specific immune cell subsets and their transcriptional profiles, offering a more detailed understanding of the autoimmune processes driving vitiligo.[24]

Oxidative Stress
Oxidative Damage in Melanocytes
- *Imbalance between reactive oxygen species production and antioxidant defenses*: Reactive oxygen species (ROS) are produced as byproducts of cellular metabolism, particularly in melanocytes during melanin synthesis. Normally, melanocytes have robust antioxidant defenses, including enzymes such as catalase, superoxide dismutase (SOD), and glutathione peroxidase, to neutralize ROS. In vitiligo, this balance is disrupted, leading to excessive ROS accumulation and oxidative stress.[25]
- *Mitochondrial dysfunction*: Mitochondria are a primary source of ROS. In vitiligo, there is evidence of mitochondrial dysfunction, characterized by decreased mitochondrial membrane potential and impaired adenosine triphosphate (ATP) production. This dysfunction exacerbates oxidative stress, leading to melanocyte apoptosis or necrosis.[26]

Environmental and Chemical Triggers
- *Phenolic compounds*: Certain chemicals, particularly phenolic compounds like monobenzyl ether of hydroquinone (MBEH), can induce depigmentation by generating ROS and directly damaging melanocytes. These compounds are structurally similar to tyrosine, a precursor in melanin synthesis, and can disrupt melanogenesis.[27]
- *Ultraviolet radiation*: Ultraviolet (UV) radiation, especially UVA and UVB, can induce oxidative stress by generating ROS in the skin. While UV light is used therapeutically in vitiligo (e.g., narrowband UVB therapy), excessive exposure can exacerbate oxidative damage, contributing to melanocyte loss.[28]

Recent Advances
- *Nuclear factor erythroid 2-related factor 2 pathway (Nrf2)*: The Nrf2 pathway plays a crucial role in cellular antioxidant defenses. Recent studies suggest that Nrf2 is downregulated in vitiligo, leading to impaired response to oxidative stress. Targeting the Nrf2 pathway to enhance antioxidant defenses represents a potential therapeutic strategy for vitiligo.[29]
- *Antioxidant therapies*: Ongoing research is exploring the efficacy of various antioxidants, such as oral or topical vitamin E, catalase, and SOD mimetics, in reducing oxidative stress and halting the progression of vitiligo.[30]

Neurogenic Factors
The neural hypothesis points to neurochemical mediators secreted from cutaneous nerve endings as responsible for the melanocytes' cytotoxic injury and death. Several clinical observations suggest this communication between the nervous system and the skin.
- Nearly dermatomal distribution of vitiligo patches in the segmental type of vitiligo.

- Vitiligo is described to develop in patients affected by transverse myelitis, diabetic neuropathy, and in demarcated areas after nerve damage.[31]
- Severe emotional stress may trigger the onset or the exacerbation of vitiligo.

Key Mechanisms of Neurogenic Factors in Etiology (Fig. 1)
- *Neuropeptides and neurotransmitters*:
  - Nerve endings in the skin release neuropeptides and neurotransmitters under stress or injury, which interact with melanocytes and other skin cells.
  - These molecules can be toxic to melanocytes or act as immune modulators, leading to inflammation and melanocyte apoptosis.
  - *Key neuropeptides and neurotransmitters involved*:
    - Substance P (SP):
      - Released by sensory nerve endings during stress or trauma.
      - Binds to melanocytes via the neurokinin-1 receptor (NK1R), inducing oxidative stress, inflammation, and apoptosis.[32]
      - Elevated levels of SP are observed in vitiligo lesions, particularly during active phases of the disease.[33]
    - Catecholamines (dopamine, norepinephrine, and epinephrine):
      - Melanocytes are capable of producing dopamine. However, excessive levels of dopamine can be cytotoxic due to its ability to generate ROS.[34]
      - Overproduction of catecholamines, triggered by stress or sympathetic nerve activity, may create a toxic microenvironment for melanocytes.[35]
    - Vasoactive intestinal peptide (VIP): Vasoactive intestinal peptide modulates immune responses and oxidative stress. Its dysregulation may contribute to melanocyte dysfunction.[36]
    - Calcitonin gene-related peptide (CGRP): Calcitonin gene-related peptide is known to enhance inflammatory responses, which may exacerbate immune-mediated melanocyte destruction.[37]
- *Neural involvement in the Koebner phenomenon*: The Koebner phenomenon, where vitiligo lesions appear at sites of trauma, is thought to involve nerve damage or irritation in the affected area. Traumatized local nerve endings release neuropeptides such as SP, which initiate inflammation, oxidative stress, and immune activation. This may serve as a trigger for melanocyte destruction.[36]
- *Stress and neurogenic pathways*: Psychological or physical stress is a common trigger for vitiligo onset or exacerbation. Stress activates the hypothalamic-pituitary-adrenal (HPA) axis and sympathetic nervous system, leading to the release of catecholamines and stress-related neuropeptides.[38] These molecules can create a hostile environment for melanocytes by:
  - Increasing oxidative stress.
  - Inducing inflammatory cytokines.
  - Amplifying immune responses against melanocytes.

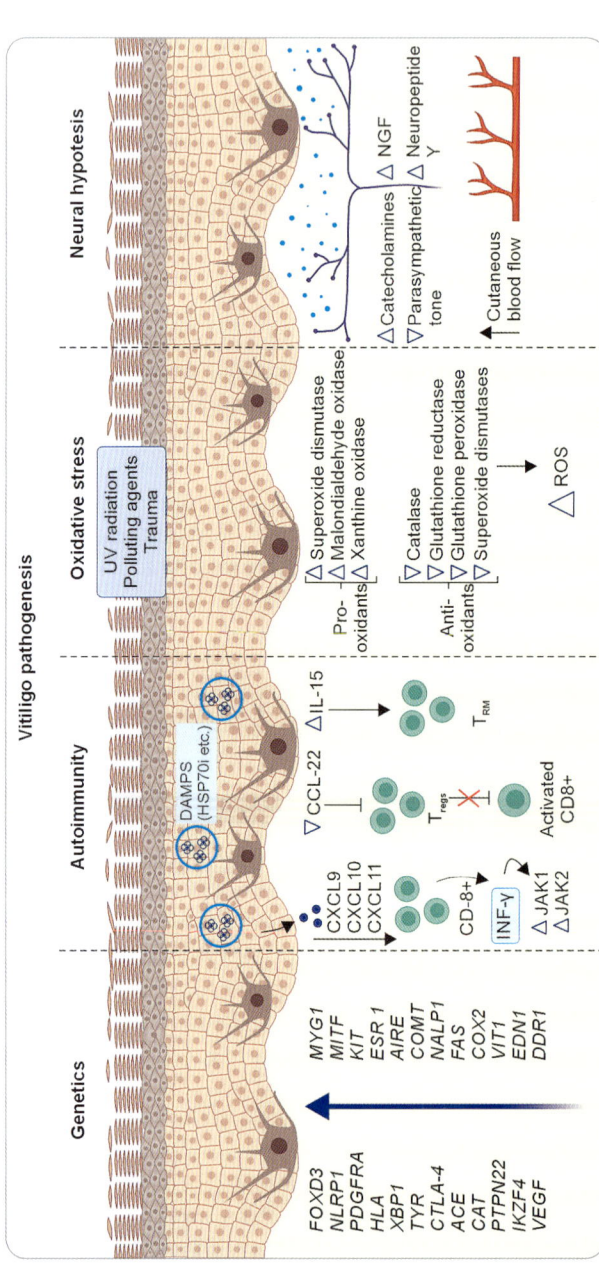

FIG. 1: Summary of the main etiological factors involved in vitiligo.

(ACE: angiotensin-converting enzyme; AIRE: autoimmune regulator; CAT: catalase; CCL22: C-C motif chemokine ligand 22; CD8: cluster of differentiation 8; COMT: catechol-O-methyltransferase; COX2: cyclooxygenase 2; CTLA-4: cytotoxic T-lymphocyte antigen 4; CXCL9-10-11: C-X-C motif chemokine ligand 9-10-11; DAMPs: damage-associated molecular patterns; EDN1: endothelin 1; ESR-1: estrogen receptor 1; FAS: Fas cell surface death receptor; FOXD3: Forkhead Box D3; HLA: human leukocyte antigen; HSP70: heat shock protein 70 kilodaltons; IFN-γ: interferon gamma; IKZF4: IKAROS family zinc finger 4; IL-15: interleukin-15; JAK1-2: Janus kinases 1 and 2; KIT: KIT proto-oncogene, receptor tyrosine kinase; MITF: melanocyte-inducing transcription factor; MYG1: MYG1 exonuclease; NALP1: nucleotide-binding oligomerization domain, leucine-rich repeat and pyrin domain containing; NGF: neural growth factor; NLRP1: NLR family pyrin domain containing 1; PDGFRA: platelet-derived growth factor receptor alpha; PTPN22: protein tyrosine phosphatase non-receptor type 22; ROS: reactive oxygen species; TREGS: regulatory T cells; TRM: resident memory T cells; TYR: tyrosinase; UV: ultraviolet; VEGF: vascular endothelial growth factor; VIT1: vacuolar iron transporter 1; XBP1: X-box binding protein-1)

Source: Adapted from https://www.mdpi.com/1422-0067/24/5/4910.

PATHOGENESIS OF VITILIGO

The above-mentioned four principal etiological factors (Genetic Factors, Autoimmunity, Oxidative Stress, and Neurogenic Factors) converge and cause destruction of "functional melanocytes." Intrinsic melanocyte defects and dysfunction play a key role in their destruction. These defects reflect an inherent vulnerability in melanocytes, making them more susceptible to oxidative stress, environmental insults, and immune attack.

Melanocytes, due to their inherent vulnerabilities, serve as the trigger for immune activation. Once the immune system is engaged, it exacerbates melanocyte dysfunction through cytokine-driven cytotoxicity, creating a vicious cycle of depigmentation.

Melanocyte Intrinsic Defects as the First Hit

The intrinsic defects in melanocytes render them fragile and predisposed to injury, which acts as the initiating event for vitiligo. These include (**Fig. 2**):
- Oxidative stress[39]
- Mitochondrial dysfunction[40]
- Endoplasmic reticulum stress[41]
- Impaired melanogenesis[39]
- Calcium dysregulation[42]

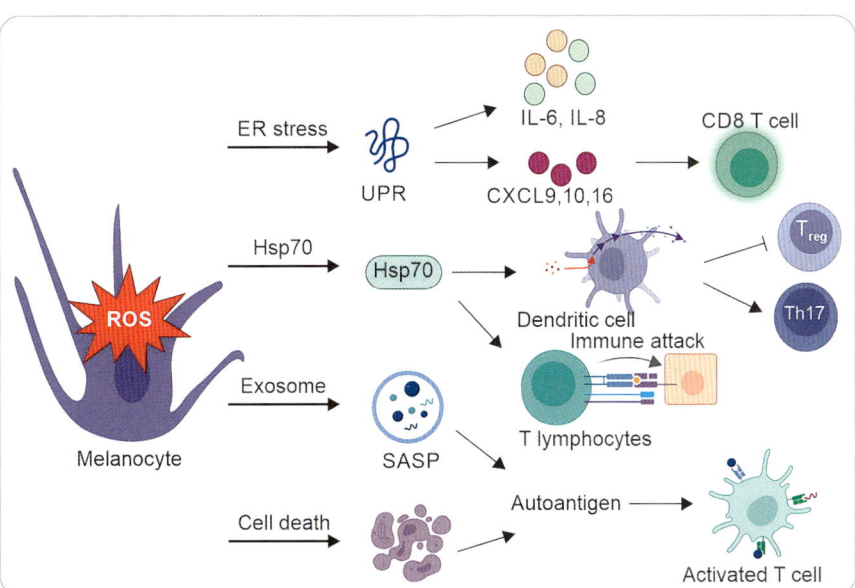

FIG. 2: Oxidative stress activates adaptive immunity through autoantigen presentation to innate immunity. Stressed melanocytes produce autoantigens in the manner of cytokines, extracellular exosomes, and cell death debris. Autoantigens can be highly immunogenic, which activates cytotoxic T cells, regulatory T (T_{reg}) cells, and T helper cells.

(CXCL: C-X-C chemokine ligand; ER: endoplasmic reticulum; Hsp70: 70-kDa heat shock protein; IL-6: interleukin-6; IL-8: interleukin-8; SASP: senescence-associated secretory phenotype; Th17: T-helper 17; UPR: unfolded protein response)

Source: https://www.mdpi.com/2073-4409/12/6/936.

Together, these processes create a microenvironment where stressed melanocytes release signals that act as danger-associated molecular patterns (DAMPs), initiating the autoimmune cascade.

Release of DAMPs and autoimmune activation:
- *Reactive oxygen species and damage markers*:
    - Oxidative stress-induced cellular damage results in the release of DAMPs such as *HMGB1 (high mobility group box 1)*, ATP, and heat shock proteins (HSPs) into the extracellular space.[43,44]
    - These molecules are recognized by innate immune cells (e.g., dendritic cells) via pattern recognition receptors (PRRs) like toll-like receptors (TLRs), marking melanocytes as "dangerous."[45]
- *Neoantigens*: Oxidative stress and impaired melanogenesis produce modified melanocyte proteins (e.g., oxidized tyrosinase) that act as neoantigens, triggering the activation of antigen-presenting cells (APCs).[46]

Autoimmune Response: The Second Hit

Once melanocytes are marked as a source of danger, the adaptive immune system engages in a targeted cytotoxic attack. This autoimmune assault further amplifies melanocyte stress and destruction.

Mechanisms of Autoimmune Response
- *Cytotoxic T cells*:
    - Activated CD8+ T cells infiltrate the skin, recognizing melanocyte antigens presented by MHC class I molecules.
    - Melanocyte-specific antigens include:
        - Tyrosinase
        - Glycoprotein 100 (gp100)
        - MART-1
    - These T cells release cytotoxic mediators such as granzyme B and perforin, directly killing melanocytes.[47]
- *Proinflammatory cytokines*:
    - CD8+ T cells and innate immune cells secrete cytokines, such as:
        - Interferon-γ:
            - Induces melanocyte apoptosis by upregulating *CXCL9* and *CXCL10*, which recruit more T cells.
            - Suppresses melanogenesis by inhibiting melanogenesis-related enzymes (e.g., tyrosinase).[47]
        - Tumor necrosis factor-α: Enhances apoptosis and perpetuates oxidative stress.[39]
        - Interleukin-17: Secreted by Th17 cells, interleukin-17 (IL-17) promotes inflammation and further disrupts melanocyte function.[48]
- *Role of regulatory T cells*: Impaired or reduced Tregs in vitiligo patients fail to suppress the autoimmune response, allowing the unchecked destruction of melanocytes.[22]

Interaction between Intrinsic Defects and Autoimmunity
Self-amplifying Feedback Loop
- *Oxidative stress enhances autoimmunity*:
  - Reactive oxygen species and melanocyte-derived DAMPs sustain the activation of dendritic cells, which continue to present melanocyte antigens to T cells.[39]
  - Persistent oxidative stress drives the generation of additional neoantigens, broadening the repertoire of immune targets.[39,46]
- *Autoimmune cytotoxicity aggravates intrinsic defects*:
  - Cytokines such as IFN-γ and TNF-α induce ROS production and endoplasmic reticulum (ER) stress in surviving melanocytes.[25]
  - Cytotoxic attacks damage mitochondrial membranes, leading to ROS leakage and apoptosis.[47]
  - Repeated immune-mediated injury disrupts calcium signaling and further impairs melanogenesis.[49]

Epitope Spreading
- As melanocytes die, they release more intracellular components, exposing additional antigens (e.g., melanosome proteins like MART-1 or gp100).
- This phenomenon, known as epitope spreading, broadens the immune response, worsening depigmentation.[50]

Loss of Immune Privilege in the Skin
Under normal conditions, melanocytes are protected by the immune privilege of the epidermis. However, in vitiligo, this privilege is disrupted:
- *Decreased expression of immune modulators*: Downregulation of HLA-G and indoleamine 2,3-dioxygenase (IDO) reduces the local immunosuppressive environment.[51]
- *Activation of local innate immunity*: Keratinocytes and fibroblasts in vitiligo lesions release proinflammatory cytokines (e.g., IL-6 and IL-1β), amplifying the immune response.[52]

CONCLUSION: A VICIOUS CYCLE OF DYSFUNCTION AND AUTOIMMUNITY

In vitiligo, melanocyte intrinsic defects (e.g., oxidative stress, mitochondrial dysfunction, and impaired melanogenesis) create a fragile cellular state, initiating autoimmune activation. Once the immune system is engaged, it exacerbates melanocyte stress and destruction through targeted cytotoxicity, proinflammatory cytokines, and epitope spreading. This self-perpetuating cycle highlights the intricate and inseparable link between melanocyte dysfunction and autoimmunity in vitiligo pathogenesis.

On the Horizon—Ongoing Research Areas in Vitiligo

Research in vitiligo pathogenesis and therapeutics have seen unprecedented pace in last two decades. Some of the ongoing research directions are:

Role of the Skin Microbiome

Dysbiosis in the skin and gut microbiome may contribute to immune dysregulation in vitiligo. Research focuses on dysbiosis patterns, effects, and means of restoring microbial balance.[53]

Interferon-γ and Janus Kinase/Signal Transducer and Activator of Transcription Pathway

Expanding use of JAK inhibitors and other small molecules to modulate immune responses. JAK3-selective ritlecitinib is under clinical trials as an oral formulation.[54]

Melanocyte Stress and Apoptosis

Enhancing melanocyte survival with Nrf2 activators and autophagy modulators.[55]

Neural Mechanisms in Segmental Vitiligo

Addressing catecholamine toxicity and neuroinflammation.

Genetic and Epigenetic Factors

Identifying susceptibility genes (e.g., *NLRP1* and *TYR*) and developing clustered regularly interspaced short palindromic repeat (CRISPR) and epigenetic therapies.[56]

T-regulatory Cells and Immune Tolerance

Promoting tolerance via low-dose of interleukin-2 (IL-2) and Treg cell infusions.[57]

Exosomes and Extracellular Vesicles

Blocking inflammatory signals and exploring exosome-based biomarkers.[58]

Skin Repigmentation and Stem Cells

Melanocyte stem-cell therapies, mesenchymal stem cells, and advanced transplantation techniques.[59]

Artificial Intelligence in Personalized Treatment

Artificial intelligence (AI)-driven models for predicting disease progression and therapy response.[60]

Novel Therapeutic Targets

Targeting interleukin-15 (IL-15)/interleukin-17 (IL-17) pathways, tyrosinase-related proteins 1/2 (TRP-1/-2) proteins, and melanocyte-specific antigens.[61,62]

REFERENCES

1. Ghalioungui P. The Ebers Papyrus. (Translated by Paul Ghalioungui.) Cairo: Academy of Scientific Research and Technology; 1987. pp. 1-10.
2. Barman S. Switra and its treatment in veda. Anc Sci Life. 1995;15:71-4.
3. Cheng Z. Chinese Medicine Archives. Traditional Chinese Medicine Compendium. Beijing: People's Medical Publishing House; 1995. pp. 120-35.
4. Jones WHS. Hippocrates. On Airs, Waters, and Places. (Translated by W.H.S. Jones.) Cambridge: Harvard University Press; 1923. pp. 91-2.
5. Westerhof W. The discovery of the human melanocyte. Pigment Cell Res. 2006;19(3):183-93.
6. Kaposi M. Pathology and treatment of diseases of the skin. New York: William Wood & Company; 1895. pp. 480-3.
7. Parrish JA, Fitzpatrick TB, Shea C, Pathak MA. Photochemotherapy of vitiligo. Use of orally administered psoralens and a high-intensity long-wave ultraviolet light system. Arch Dermatol. 1976;112(11):1531-4.
8. Westerhof W, Nieuweboer-Krobotova L. Narrowband UVB therapy for vitiligo: Efficacy and safety. J Invest Dermatol. 1983;81(6):522-6.
9. Le Poole IC, van den Wijngaard RM, Westerhof W, Das PK. Presence of T cells and macrophages in inflammatory vitiligo skin parallels melanocyte disappearance. Am J Pathol. 1996;148(4):1219-28.
10. Schallreuter KU, Wood JM, Berger J. Low catalase levels in the epidermis of patients with vitiligo. J Invest Dermatol. 1991;97(6):1081-5.
11. Spritz RA. The genetics of generalized vitiligo and associated autoimmune diseases. J Dermatol Sci. 2006;41(1):3-10.
12. Rashighi M, Harris JE. Interfering with the IFN-γ/CXCL10 pathway to develop new targeted treatments for vitiligo. Ann Transl Med. 2015;3(21):343.
13. Majumder PP, Das SK, Li CC. A genetical model for vitiligo. Am J Hum Genet. 1988;43(2):119-25.
14. Alkhateeb A, Fain PR, Thody A, Bennett DC, Spritz RA. Epidemiology of vitiligo and associated autoimmune diseases in Caucasian probands and their families. Pigment Cell Res. 2003;16(3):208-14.
15. Jin Y, Andersen G, Yorgov D, Ferrara TM, Ben S, Brownson KM, et al. Genome-wide association studies of autoimmune vitiligo identify 23 new risk loci and highlight key pathways and regulatory variants. Nat Genet. 2016;48(11):1418-24.
16. Šahmatova L, Tankov S, Prans E, Aab A, Hermann H, Reemann P, et al. MicroRNA-155 is Dysregulated in the Skin of Patients with Vitiligo and Inhibits Melanogenesis-associated Genes in Melanocytes and Keratinocytes. Acta Derm Venereol. 2016;96(6):742-7.
17. Pu Y, Chen X, Chen Y, Zhang L, Chen J, Zhang Y, et al. Transcriptome and differential methylation integration analysis identified important differential methylation annotation genes and functional epigenetic modules related to vitiligo. Front Immunol. 2021;12:587440.
18. Kemp EH, Waterman EA, Hawes BE, O'Neill K, Gottumukkala RV, Gawkrodger DJ, et al. The melanin-concentrating hormone receptor 1, a novel target of autoantibody responses in vitiligo. J Clin Invest. 2002;109(7):923-30.
19. Wu J, Zhou M, Wan Y, Xu A. CD8+ T cells from vitiligo perilesional margins induce autologous melanocyte apoptosis. Mol Med Rep. 2013;7(1):237-41.
20. Custurone P, Di Bartolomeo L, Irrera N, Borgia F, Altavilla D, Bitto A, et al. Role of cytokines in vitiligo: Pathogenesis and possible targets for old and new treatments. Int J Mol Sci. 2021;22(21):11429.
21. Rashighi M, Agarwal P, Richmond JM, Harris TH, Dresser K, Su MW, et al. CXCL10 is critical for the progression and maintenance of depigmentation in a mouse model of vitiligo. Sci Transl Med. 2014;6(223):223ra23.
22. Dwivedi M, Kemp EH, Laddha NC, Mansuri MS, Weetman AP, Begum R. Regulatory T cells in vitiligo: Implications for pathogenesis and therapeutics. Autoimmun Rev. 2015;14(1):49-56.

23. Billon E, Walz J, Brunelle S, Thomassin J, Salem N, Guerin M, et al. Vitiligo adverse event observed in a patient with durable complete response after nivolumab for metastatic renal cell carcinoma. Front Oncol. 2019;9:1033.
24. Gellatly KJ, Strassner JP, Essien K, Refat MA, Murphy RL, Coffin-Schmitt A, et al. scRNA-seq of human vitiligo reveals complex networks of subclinical immune activation and a role for CCR5 in Treg function. Sci Transl Med. 2021;13(610):eabd8995.
25. Chang WL, Ko CH. The role of oxidative stress in vitiligo: An update on its pathogenesis and therapeutic implications. Cells. 2023;12(6):936.
26. Lin Y, Ding Y, Wu Y, Yang Y, Liu Z, Xiang L, et al. The underestimated role of mitochondria in vitiligo: From oxidative stress to inflammation and cell death. Exp Dermatol. 2024;33(1):e14856.
27. van den Boorn JG, Melief CJ, Luiten RM. Monobenzone-induced depigmentation: from enzymatic blockade to autoimmunity. Pigment Cell Melanoma Res. 2011;24(4):673-9.
28. Laddha NC, Dwivedi M, Mansuri MS, Gani AR, Ansarullah M, Ramachandran AV, et al. Vitiligo: interplay between oxidative stress and immune system. Exp Dermatol. 2013;22:245-50.
29. Jian Z, Li K, Song P, Zhu G, Zhu L, Cui T, et al. Impaired activation of the Nrf2-ARE signaling pathway undermines H_2O_2-induced oxidative stress response: A possible mechanism for melanocyte degeneration in vitiligo. J Invest Dermatol. 2014;134(8):2221-30.
30. Speeckaert R, Bulat V, Speeckaert MM, van Geel N. The impact of antioxidants on vitiligo and melasma: A scoping review and meta-analysis. Antioxidants (Basel). 2023;12(12):2082.
31. Diotallevi F, Gioacchini H, De Simoni E, Marani A, Candelora M, Paolinelli M, et al. Vitiligo, from Pathogenesis to Therapeutic Advances: State of the Art. Int J Mol Sci. 2023;24:4910.
32. Wu H, Zhao Y, Huang Q, Cai M, Pan Q, Fu M, et al. NK1R/5-HT1AR interaction is related to the regulation of melanogenesis. The FASEB J. 2018;32:3193-214.
33. Wu CS, Yu HS, Chang HR, Yu CL, Yu CL, Wu BN. Cutaneous blood flow and adrenoceptor response increase in segmental-type vitiligo lesions. J Dermatol Sci. 2000;23(1):53-62.
34. Chu CY, Liu YL, Chiu HC, Jee SH. Dopamine-induced apoptosis in human melanocytes involves generation of reactive oxygen species. Br J Dermatol. 2006;154(6):1071-9.
35. Morrone A, Picardo M, de Luca C, Terminali O, Passi S, Ippolito F. Catecholamines and vitiligo. Pigment Cell Res. 1992;5(2):65-9.
36. Al'Abadie MS, Senior HJ, Bleehen SS, Gawkrodger DJ. Neuropeptide and neuronal marker studies in vitiligo. Br J Dermatol. 1994;131(2):160-5.
37. Zhou J, Feng JY, Wang Q, Shang J. Calcitonin gene-related peptide cooperates with substance P to inhibit melanogenesis and induces apoptosis of B16F10 cells. Cytokine. 2015;74(1):137-44.
38. Cao C, Lei J, Zheng Y, Xu A, Zhou M. The brain-skin axis in vitiligo. Arch Dermatol Res. 2024;316(8):607.
39. Xuan Y, Yang Y, Xiang L, Zhang C. The role of oxidative stress in the pathogenesis of vitiligo: A culprit for melanocyte death. Oxid Med Cell Longev. 2022;2022:8498472.
40. Kaushik H, Kumar V, Parsad D. Mitochondria-Melanocyte cellular interactions: An emerging mechanism of vitiligo pathogenesis. J Eur Acad Dermatol Venereol. 2023;37(11):2196-207.
41. Jadeja SD, Mayatra JM, Vaishnav J, Shukla N, Begum R. A concise review on the role of endoplasmic reticulum stress in the development of autoimmunity in vitiligo pathogenesis. Front Immunol. 2021;11:624566.
42. Li S, Zhu G, Yang Y, Ge L, Bi Y, Han R, et al. Dysfunction of calcium and calcium-related signaling pathways in vitiligo pathogenesis. Front Cell Dev Biol. 2021;9:642112.
43. Kang P, Zhang W, Chen X, Yi X, Song P, Chang Y, et al. TRPM2 mediates mitochondria-dependent apoptosis of melanocytes under oxidative stress. Free Radic Biol Med. 2018;126:259-68.
44. Wang J, Pan Y, Wei G, Mao H, Liu R, He Y. Damage-associated molecular patterns in vitiligo: igniter fuse from oxidative stress to melanocyte loss. Redox Rep. 2022;27(1):193-9.
45. Roh JS, Sohn DH. Damage-associated molecular patterns in inflammatory diseases. Immune Netw. 2018;18(4):e27.

46. Hlača N, Žagar T, Kaštelan M, Brajac I, Prpić-Massari L. Current concepts of vitiligo immunopathogenesis. Biomedicines. 2022;10(7):1639.
47. Yang L, Wei Y, Sun Y, Shi W, Yang J, Zhu L, et al. Interferon-gamma inhibits melanogenesis and induces apoptosis in melanocytes: A pivotal role of CD8+ cytotoxic T lymphocytes in vitiligo. Acta Derm Venereol. 2015;95(6):664-70.
48. Singh RK, Lee KM, Vujkovic-Cvijin I, Ucmak D, Farahnik B, Abrouk M, et al. The role of IL-17 in vitiligo: A review. Autoimmun Rev. 2016;15(4):397-404.
49. Xie H, Zhou F, Liu L, Zhu G, Li Q, Li C, et al. Vitiligo: How do oxidative stress-induced autoantigens trigger autoimmunity? J Dermatol Sci. 2016;81(1):3-9.
50. Mandelcorn-Monson RL, Shear NH, Yau E, Sambhara S, Barber BH, Spaner D, et al. Cytotoxic T lymphocyte reactivity to gp100, MelanA/MART-1, and tyrosinase, in HLA-A2-positive vitiligo patients. J Invest Dermatol. 2003;121(3):550-6.
51. Speeckaert R, Belpaire A, Speeckaert M, van Geel N. The delicate relation between melanocytes and skin immunity: A game of hide and seek. Pigment Cell Melanoma Res. 2022; 35(4):392-407.
52. Touni AA, Shivde RS, Echuri H, Abdel-Aziz RTA, Abdel-Wahab H, Kundu RV, et, al. Melanocyte-keratinocyte cross-talk in vitiligo. Front Med (Lausanne). 2023;10:1176781.
53. Nigro A, Osman A, Suryadevara P, Cices A. Vitiligo and the microbiome of the gut and skin: a systematic review. Arch Dermatol Res. 2025;317(1):201.
54. Inouea S, Suzukib T,·Sanoc S, Katayamad I. JAK inhibitors for the treatment of vitiligo. J Dermatol Sci. 2024;113(3):86-92.
55. Frantz MC, Rozot R, Marrot L. NRF2 in dermo-cosmetic: From scientific knowledge to skin care products. BioFactors. 2023;49(1):32-61.
56. Bajpai VK, Swigut T, Mohammed J, Naqvi S, Arreola M, Tycko J, et al. A genome-wide genetic screen uncovers determinants of human pigmentation. Science. 2023;381(6658):eade6289.
57. Tahvildari M, Dana R. Low-dose IL-2 therapy in transplantation, autoimmunity, and inflammatory diseases. J Immunol. 2019;203:2749-55.
58. Li W, Pang Y, He Q, Song Z, Xie X, Zeng J, et al. Exosome-derived microRNAs: emerging players in vitiligo. Front. Immunol. 2024;15:1419660.
59. Paino F, Ricci G, De Rosa A, D'Aquino R, Laino L, Pirozzi G, et al. Ecto-mesenchymal stem cells from dental pulp are committed to differentiate into active melanocytes. Eur Cell Mater. 2010;20:295-305.
60. Wang Z, Xue Y, Liu Z, Wang C, Xiong K, Lin K, et al. AI fusion of multisource data identifies key features of vitiligo. Sci Rep. 2024;14:24278.
61. Bhardwaj S, Bhatia A, Kumaran MS, Parsad D. Role of IL-17A receptor blocking in melanocyte survival: A strategic intervention against vitiligo. Exp Dermatol. 2019;28(6):682-9.
62. Zou DP, Chen YM, Zhang LZ, Yuan XH, Zhang YJ, Inggawati A, et al. SFRP5 inhibits melanin synthesis of melanocytes in vitiligo by suppressing the Wnt/β-catenin signaling. Genes Dis. 2020;8(5):677-88.

3 CHAPTER

Clinical Presentation and Diagnosis
Classifying Vitiligo: Types and Patterns; Diagnostic Tools and Criteria

Madhulika Mhatre, Aseem Sharma

INTRODUCTION

Vitiligo is an acquired disorder of hypopigmentation characterized by progressive deprivation of melanocytes in the epidermis, hair bulb, mucous membrane, and eyes. It is widely considered to be a complex reaction pattern—a multifactorial disease with numerous genetic inherited factors and environmental triggers with strong evidence to consider it an autoimmune disease or syndrome. There is literature supporting the presence of antibodies to melanocytes in serum. There are several ways to classify vitiligo depending upon the distribution, extent, color, and symmetry. Classification of vitiligo is primarily clinical. There is a need to classify vitiligo on the basis of pathophysiology and diagnosis, but this warrants further research and high-level evidence. The global incidence of vitiligo is 0.5–1%.[1] The most common age of presentation is between 5 and 30 years of age. 10–70% of patients have some underlying stressful stimuli leading to the development of vitiligo.[1] However, the onset of vitiligo is variable among different studies but widely agreed as prior to 30 years of age. Of the clinical types, segmental vitiligo (SV) is the most prevalent in the pediatric age-group. Vitiligo also has a huge impact on quality of life. The profound psychological and social burden of the disease extends far beyond its physical manifestation.[2]

CURRENT REVISED CLASSIFICATION: VITILIGO GLOBAL ISSUES CONSENSUS CONFERENCE, VITILIGO EUROPEAN TASK FORCE

Classification[3,4]
Refer to **Table 1**.

Further Simplified Classification (Table 1)
- Segmental vitiligo
- Nonsegmental vitiligo (NSV)

TABLE 1: Classifications of vitiligo.		
Type of vitiligo	**Subtypes**	**Remarks**
Nonsegmental vitiligo (NSV)	Focal,[a] mucosal, acrofacial, generalized, and universal	Subtyping may not reflect a distinct nature, but useful information for epidemiologic studies
Segmental vitiligo (SV)	Focal,[b] mucosal, unisegmental, bi- or multisegmental	Further classification according to distribution pattern possible, but not yet standardized
Mixed (NSV + SV)	According to severity of SV	Usually, the SV part in mixed vitiligo is more severe
Unclassified	Focal at onset, multifocal asymmetrical nonsegmental, and mucosal (only one site)	This category is a means to allow, after sufficient observation time (and if needs investigations), for a definitive classification

[a]Possible onset of NSV.
[b]See text for discussion.

- Mixed
- Unclassified

Segmental vitiligo includes:
- Mucosal
- Focal
- Unisegmental
- Bisegmental or multisegmental

Nonsegmental vitiligo includes:
- Mucosal
- Universal
- Generalized
- Acrofacial

Nonsegmental Vitiligo

It is classified as an umbrella term for all types of vitiligo that is nonsegmental—acrofacial, mucosal (multifocal), generalized, and universal subtypes. There is another way of classifying—bilateral and unilateral[5] but this remains inconclusive. NSV usually occurs between 20 and 30 years of age.[6] It classically presents as a depigmented macule of varying sizes with a propensity to be bilaterally symmetrical. Wood's lamp remains an important diagnostic and evaluation tool to assess this depigmented macule. Vitiligo minor is rare form of NSV.[4] This entity mainly encountered in dark skin types where "minor" represents a partial defect in pigmentation. Follicular vitiligo is a subtype seen in young dark-skinned patients which manifests with a predominant involvement of hair follicle and limited skin involvement.

Acrofacial Vitiligo

This entity is characterized by lesions involving acral part on the limbs, and around body orifices. Digital tip involvement lowers the prognosis as compared to that of nonfingertip lesions. Only 50% patients with acrofacial vitiligo and "lip-tip involvement" respond to melanocyte transplantation.

Focal Vitiligo
This type is diagnosed after careful elimination of other subtypes. The natural course of focal vitiligo can be classified into generalized or segmental types. A typical lesion fits neither into a typical segmental type nor progresses to NSV, and other causes of localized depigmentation have been ruled out.

Mucosal Vitiligo
This refers to the involvement of oral and genital mucous membranes. If genital mucosa is involved in isolation, a differential diagnosis of lichen sclerosis must be considered.[7] However, conjoint association of the conditions have been reported. Unclassified mucosal vitiligo must present with a duration of >2 years, absence of other bodily lesions, and restriction to dry labial mucosa (lip lesions) according to Prasad et al. and the Vitiligo Global Issues Consensus Conference (VGICC) classification.[8] That being said, there is a case report on extension of lip vitiligo to wet labial mucosa.[9] The lip-tip pattern of acrofacial vitiligo is another example of mucosal vitiligo.

Universal Vitiligo
When vitiligo causes complete or near complete depigmentation, it is termed as vitiligo universalis. Scalp hair involvement is frequently observed in this subtype but is a marker of advanced disease where axillary and pubic regions are also involved. Small, perifollicular, discrete, or coalescent pigmentation may persist in sun-exposed areas. The distinction between universal vitiligo (UV) and fulminant vitiligoid conditions affecting melanocytes of ear and eyes as part of Vogt–Koyanagi–Harada syndrome is still in a shroud. It is discerning to differentiate between monobenzone-induced depigmentation and spontaneous depigmentation.

Mixed Vitiligo
A pediatric case was reported wherein generalized vitiligo responded to treatment, leaving behind an SV patch. This is the first known case of mixed vitiligo.[10] Additional cases were successively reported fulfilling the definition criteria.[11,12] This unique association may be viewed as an example of superimposed segmental manifestation of a generalized polygenic disorder, in which segmental involvement precedes disease generalization and is more resistant to treatment.[13] However, the important risk factors for development of mixed vitiligo are attributed to development of halo nevi and leukotrichia.[14] Recent clinical reports of mixed vitiligo, SV and NSV, have challenged the concept of binary representation of vitiligo. Mulekar et al. are credited with the nomenclature of mixed vitiligo.[11]

Segmental Vitiligo
This term was used by Koga and Tango for the first time. It has three distinct subtypes: mono-, bi-, and multisegmental. Each has a specific morphological pattern. SV has an early age of onset. It becomes clinically stable quite early in

the course of the disease and does not convert into NSV. In addition to its limited distribution, SV has distinguishing characteristics when compared to NSV.[10] The common sites of predilection are the face and neck.[15] The average length of stability is 6 months. It yields a relative resistance to medical therapy and a favorable response to surgical therapies. This is due to the melanocyte reservoir, which is located in hair follicle. Poliosis, or circumscribed patch of white hair, is known to set in early in the course of SV. The results of Van Geel demonstrate that distribution of SV is not similar to any other skin disease pattern and may be a result of mosaicism. Furthermore, evidence of inflammation has been demonstrated in some cases of early SV, suggesting that NSV and SV may both involve inflammatory or immune-related etiologies **(Table 2)**.[16]

Occupational/Contact Vitiligo

The term "contact vitiligo (CV) or occupational vitiligo" is a distinct entity due to persistent occupation-related exposure to certain toxic chemicals such as aromatic and aliphatic derivative of phenol and catechol. While depigmentation initially starts at sites of exposure, the development of remote lesions with progression to a more widespread, typical pattern is common.[17] However, there are lacunae among causative factors and a clearcut definition of CV has not been formed. In effect, chemical agents serve as uncommon environmental triggers or haptens for the induction of what in fact is typical vitiligo and not chemical leukoderma. The opinion of the VGICC participants was that CV requires clearer definition by case studies and epidemiological investigation in at-risk populations to further establish this entity.

Other Unclassified or Poorly Classified Generalized Vitiligoid Conditions

Many conditions do not classically fit into the binary domain of SV or NSV or even mixed vitiligo. Few conditions such as punctate vitiligo, idiopathic guttate melanosis, and progressive macular hypomelanosis are conditions that resemble

TABLE 2: Difference between segmental and nonsegmental vitiligo.	
Segmental vitiligo	**Nonsegmental vitiligo**
Usually asymmetrical	Symmetrical
Nonconfluent, depigmented, unilateral, cutaneous macule, does not cross midline	Bilateral, symmetrical, and depigmented macule
Mosaic genetic skin disorder	Multifactorial with an immune-mediated melanocytic destruction
Rapid onset	Slow onset
Leukotrichia present usually	Body hair pigmentation usually remains, and pigment loss is noticed during progression
Incidence of Koebner's phenomenon is noticed	Koebner's phenomenon is controversial
Better response to surgical therapy	Responds to both

vitiligo closely and not defined in detail. Punctate vitiligo refers to depigmented macules which may involve any area of the body. When these lesions coexist with classical macules of vitiligo, it is best to classify as NSV.

MORPHOLOGICAL FORMS OF VITILIGO

- *Trichrome:* A central depigmented area which is surrounded by a relative intermediate hypopigmented zone with a peripheral rim of hyperpigmentation separating this zone from normal skin. Cockade-like vitiligo is a variant of trichrome-like vitiligo.
- *Quadrichrome:* Features of trichrome vitiligo also show additional feature of perifollicular pigmentation which is a sign of therapeutic response.
- *Pentachrome:* It is described as presence of five shades of colors seen in a vitiliginous macule—white, tan, medium brown, dark brown, and black.
- *Blue vitiligo:* The blue discoloration of vitiligo lesion is seen in skin affected by prior postinflammatory hyperpigmentation. On scattering of light, the longer wavelength, yellow and red, tends to penetrate whereas blue light scatters leading to appearance of a bluish hue, as per Tyndall effect.

RECENT UPDATES IN CLINICAL EVALUATION

Till date, there is no joint consensus on clinical assessment criteria for a vitiliginous patch. Wood's lamp is a vital clinical evaluatory tool to gauge infraclinical changes.[18] The appearance of a macule with detailed clinical examination of the margin is critical. Different descriptive factors for clinical evaluation are inflammatory lesions with raised borders, morphological color (trichrome, quadrichrome, pentachrome, and blue), hypomelanotic macules with poorly defined borders, and amelanotic macules with sharply demarcated borders. The size and the number of the lesion is an essential part of clinical examination with good clinical photographic image for record. Additionally, if there is no increase in size of existing lesions or any new lesion in 1 year, then it may be considered as "stable" (type S) vitiligo and conversely as "active" (type A) vitiligo. The incidence of Koebner's isomorphic phenomenon (as a negative marker of stability) in NSV has been reported to be from 15 to 70% and is considered controversial in SV. Recently, the predictive value of Koebner's has been put to test by history (Kb-h) or by experimental induction (Kb-e).[18,19] Histologically, stability of the lesion correlates with significant absence of melanin in the depigmented epidermis on the border, and larger than normal melanocytes, with long dendritic process.[18] Additionally, dermoscopy is an important tool to assess clinical activity of the disease. Depending on the retention or loss of perifollicular pigment, one can assess the activity of the disease by means of a dermoscope with perifollicular pigmentation corresponding with unstable spectrum of the disease.[20]

ASSESSMENT OF VITILIGO ACTIVITY (STABILITY)

This faction of vitiligo diagnosis heavily impacts management and has always been a bone of contention.

Duration

There is a wide dispute about the time duration following which it has to be labeled as stable vitiligo. Additionally, there are variable reports depicting minimum duration for clinical stability from 3 months to 4 years.[21] However, in this regard, the broad consensus is 1 year.

As mentioned earlier, vitiligo is primarily a clinical diagnosis. The same fundamental translates to stability assessment as well. Clinical pointers to evaluate stability include (the same has been summarized in **Table 3**):

- History and evidence of new lesions
- Extension of existing lesions and Koebner's phenomenon.[22]
- *Minigraft testing*: Apart from clinical stability, there is also the concept of "surgical stability" or cellular stability. A few test grafts placed in the center of the lesion and assessment of perigraft repigmentation is carried out to assess stability, as described by Falabella et al.[19,21]
- *Standardized serial photography* may also be employed to gauge stability. This should be used in conjunction with a scoring system:
  - Vitiligo disease activity (ViDA)
  - Vitiligo Area Severity Index (VASI)
  - Vitiligo European Task Force (VETF) score
- *Dermoscopy* has evolved from a diagnostic luxury to a multipronged aid in assessing vitiligo activity. Dermoscopic markers for unstable vitiligo include:[20]
  - Altered pigmentary network
  - White dots, clods, and globules
  - Starburst depigmentation pattern

At the other spectrum, stable vitiliginous macules show the following dermoscopic pattern(s):[20]
  - *Untreated lesion*:
    – Perifollicular depigmentation
    – Leukotrichia
  - *Treated: repigmenting lesion—*
    – Perifollicular repigmentation
    – Marginal (perilesional) repigmentation
    – Sharp, contained borders

TABLE 3: Salient markers of stability.	
History	• New lesions • Extension of existing lesions • Koebner's phenomenon
Minigraft testing	
Standardized serial photography	With or without grading systems: • ViDA[a] • VASI[b] • VETF[c]
Dermoscopy	Proposed criteria as mentioned

[a]Vitiligo disease activity.
[b]Vitiligo area severity index.
[c]Vitiligo European Task Force score.

- *Biochemical markers*: Another set of markers for vitiligo activity is biochemical and serological markers. These are considered cross-sectional, and hence, do not elucidate their correlation with the course and prognosis of the disease.[19,23] The biochemical markers include the following:
    - Catalase
    - Glutathione peroxidase (GSH)
    - Superoxide dismutase (SOD)
    - Catecholamines

  Another marker that has recently come to the forefront is the S100B serum levels. At present, the evidence is contradictory with a few reports suggesting its strong correlation with disease activity and others not finding an association with VIDA or VASI scores.[24,25]
- *Histological* aid is sought for stability in two ways: First, as mentioned in the previous section, and secondly for enzymological assessment on tissue. Immunohistochemistry may be performed on the biopsy sample for calculating cytotoxic T-cell lymphocytes, CD45 RO memory T-cell and even CD4/CD8 ratio estimation.[23] Akin to biochemical markers, there is no consensus for use of patterns for these tests.

There is also the concept of the different paradigms of stability—lesional stability (lesion), regional stability (local area), or overall stability (most widely accepted). In a multicentric trial, it was observed that lesional stability is also important and it was found that patients with overall stability of >6 months, but a lesional stability of >1 year had comparable results to another group of patients with overall stability of >1 year duration. This observation is extremely important in patients who are time-bound due to social crises and need care at the earliest.[21] Thus lesional stability seems to be more significant for surgical intervention in vitiligo.

Such cases need not wait for surgical treatment just because their disease has not been stable for over a 1 year. A recent study performed in patients with varying durations of stability where suction blister grafting was done. Repigmentation of 28.5% cases was noted in patients with stable period between 3 months and 1 year, 37.5% in 1–2 years group, and 77.8% when stability exceeded 2 years **(Table 4)**.

TABLE 4: Scoring system used to assess repigmentation.[19]		
Clinical observation	**Score given**	**Response assessment**
No change in the depigmented area	0	Poor
Specks of repigmentation or concavity of margins	1	Poor
Area of repigmentation less than the residual depigmented area	2	Poor
Area of repigmentation almost equal to that of residual depigmentation	3	Good
Area of repigmentation more than the residual depigmented area	4	Good
Some specks of depigmentation left	5	Excellent
Near-complete repigmentation	6	Excellent

The consensus on minimum duration of stability before surgery continues to change, be unchanged, and rechange.[26] The psychological impact of the devastating disease is also related to the site of lesion. The avoidance behavior and decreased social interaction due to the disease warrants extensive research to prognosticate the stability of the disease in an implied way.[27]

CONCLUSION

Vitiligo is a complex disorder which wields a stigma and runs deeper to the integument. The basis of classification has changed over the years to include clearly defined subtypes with distinct management protocols. And even though the diagnosis and prognosis remain clinical, many aids have been employed to assess vitiligo activity ranging from dermoscopy to histopathology and from serology to immunohistochemistry. Stability has always been a matter of debate and continues to be so, till date. Lesional stability is emerging as a more reliable marker than overall stability.

REFERENCES

1. Speeckaert R, van Geel N. Vitiligo: An Update on Pathophysiology and Treatment Options. Am J Clin Dermatol. 2017;18(6):733-44.
2. Lai YC, Yew YW, Kennedy C, Schwartz RA. Vitiligo and depression: a systematic review and meta-analysis of observational studies. Br J Dermatol. 2017;177(3):708-18.
3. Taïeb A, Picardo M; VETF Members. The definition and assessment of vitiligo: a consensus report of the Vitiligo European Task Force. Pigment Cell Res. 2007;20(1):27-35.
4. Ezzedine K, Lim HW, Suzuki T, Katayama I, Hamzavi I, Lan CC, et al. Revised classification/nomenclature of vitiligo and related issues: the Vitiligo Global Issues Consensus Conference. Pigment Cell Melanoma Res. 2012;25(3):E1-13.
5. Bishnoi A, Parsad D. The Concept of Stability of Vitiligo and Stabilization Therapies. In: Gupta S, Olsson MJ, Parsad D, Lim HW, van Geel N, Pandya AG (Eds). Vitiligo: Medical and Surgical Management. United States: John Wiley & Sons Ltd; 2018. pp. 81-90.
6. Ezzedine K, Eleftheriadou V, Whitton M, van Geel N. Vitiligo. Lancet. 2015;386(9988):74-84.
7. Ortonne JP. Depigmentation of hair and mucous membrane. In: Hann SK, Nordlund JJ (Eds). Vitiligo. Oxford: Blackwell Publishing Ltd; 2000. pp. 76-80.
8. Parsad D. Mucosal vitiligo. In: Picardo M, Taïeb A (Eds). Vitiligo. Berlin, Heidelberg: Springer; 2010. pp. 57-9.
9. Andrade SA, Baeta IGR, Ribeiro MM, Pratavieira S, Bagnato VS, Varotti FP. Mucosal vitiligo in angles of the mouth: clinical and fluorescence aspects. Rev Assoc Med Bras. 2019;65(3):330-2.
10. Gauthier Y, Cario Andre M, Taïeb A. A critical appraisal of vitiligo etiologic theories. Is melanocyte loss a melanocytorrhagy? Pigment Cell Res. 2003;16(4):322-32.
11. Mulekar SV, Al Issa A, Asaad M, Ghwish B, Al Eisa A. Mixed vitiligo. J Cutan Med Surg. 2006;10(2):104-7.
12. Ezzedine K, Gauthier Y, Léauté-Labrèze C, Marquez S, Bouchtnei S, Jouary T, et al. Segmental vitiligo associated with generalized vitiligo (mixed vitiligo): a retrospective case series of 19 patients. J Am Acad Dermatol. 2011;65(5):965-71.
13. Happle R. Superimposed segmental manifestation of polygenic skin disorders. J Am Acad Dermatol. 2007;57(4):690-9.
14. Ezzedine K, Diallo A, Léauté-Labrèze C, Séneschal J, Prey S, Ballanger F, et al. Halo naevi and leukotrichia are strong predictors of the passage to mixed vitiligo in a subgroup of segmental vitiligo. Br J Dermatol. 2012;166(3):539-44.

15. Van Geel N, Bosma S, Boone B, Speeckaert R. Classification of segmental vitiligo on the trunk. Br J Dermatol. 2014;170:322-7.
16. van Geel NA, Mollet IG, De Schepper S, Tjin EP, Vermaelen K, Clark RA, et al. First histopathological and immunophenotypic analysis of early dynamic events in a patient with segmental vitiligo associated with halo nevi. Pigment Cell Melanoma Res. 2010;23(3): 375-84.
17. Rodrigues M, Ezzedine K, Hamzavi I, Pandya AG, Harris JE; Vitiligo Working Group. New discoveries in the pathogenesis and classification of vitiligo. J Am Acad Dermatol. 2017; 77(1):1-13.
18. Benzekri L, Gauthier Y, Hamada S, Hassam B. Clinical features and histological findings are potential indicators of activity in lesions of common vitiligo. Br J Dermatol. 2013;168(2): 265-71.
19. Sahni K, Parsad D. Stability in vitiligo: Is there a perfect way to predict it? J Cutan Aesthet Surg. 2013;6:75-8.
20. Jha AK, Sonthalia S, Lallas A. Dermoscopy as an evolving tool to assess vitiligo activity. J Am Acad Dermatol. 2018;78(5):1017-9.
21. Majid I, Mysore V, Salim T, Lahiri K, Chatterji M, Khunger N, et al. Is lesional stability in vitiligo more important than disease stability for performing surgical interventions? results from a multicentric study. J Cutan Aesthet Surg. 2016;9:13-9.
22. Mulekar SV, Al Eissa A, Asaad M. Koebnerization of donor site in unilateral vitiligo patients, treated successfully by autologous, noncultured melanocyte-keratinocyte (MK) cell transplantation. Clin Exp Dermatol. 2005;30(4):445-6.
23. Gupta S. Stability in vitiligo: Why such a hullabaloo? J Cutan Aesthet Surg. 2009;2(1):41.
24. Badran AY, Gomaa AS, El-Mahdy RI, El Zohne RA, Kamal DT, Abou-Taleb DAE. Serum level of S100B in vitiligo patients: Is it a marker of disease activity? Australas J Dermatol. 2021; 62(1):e67-e72.
25. Speeckaert R, Voet S, Hoste E, van Geel N. S100B Is a Potential Disease Activity Marker in Nonsegmental Vitiligo. J Invest Dermatol. 2017;137(7):1445-53.
26. Rao A, Gupta S, Dinda AK, Sharma A, Sharma VK, Kumar G, et al. Study of clinical, biochemical and immunological factors determining stability of disease in patients with generalized vitiligo undergoing melanocyte transplantation. Br J Dermatol. 2012;166:1230-6.
27. Florez-Pollack S, Jia G, Zapata L Jr, Rodgers C, Hernandez K, Hynan LS, et al. Association of Quality of Life and Location of Lesions in Patients With Vitiligo. JAMA Dermatol. 2017; 153(3):341-2.

CHAPTER 4

Stability of Vitiligo: Recommendations and Controversies

Koushik Lahiri, Abhijit Saha

INTRODUCTION

Concept of stability of vitiligo is of utmost importance as far as treatment planning and prognosis of patient is concerned. In spite of considerable amount of improvement in medical management of vitiligo not all patients respond in a predictable manner. In those medical management failure cases, transplantation techniques are the only viable options to replenish lost melanocytes. A number of surgical modalities have been developed in the last few decades. Success of any surgical modality depends upon proper selection of cases. The specific criteria for selection have been well defined.[1]

Principles for selection are based on one single criterion, i.e., stability of the disease. It is taken as the most important parameter before opting for any transplantation technique to treat vitiligo.[2] But, the most decisive factor still remains elusive on several grounds. Better understanding of vitiligo pathophysiology over the years has prompted researchers to look into ultrastructural, biochemical, and serological parameters in addition to clinical parameters to define stability.

There are several issues to be considered while defining stability. These include:
- Defining minimum duration of stability
- Is stability area-specific?
- Validity of test graft (TG)
- How long does stability last?
- Any role of dermatoscope in defining stability
- Concept of cellular stability

MINIMUM DURATION OF STABILITY

The basic fundamental requirement "optimal duration" of the concept of stability lacks unanimity among researchers even after four decades of experience in vitiligo surgery. Lack of consensus among workers could be attributed to lack of evidence behind and subjective bias. Different periods of stability have been mentioned by different authors which range from 4 months to 3 years.[3] Even same author has considered different periods of stability in different articles.[3-5] The Indian Association of Dermatologists, Venereologists and Leprologists (IADVL) task force came forward to solve this issue. In recent past, in their consensus recommendations, the IADVL task force for standard guidelines of care for dermatosurgical procedures attempted to provide a clear definition of stability as "a patient reporting no new lesions, no progression of existing lesions, and absence of Koebner phenomenon during the past 1 year."[6] In the absence of further clarification, this recommendation holds good before opting for surgical intervention. Rao et al. compared successes of suction blister grafting in patient with different periods of stability. Successful repigmentation (>75%) was achieved in 0% of patients in 3 months to 1 year group, 37.5% in 1–2 years group and 77.8% in >2 years group ($p = 0.005$).[7]

A recent cross-sectional study by Taneja et al. further adds to the confusion.[8] They found no association between period of stability (inactivity) and risk of reactivation in case of nonsegmental vitiligo. Longitudinal cohort study using parameters beyond clinical has been suggested in this regard.

IS STABILITY AREA-SPECIFIC?

Results are extremely variable following repigmentation of depigmented area. Simultaneous depigmentation and repigmentation have been observed in different areas of the same patient.[9]

Depigmentation of grafts was documented in herpes labialis-induced lip leukoderma.[10-16] Concurrent donor site repigmentation and depigmentation of grafts at the recipient site or vice versa have also been noticed.[5,9,17] Simultaneous perigraft spread of pigment in one area and spread of vitiligo in another area can be found in the same patient. Parallel concurrence of surgical repigmentation from the grafts and increase in size of an existing lesion in the same anatomical location was also observed. This area-based variable status of stability is neither related to the conventional refractory behavior of vitiligo, typically seen in the so-called "resistant" anatomical sites such as palms, soles, lips, nipples, areola, glans penis, and bony prominences nor it is related to the type of vitiligo such as unilateral (segmental/focal) or bilateral (symmetric, vulgaris, or generalized).

A holistic approach to the assessment of stability was conferred by Falabella[1,5] which comprises the following:
- Lack of progression of old lesions within the past 2 years (in unilateral vitiligo may be shorter, and in bilateral vitiligo, stability establishes after several years)
- No new lesions developing within the same period
- Absence of a recent Koebner phenomenon (either from history or experimentally produced)
- Repigmentation of depigmented areas by medical treatment or sometimes spontaneous repigmentation
- A positive minigrafting test
- Lack of Koebnerization at donor site

VALIDITY OF TEST GRAFT

Introduction of minigrafting test by Falabella in 1995 added an objective dimension to the concept of stability than just arbitrarily depending upon subjective assumption of duration of stability (inactivity).[5] In the original suggested procedure, a few grafts (1.0–1.2 mm) were placed in the center of the depigmented lesion to be scrutinized. Dressing was done by Micropore® adhesive tape and kept for a couple of weeks. After removal of the tape, the area was exposed to sunlight for 15 minutes daily for a period of 3 months. No treatment was permitted during this test period. All test sites are visualized under Wood's light. The test was considered positive if unequivocal repigmentation takes place beyond 1 mm from the border of the implanted grafts. On the other hand, if <1 mm or no repigmentation was observed, the test was considered as negative. This test was further renamed as test grafting in few successive studies and found to be more realistic than arbitrary period of stability.[14,15,18]

Though TG gained popularity as a reliable method to assess stability over the years, but was not beyond criticism.

In the original article, no mention was there about the donor site. Inclusion of the outcome of the donor site will provide much comprehensive idea about stability.[19] Many researchers raised question about reliability and validity of TG as a predictor of successful repigmentation in each and every case being grafted.[18,20] Some researchers expressed their faith on availability of method of identification and isolation of skin-homing melanocyte-specific cytotoxic T-cell.[21]

None other than Falabella himself expressed his doubts about the comprehensiveness of minigraft test. He observed that even when the minigrafting test is positive, "depigmenting activity" may still be present and prevent satisfactory repigmentation.[4]

Few years later, Njoo et al. came up with their work to establish relationship between experimentally induced Koebner phenomenon (KP-e) and Koebner phenomenon by history (KP-h) and the responsiveness to ultraviolet light therapy [ultraviolet A (UVA) plus fluticasone propionate or narrowband ultraviolet B (NB-UVB)] in 61 patients who were off any topical or systemic therapies for at least 6 months. KP-e was assessed by inducing an injury by taking a 2-mm punch biopsy specimen from clinically uninvolved skin scar or depigmentation of the biopsy site after 3 months was considered as KP-e positive. A substantial difference was noted between KP-h and KP-e and the positive and negative predictive value, respectively, of KP-h was found to be 89 and 52%, respectively. Surprisingly, the responsiveness to UVB (311 nm) therapy among KP-e-positive or KP-e-negative patients did not show any statistically significant difference ($p = 0.66$). However, in the fluticasone propionate plus UVA group, KP-e-positive patients showed a better response than did KP-e-negative patients ($p = 0.01$).[22]

Vitiligo disease activity (VIDA) score was described by the same worker to grade the level of activity of disease in individual vitiligo patients who were without any therapies for at least 6 months. Scores were given from +4 to –1 depending upon decrease in disease activity. It was observed that patients with VIDA scores

of +1 and +2 did not necessarily show a positive KP-e. However, all the patients with VIDA scores of +3 and +4 showed a positive KP-e. They concluded:
- The VIDA score did not always predict a positive KP-e.
- The KP-e may function well as a clinical factor to assess present disease activity and may also predict the responsiveness to fluticasone propionate plus UVA therapy but not to UVB (311 nm) therapy.

It this context, it can be concluded that KP or TG should not be considered as full proof of disease activity. Because what these two reveal is the apparent clinical stability only and that may not be the true reflection of stability status of the disease at the cellular level.[18]

HOW LONG DOES STABILITY LAST?

It is often hard to predict how long the disease will remain stable or on the other way round when it will start to become unstable. Repigmentation in previous graft failure cases with NB-UVB (311 nm) phototherapy has been documented.[16] Proposed mechanism of action of NB-UVB might stabilize the disease by promoting apoptosis of the perilesional and circulating melanocyte-specific cytotoxic CD8 cells.[23] The observation of spontaneous repigmentation points toward a possible release of fresh cytokines from the donor skin not only stimulate the vitiliginous patches and hair follicles of the grafted sites but also repigment distant sites by local absorption.[24-26] Another theory was the immunogenic mechanism which was originally responsible for the development of vitiligo may have lost its antigenicity due to the autologous grafts.[23] Successful split-thickness skin graft (STSG) in PG failure cases further complicates the picture.[27] Period of stability of repigmentation has been proposed as 1 year. That means, to qualify as stable, the repigmented status must be maintained for a period of not <1 year.[28]

ROLE OF DERMATOSCOPE IN DEFINING STABILITY

Recently, dermatoscope has emerged as a powerful tool to assess stability of vitiligo. Perifollicular and perilesional hyperpigmentation point toward stable vitiligo whereas trichome border, satellite lesions, and micro-Koebner phenomenon is strongly associated with instability.[29]

CONCEPT OF CELLULAR STABILITY

The exact pathomechanism of stability is still an enigma. The incompletely understood mechanism involves many theories and hypothesis. The only definite and certain factor is the absence of melanocytes in the lesion. So, it can be concluded that destruction of melanocytes is the key factor for unfolding of the disease process. Classically, there have been three hypotheses to elucidate vitiligo: the neural hypothesis, the self-destruct hypothesis, and the immune hypothesis of which the last one is gaining grounds. Aberrations of both humoral and cell-mediated immunity have been noticed. Most of the patients with generalized vitiligo were found to have circulating antibodies to cell surface antigens on normal human melanocytes; these antibodies were cytotoxic to normal melanocytes and to melanoma cells in tissue culture. Humoral immunity does not appear to be fundamental for the pathogenesis of vitiligo, as serum titers of melanocyte-reactive antibodies do not correlate with disease activity,[30] and the uniform distribution of circulating antibodies cannot explain the patchy appearance of vitiligo lesions.[31] Perilesional and circulating T-cells strongly suggest that melanocyte-specific cytotoxic T cells are involved. And now it is known that UVB therapy promotes this T-cell apoptosis. Repigmentation has been successfully induced in previous graft failure cases under NB-UVB (311 nm) phototherapy.[32]

Recent updates on pathogenesis in vitiligo focus on few important points:
- Resident memory T cells (T_{RM}) play a crucial role in the persistence and relapse of vitiligo. They (a type of CD8+ T cells expressing CD69, CD103, and CD49a) have the ability to remain in tissues and induce early immune responses.[33] A large population of T_{RM} cells reside in vitiligo skin and are involved in relapse promoting recruitment and proliferation of circulating CB8+ T cells through the release of interferon (IFN) pathway cytokines.[34] Interleukin-15 (IL-15) has a central role in the maintenance and function of T_{RM} cells. CD8+ T cells secrete IFN-γ, which induces the production of chemokines CXCL9 and CXCL10 by keratinocytes.[35] These chemokines bind to the T-cell receptor CXCR3, increasing T-cell recruitment, thereby leading to the initiation, progression, and maintenance of vitiligo lesions.[36] Tregs play a pivotal role in maintaining self-tolerance by suppressing the activity of autoreactive effector T cells. IL-2 is essential for Tregs survival and functionality in peripheral tissues.
- In one study, significant increases in CD3+, CD4+, and CD8+ T cells were found in margin of vitiligo lesions and these cells were mostly activated CD45RO+ cells of the memory subset. Most intense infiltration was present within 0.6 mm of the edge of the lesion.[37]
- The detection of melanocyte-reactive cytotoxic T cells in the peripheral blood of vitiligo patients and the observed correlation between perilesional T-cell infiltration and melanocyte loss in situ suggest the important role of cellular autoimmunity in the pathogenesis of this disease. T cells have been isolated from both perilesional and nonlesional skin biopsies of vitiligo patients, then cloned and their profile of cytokine production analyzed. Perilesional T-cell clones (TCC) derived from patients with vitiligo revealed a predominant type-1-like cytokine secretion profile, but the degree of type-1 polarization in uninvolved skin-derived TCC correlated with the process of microscopically observed melanocyte destruction in situ. Furthermore, CD8+ TCC derived from two patients also were analyzed for reactivity against autologous melanocytes. The antimelanocyte cytotoxic reactivity was observed among CD8+ TCC isolated from perilesional biopsies of patients with vitiligo.[38]
- Expression of CCL22, a skin-homing chemokine for Treg (regulatory T cells), has been found to be deficient in vitiligo skin on immunohistochemistry. This was hypothesized to explain the failure of circulating functional Treg to

home to the skin in vitiligo. Absence of Treg cells at the place of occurrence perpetuate antimelanocyte reactivity in progressive disease.[39]
- Rao et al. studied the correlation of results of repigmentation following suction blister grafting in vitiligo with serum catalase levels and lesional immunohistochemistry for CD4, CD8, CD45RO, CD45RA, and FoxP3. No correlation of serum catalase levels with either the period of stability or the results of surgical repigmentation was found. Similarly, CD45RA, CD4, and Fox P3 were also not found to correlate with response to surgical treatment. However, CD8 T-cell counts were found to be lower in responders [median 1% (range 0–4%)] as compared to the nonresponders [median 3% (range 1–7%)] ($p = 0.04$). Higher percentage of CD8+ cells is associated with lower percentage of repigmentation. CD45RO cells were found to be completely absent in responders while some nonresponders showed their presence. Along with CD8 cells, CD45RO cells contribute significantly for propagation and persistence of cytokine milieu which are responsible for instability.[7]
- A recent study evaluated potential biomarkers to assess stability of vitiligo and success of surgical transplantation. CXCL9 and CXCL10 levels in blister fluid sample of stable and active vitiligo were measured. Outcome of the cultured pure melanocyte transplantation (CMT) was evaluated after 6 months. CXCL9 and CXCL10 levels were found to be sensitive and specific markers of active vitiligo. CXCL9 and CXCL10 levels were significantly lower in stable vitiligo. Effectiveness of CMT was determined by CXCL9 level.[40]

CONCLUSION

It is obvious that before any attempt to predict the outcome of any vitiligo surgery, along with the clinical stability, assessment of "cellular" stability is of utmost importance. Before embarking upon any surgical alternative, no preconceived, biased, and arbitrary formulae should guide us to assess stability of vitiligo. Till those unexplored areas are charted and the cellular parameters come into real practice, we should not step back from surgical options rather we should continue surgical interventions based on logical application of our clinical knowledge. Also, so far these tests are only research tools available in very few centers and extensive work needs to be done to make these tests sufficiently reliable, cheap, and widely available. Lesional stability as a concept needs to be investigated in depth. In addition, there is a need to set uniform clinical criteria for defining stability before embarking on biochemical and other investigative findings so as to be able to compare results between studies and draw definitive conclusions.

REFERENCES

1. Falabella R. Grafting and transplantation of melanocytes for repigmenting vitiligo and other types of leucodermas. Int J Dermatol. 1989;28:363-9.
2. Olsson MJ, Juhlin L. Long-term follow-up of leucoderma patients treated with transplants of autologous cultured melanocytes, ultrathin epidermal sheets and basal cell layer suspension. Br J Dermatol. 2002;147:893-904.
3. Lahiri K, Malakar S. The concept of stability of vitiligo: A reappraisal. Indian J Dermatol. 2012; 57:83-9.

4. Falabella R, Escobar C, Borrero I. Treatment of refractory and stable vitiligo by transplantation of in vitro cultured epidermal autografts bearing melanocytes. J Am Acad Dermatol. 1992; 26:230-6.
5. Falabella R, Arrunategui A, Barona MI, Alzate A. The minigrafting test for vitiligo: Detection of stable lesions for melanocyte transplantation. J Am Acad Dermatol. 1995;32:228-32.
6. Parsad D, Gupta S; IADVL Dermatosurgery Task Force. Standard guidelines of care for vitiligo surgery. Indian J Dermatol Venereol Leprol. 2008;74:S37-45.
7. Rao A, Gupta S, Dinda AK, Sharma A, Sharma VK, Kumar G, et al. Study of clinical, biochemical and immunological factors determining stability of disease in patients with generalized vitiligo undergoing melanocyte transplantation. Br J Dermatol. 2012;166:1230-6.
8. Taneja N, Sreenivas V, Sahni K, Gupta V, Ramam M. Disease stability in segmental and non-segmental vitiligo. Indian Dermatol Online J. 2022;13:60-3.
9. Falabella R. Surgical treatment of vitiligo: why, when and how. J Eur Acad Dermatol Venereol. 2003;17:518-20.
10. Malakar S, Dhar S. Rejection of punch grafts in three cases of herpes labialis induced lip leucoderma, caution and precaution. Dermatology. 1997;195:414.
11. Malakar S, Dhar S. Acyclovir can abort rejection of punch grafts in herpes-simplex induced lip leucoderma. Dermatology. 1999;199:75.
12. Malakar S, Lahri K. Successful repigmentation of six cases of Herpes labialis induced lip leucoderma by micropigmentation. Dermatology. 2001;203:194.
13. Lahiri K, Malakar S. Herpes simplex induced lip leucoderma: Revisited. Dermatology. 2004; 208:182.
14. Malakar S, Dhar S. Treatment of stable and recalcitrant vitiligo by autologous mimiature punch grafting: A prospective study of 1,000 patients. Dermatology. 1999;198:133-9.
15. Malakar S, Lahiri K. Punch grafting for lip leucoderma. Dermatology. 2004;208:125-8.
16. Lahiri K, Malakar S, Sarma N, Banerjee U. Repigmentation of vitiligo with punch grafting and NB UVB (311 nm) - a prospective study. Int J Dermatol. 2006;45:649-55.
17. Malakar S, Lahiri K. How unstable is the concept of stability in surgical repigmentation of vitiligo? Dermatology. 2000;201:182-3.
18. Lahiri K, Malakar S, Banerjee U, Sarma N. Clinico-cellular stability of vitiligo in surgical repigmentation: An unexplored frontier. Dermatology 2004;209:170-1.
19. Westerhof W, Boersma B. The minigrafting test for vitiligo: Detection of stable lesions for melanocyte transplantation. J Am Acad Dermatol. 1995;33:1061.
20. Lahiri K. Stability in vitiligo? What's that? J Cutan Aesthet Surg. 2009;2:38-40.
21. Juhlin L. How unstable is the concept of stability in surgical repigmentation of vitiligo. Dermatology. 2000;201:183.
22. Njoo MD, Das PK, Bos JD, Westerhof W. Association of the Köbner phenomenon with disease activity and therapeutic responsiveness in vitiligo vulgaris. Arch Dermatol. 1999;135(4): 407-13.
23. van den Wijngaard RM, Aten J, Scheepmaker A. Expression and modulation of apoptosis regulatory molecules in human melanocytes: Significance in vitiligo. Br J Dermatol. 2000; 143:573-81.
24. Malakar S. Spontaneous repigmentation of vitiligo patches other than the grafted site. Indian J Dermatol. 1997;472:68-70.
25. Malakar S, Dhar S. Spontaneous repigmentation of vitiligo patches distant from the autologous skin graft sites: A remote reverse Koebner's phenomenon? Dermatology. 1998; 197:274.
26. Malakar S, Lahiri K. Spontaneous repigmentation in vitiligo: Why it is important. Int J Dermatol. 2006;45:478-9.
27. Malakar S. Successful split thickness skin graft in stable vililigo not responding to autologous miniature punch grafts. Indian J Dermatol. 1997;42:215-8.
28. Parsad D, Pandhi R, Dogra S, Kumar B. Clinical study of repigmentation patterns with different treatment modalities and their correlation with speed and stability of repigmentation in 352 vitiliginous patches. J Am Acad Dermatol. 2004;50:63-7.

29. Sindhuri G, Karim S, Patel P, Nadkarni N, Patil S, Godse K. Dermatoscope as a tool to determine the stability of vitiligo. IP Indian J Clin Exp Dermatol. 2024;10(2):187-91.
30. Kroon MW, Kemp EH, Wind BS, Krebbers G, Bos JD, Gawkrodger DJ, et al. Melanocyte antigen-specific antibodies cannot be used as markers for recent disease activity in patients with vitiligo. J Eur Acad Dermatol Venereol. 2013;27(9):1172-5.
31. Katz EL, Harris JE. Translational Research in Vitiligo. Front Immunol. 2021;12:624517.
32. Lahiri K, Malakar S, Sarma N, Banerjee U. Inducing repigmentation by regrafting and phototherapy (311 nm) in punch grafting failure cases of lip vitiligo: a pilot study. Indian J Dermatol Venereol Leprol. 2004;70(3):156-8.
33. Tokura Y, Phadungsaksawasdi P, Kurihara K, Fujiyama T, Honda T. Pathophysiology of Skin Resident Memory T Cells. Front Immunol. 2021;11:618897.
34. Richmond JM, Strassner JP, Rashighi M, Agarwal P, Garg M, Essien KI, et al. Resident Memory and Recirculating Memory T Cells Cooperate to Maintain Disease in a Mouse Model of Vitiligo. J Invest Dermatol. 2019;139(4):769-78.
35. Wang XX, Wang QQ, Wu JQ, Jiang M, Chen L, Zhang CF, et al. Increased expression of CXCR3 and its ligands in patients with vitiligo and CXCL10 as a potential clinical marker for vitiligo. Br J Dermatol. 2016;174(6):1318-26.
36. Richmond JM, Bangari DS, Essien KI, Currimbhoy SD, Groom JR, Pandya AG, et al. Keratinocyte-Derived Chemokines Orchestrate T-Cell Positioning in the Epidermis during Vitiligo and May Serve as Biomarkers of Disease. J Invest Dermatol. 2017;137(2):350-8.
37. Badri AM, Todd PM, Garioch JJ, Gudgeon JE, Stewart DG, Goudie RB. An immunohistological study of cutaneous lymphocytes in vitiligo. J Pathol. 1993;170:149-55.
38. Wankowicz-Kalinska A, van den Wijngaard RM, Tigges BJ, Westerhof W, Ogg GS, Cerundolo V, et al. Immunopolarization of CD4+ and CD8+ T cells to Type-1-like is associated with melanocyte loss in human vitiligo. Lab Invest. 2003;83:683-95.
39. Klarquist J, Denman CJ, Hernandez C, Wainwright DA, Strickland FM, Overbeck A, et al. Reduced skin homing by functional treg in vitiligo. Pigment Cell Melanoma Res. 2010;23: 276-86.
40. Lin F, Hu W, Xu W, Zhou M, Xu AE. CXCL9 as a key biomarker of vitiligo activity and prediction of the successes of cultured melanocyte transplantation. Sci Rep. 2021;11(1):18298.

CHAPTER 5

Topical Treatments

Deepak Mohana

INTRODUCTION

Vitiligo is a psychologically devastating condition. Topical therapy is employed as first-line treatment in localized vitiligo **(Table 1)**. Currently, several topical agents are available in many forms, viz., methoxsalen (solution and cream), trioxsalen (solution), corticosteroids (gel, cream, ointment, and solution) and calcineurin inhibitors (ointment and cream). Although topical therapy has an important position in vitiligo treatment, side effects or poor efficacy affect their utility and patient compliance. Novel drug delivery strategies can play a pivotal role in improving the topical delivery of various drugs by enhancing their epidermal localization with a concomitant reduction in their side effects and improving their effectiveness.

VITILIGO TREATMENT BY TOPICAL THERAPIES

The goal of vitiligo treatment is to control the autoimmune damage to melanocytes and stimulate their migration from surrounding skin and adnexal reservoirs.

TABLE 1: Types of topical therapies.	
Topical therapies	<ul><li>Corticosteroids</li><li>Intralesional corticosteroids</li><li>Pulsed steroids</li><li>Vitamin D analogs (tacalcitol and calcipotriol)</li><li>Calcineurin inhibitors (tacrolimus and pimecrolimus)</li><li>Khellin</li><li>Pseudocatalase</li><li>Other [melagenina, topical antioxidant gel containing pseudocatalase, superoxide, glutathione coenzyme Q10, carotenoids, vitamins A, E, C, and selenium, plant-based topical catalase/dismutase superoxide, tetrahydrocurcuminoid cream, and 5 fluorouracil (5-FU) cream]</li><li>Topical JAK inhibitors</li></ul>

TABLE 2: Drugs, their actions, and side effect of use in topical treatments.

Treatment modality	Drugs	Mechanism of actions	Side effects
Topical treatments	Calcineurin inhibitors	Immunomodulation	Burning sensation, erythema, transient pruritus; risk of malignancies?
	Calcipotriol	Repigmentation and immunosuppression	Transient burning or irritation
	Corticosteroids	Immunomodulation	Epidermal atrophy, striae, telangiectasia, glaucoma, tachyphylaxis, hypothalamus-pituitary axis suppression, Cushing's syndrome, and growth retardation

Treatment may be divided into pharmacological, surgical, and physical, which can sometimes be combined.
- Pharmacological treatment
    - Topical **(Table 2)**
    - Systemic
- Physical treatment
- Surgical treatment

Corticosteroids

Topical corticosteroid therapy is considered as a first-line treatment of vitiligo since its cost is low and is easy to apply. It is limited by the risk of local adverse effects, such as atrophy, striae and telangiectasias and also systemic side effects. Thus, the use of high-potency topical corticosteroids is more suitable to treat small-affected areas, being more effective on the face, elbows, and knees, although some authors prefer to use low-power corticosteroids on the face and flexural areas.

A meta-analysis demonstrated that class 3 topic corticosteroids had higher efficacy in the treatment of localized vitiligo, compared to class 4 and intralesional corticosteroids, also showing higher incidence of atrophy in class 4 drugs.

A retrospective study compared the use of high and moderate power topical corticosteroids in 101 children—both groups showed repigmentation in 64% of cases, stabilization in 24%, and worsening in 11%. In the stratified analysis according to corticosteroid potency, no difference was found between the moderate and high-power drugs ($p = 0.03$), nor in the incidence of local adverse events ($p = 0.3$).

Although studies recommend the use of high-power topical corticosteroids in localized vitiligo, its use should be limited to 2–4 months periods, as low-power corticosteroids or the use of other immunomodulators should be considered in order to decrease the risk of adverse events. If no clinical response is seen with topical corticosteroids in 3–4 months, their application should be suspended.

Calcineurin Inhibitors

Initially used in transplant patients, calcineurin inhibitors are immunosuppressants, the first of which, cyclosporine, is not used topically due to the lack of good cutaneous absorption. Subsequently, tacrolimus and pimecrolimus, other calcineurin inhibitors, demonstrated good absorption when used topically.

Corticosteroids inhibit collagen synthesis, leading to an increased risk of skin atrophy, especially during prolonged use. An advantage of calcineurin inhibitors is that neocollagenesis does not depend on calcineurin; hence, there is no risk of atrophy.

Topical tacrolimus is a calcineurin inhibitor that controls the activity of T lymphocytes through the inhibition of proinflammatory cytokines, blocking the transcription of the *IL-2* genes which are important for the proliferation of cytotoxic T lymphocytes, and also inhibiting the transcription and production of IL-4, IL-5, IL-10, IFN-γ, and TNF-α. In an open-label, noncomparative study, 42 patients were treated with 0.1% tacrolimus, twice a day for 6 months, with 76.09% achieving some degree of repigmentation. Children showed higher response rates than adults and the clinical forms with best response were vulgaris and focal.

In a randomized, double-blind study, the use of 0.1% tacrolimus was as effective as 0.5% clobetasol propionate, when applied twice a day for 60 days in children ($p > 0.05$). Both treatments achieve the highest response rates on facial areas or those with high density of hair follicles. Atrophy and telangiectasia were only observed in the clobetasol group.

In a prospective study, 1% pimecrolimus was compared to 0.5% clobetasol propionate with results being assessed in lesions on parasagittal planes. The results showed no statistical difference in repigmentation.

The association of a topical immunosuppressive drug with a physical treatment was investigated in a comparative, randomized, single-blinded study that showed better therapeutic response in groups treated by excimer laser (308 nm) associated with 1% topical pimecrolimus when compared to LASER (light amplification by stimulated emission of radiation) used alone.

Calcineurin inhibitors have demonstrated efficacy similar to topical corticosteroids, without the risk of cutaneous atrophy in the long-term use.

Calcipotriol

Calcipotriol is a vitamin D3 analog that might be effective on immunomodulatory systems, inflammatory mediators, and melanocytes. Tomita et al. showed that vitamin D3-induced features similar to those noted in UV-radiated skin (such as swelling of melanocytes in the epidermis and increased tyrosinase activity resulting in a deposition of melanin in the epidermis).

Kumaran et al. conducted a randomized trial that studied the effect of 0.005% topical calcipotriol, 0.05% betamethasone dipropionate and their combination in the treatment of localized vitiligo. When used individually, the betamethasone dipropionate and the calcipotriol were found to be equally effective but the combination of the two appeared to give a significantly faster onset of repigmentation along with better stability of the achieved pigmentation and with lesser number of side effects.

Ameen et al. conducted an open study to investigate the efficacy and tolerability of calcipotriol cream as monotherapy and in combination with psoralen plus ultraviolet A (PUVA) therapy. They found that topical calcipotriol appears to be an effective and well-tolerated treatment for vitiligo and can be safely used in combination with PUVA. Chiavérini et al. performed a prospective, right-left comparative, open study, and examined the efficiency of topical calcipotriol as a monotherapy for the treatment of vitiligo. They concluded that it was not effective.

Pseudocatalase Cream

One study showed that patients with vitiligo have low catalase levels in their epidermis in association with accumulation of hydrogen peroxide (H_2O_2). A topical pseudocatalase cream and calcium used twice daily with UVB therapy, twice weekly, resulted in repigmentation in the majority of cases in a case study with 33 patients after 2–4 months. However, it was not known whether the repigmentation was due to the UVB or the pseudocatalase. Sanclemente et al. compared the effect of topical 0.05% betamethasone valerate versus catalase/dismutase superoxide (C/DSO) and concluded that vitiligo repigmentation with topical C/DSO at 10 months is similar to repigmentation with topical 0.05% betamethasone valerate.

More studies on the use of pseudocatalase cream in the treatment of vitiligo are necessary to prove its possible therapeutic effect.

Beta-fibroblast Growth Factor

Topical beta-fibroblast growth factor (β-FGF) is a therapy with a promising role in stable vitiligo. β-FGF is safe and effective in inducing repigmentation of vitiligo lesions. Combination therapy of β-FGF with other topical therapies, phototherapy, and surgical procedures can be beneficial in patients of vitiligo.

Prostaglandins and Analogs

Prostaglandins act on numerous cells in human skin, namely keratinocytes, Langerhans cells, and melanocytes, which contributes to the increased stimulation of melanocytes and the neural response to stimulation. Additionally, prostaglandins may stimulate the activity and expression of tyrosinase, which is an enzyme limiting the pace of melanin synthesis. As mentioned earlier, oxidative stress has been identified in vitiligo skin. Furthermore, it leads to the reduced synthesis of prostaglandin E2 (PGE2) along with the antagonizing prostaglandin F2 (PGF2α) synthetized in skin. PGF2α has been a known marker of oxidative stress and has been recently shown to be elevated (its expression) in vitiligo skin.

An original preclinical hypothesis was that the use of PGE may cause repigmentation. However, since the discovery of periocular hyperpigmentation caused by PGF2α during therapy of glaucoma, the researchers focused on the possible role of the latter prostaglandin in the clinical studies. In numerous studies, analogs of PGF2α, topical latanoprost and bimatoprost, proved to be an effective additional method of treatment of vitiligo when combined with other methods, narrow-band ultraviolet B (NB-UVB), microneedling, and mometasone.

The Use of Janus Kinase Inhibitors in Vitiligo Treatment

Janus kinase (JAK) inhibitors have been shown to block IFN-γ signaling, contributing to repigmentation in individuals with vitiligo. Tofacitinib (Pfizer, New York, NY, USA), ruxolitinib (Celgene, Summit, NJ, USA), and baricitinib (Indianapolis, IN, USA) are the three most commonly reported JAK inhibitors used in vitiligo treatment.

Ruxolitinib

Ruxolitinib is a small-molecule inhibitor that selectively targets JAK1 and JAK2. The oral form of ruxolitinib was first approved in 2011 to treat polycythemia vera, essential thrombocythemia, and myelofibrosis. Although oral ruxolitinib has been shown to improve skin conditions, such as alopecia areata, topical administration of ruxolitinib resulted in higher concentrations in both the epidermis and dermis with minimal deleterious systemic effects versus oral administration, demonstrating sustained and near-complete blockage of the JAK/STAT signaling pathway in the tissues to which it was applied, with negligible plasma concentrations. Therefore, more studies have been conducted on ruxolitinib cream to investigate its efficacy in treating inflammatory skin disorders, such as alopecia areata, atopic dermatitis, lichen planus, and psoriasis.

Rapid skin repigmentation was observed in male patients with vitiligo and alopecia areata treated with oral ruxolitinib, with marked declines in serum CXCL10 levels after administration, indicating that ruxolitinib's mechanism of action may involve disruption of IFN-γ signaling and JAKs. The role of IFN-γ- and CD8+ T-cell-dependent cytokine activity, which is implicated in the pathogenesis of alopecia areata, may thus also play a role in the pathogenesis of vitiligo. Although the mechanism of action of ruxolitinib cream in the treatment of vitiligo is still unclear, studies on mice and human tissues have found that in addition to blocking IFN-γ and its downstream effector, JAKs, ruxolitinib also inhibited the differentiation and migration of human dendritic cells (DCs) ex vivo. This reduced DC-induced antigen-specific CD4+ and CD8+ T-cell responses and the induction of CD8+ cytotoxic T-cell responses, which are the key cell responses that are hypothesized to participate in the pathogenesis of vitiligo, in vivo. An ongoing phase 2 study, sponsored by the Incyte Corporation, is currently in the recruitment stage. This study aimed to investigate the mechanism of action of ruxolitinib cream in treating patients with vitiligo by evaluating changes in immune biomarkers, including CXCL10.

Based on preliminary findings in mice and human tissues, clinical trials with topical ruxolitinib have been conducted. In a 20-week, open-label, phase 2 trials, 12 patients received topical 1.5% ruxolitinib cream applied to vitiligo lesions twice daily. Compared with baseline, four patients showed significant improvement in facial lesions, and all patients showed a 23% average decrease in the Vitiligo Area Scoring Index (VASI). A 32-week extension study followed, but no improvement was found in skin lesions that were previously nonresponsive to ruxolitinib. However, five patients followed up after the trial maintained their response to treatment for up to 6 months after treatment discontinuation.

Tofacitinib

Tofacitinib is a selective JAK1 and JAK3 inhibitor approved to treat moderate and severe rheumatoid arthritis. Both oral and topical forms of tofacitinib have shown efficacy in treating immune-mediated skin disorders, including plaque psoriasis, atopic dermatitis, and alopecia areata. Oral administration of tofacitinib was first used in a female patient with vitiligo who had approximately 10% depigmentation in her total body surface area, which was unresponsive to the traditional application of topical corticosteroid ointment and tacrolimus ointment. Given the hypothesized common pathogenesis in alopecia areata and vitiligo, the patient was prescribed 5 mg of oral tofacitinib citrate on alternate days, which was increased to 5 mg daily from week 4. After 5 months of treatment, only 5% of the patient's total body surface area remained depigmented. No side effects were reported during the treatment period.

In a retrospective study of 10 tofacitinib-treated patients with vitiligo, changes in their autoimmune responses were evaluated through suction blister sampling. 10 patients underwent tofacitinib therapy at a dosage of 5–10 mg daily or twice daily for an average of 9.9 months, with only half of the patients achieving repigmentation that occurred in sun-exposed areas or areas that received phototherapy only. Flow cytometry revealed a decline in the number of CD8+ T cells after tofacitinib treatment, but there was no change in the percentage of melanocyte-specific T cells. In addition, chemokines, such as CXCL9 and CXCL10, were reduced and became undetectable after tofacitinib treatment. These findings indicate that repigmentation of vitiligo lesions may require both JAK inhibitors (to inhibit local inflammation) and light exposure (to stimulate melanocytes), which is consistent with the finding that sun-exposed areas, such as the hands and face, are more responsive to topical ruxolitinib treatment.

Topical 2% tofacitinib cream was also administered to 16 patients with vitiligo, including 11 patients with generalized vitiligo. Consistent with previous studies, more significant responses were noted for facial lesions and patients with darker skin types, while no superior responses were observed in those who received concomitant phototherapy, which contrasts with previously reported results. There are no registered clinical trials currently being performed to investigate the use of tofacitinib in vitiligo treatment, and further research is necessary to determine its safety and efficacy, as well as the role of phototherapy in combination with tofacitinib.

MAINTENANCE THERAPY TO PREVENT RECURRENCE OF THE DISEASE

As previously discussed, vitiligo is a chronic inflammatory skin disease that needs a careful follow-up for optimal maintenance therapy. Recurrence of the disease is mediated by autoreactive tissue-resident memory T (T_{RM}) cells located close to replenished melanocytes. To date, a prospective randomized study showed that a twice-weekly application of topical calcineurin inhibitors is an effective treatment strategy to prevent vitiligo relapses by supporting the need to continuously inhibit the immune system to maintain repigmentation. Therefore, with the development of targeted therapies, the use of topical JAK inhibitors could be a reliable treatment in this context. As T_{RM} maintenance in the skin is dependent on IL-15, targeting IL-15 could be another potential treatment strategy. We have recently shown that matrix metalloproteinase (MMP)-9 released by keratinocytes in vitiligo lesional skin could induce the cleavage of E-cadherin, leading to the detachment of epidermal melanocytes. Consequently, MMP-9 inhibition could also be an interesting strategy for stabilizing melanocytes in the basal layer of the epidermis and prevent their loss.

NANODRUG DELIVERY SYSTEM

Therapeutic aim is to control immunoreaction by relieving oxidative stress. Unfortunately, the cuticle barrier function and lack of specific accumulation lead to unsatisfactory therapeutic outcomes and side effects. The introduction and innovation of nanotechnology offers inspiration and clues for the development of new strategies to treat vitiligo. However, not many studies have been done to interrogate how nanotechnology can be used for vitiligo treatment. In this review, we summarize and analyze recent studies involving nanodrug delivery systems for the treatment of vitiligo, with a special emphasis on liposomes, niosomes, nanohydrogel, and nanoparticles. These studies made significant progress by either increasing drug loading efficiency or enhancing penetration. Based on these studies, there are three proposed principles for topical nanodrug delivery systems treatment of vitiligo including the promotion of transdermal penetration, enhancement of drug retention, and facilitation of melanin regeneration. The presentation of these ideas may provide inspirations for the future development of topical drug delivery systems that will conquer vitiligo **(Fig. 1)**.

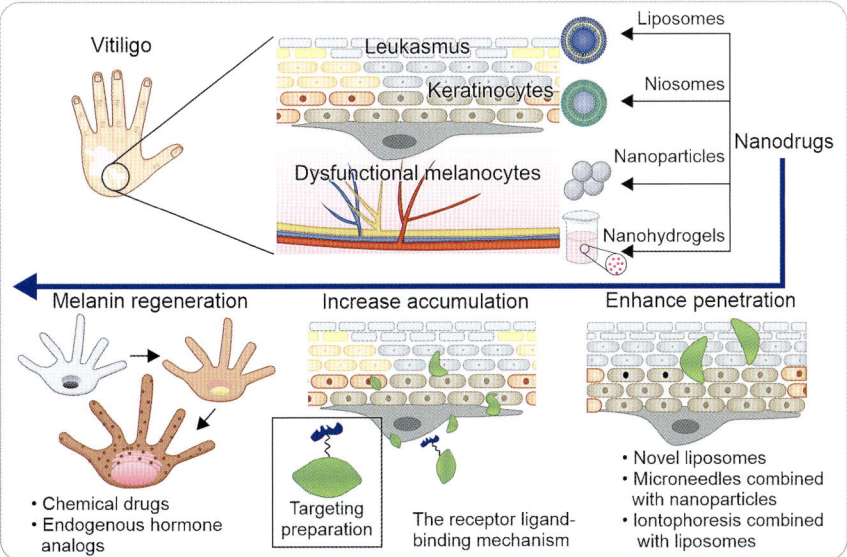

FIG. 1: Nanodrug delivery system mechanisms.

CONCLUSION

According to the current guidelines, a <2-month trial of potent or very potent topical corticosteroids or topical calcineurin inhibitors may be used for therapy of localized vitiligo (<20% skin surface area). Combinations of topical corticosteroids with excimer laser and UVA seem to be more effective than steroids alone. Pseudocatalase plus NB-UVB does not seem to be more effective than placebo with NB-UVB. Combinations of vitamin D analogs have varied efficacy based on which type is used and the type of UV light. Efficacy of calcineurin inhibitor combinations also varies based on the type used and UV light combined with tacrolimus being more effective with excimer laser. Pimecrolimus has been effective with NB-UVB and excimer laser on facial lesions, and microdermabrasion on localized areas. Recently, JAK inhibitors such as tofacitinib and ruxolitinib are showing promising results in vitiligo.

SUGGESTED READINGS

1. Kwinter J, Pelletier J, Khambalia A, Pope E. High-potency steroid use in children with vitiligo: a retrospective study. J Am Acad Dermatol. 2007;56:236-41.
2. Lotti T, Berti S, Moretti S. Vitiligo therapy. Expert Opin Pharmacother. 2009;10:2779-85.
3. Njoo MD, Spuls PI, Bos JD, Westerhof W, Bossuyt PM. Nonsurgical repigmentation therapies in vitiligo. Meta-analysis of the literature. Arch Dermatol. 1998;134:1532-40.
4. Falabella R, Barona MI. Update on skin repigmentation therapies in vitiligo. Pigment Cell Melanoma Res. 2009;22:42-65.
5. Kostovic K, Pasic A. New treatment modalities for vitiligo: focus on topical immunomodulators. Drugs. 2005;65:447-59.
6. Udompataikul M, Boonsupthip P, Siriwattanagate R. Effectiveness of 0.1% topical tacrolimus in adult and children patients with vitiligo. J Dermatol. 2011;38:536-40.
7. Lepe V, Moncada B, Castanedo-Cazares JP, Torres-Alvarez MB, Ortiz CA, Torres-Rubalcava AB. A double-blind randomized trial of 0.1% tacrolimus vs 0.05% clobetasol for the treatment of childhood vitiligo. Arch Dermatol. 2003;139:581-5.
8. Coskun B, Saral Y, Turgut D. Topical 0.05% clobetasol propionate versus 1% pimecrolimus ointment in vitiligo. Eur J Dermatol. 2005;15:88-91.
9. Hui-Lan Y, Xiao-Yan H, Jian-Yong F, Zong-Rong L. Combination of 308-nm excimer laser with topical pimecrolimus for the treatment of childhood vitiligo. Pediatr Dermatol. 2009;26:354-6.
10. Travis LB, Silverberg NB. Calcipotriene and corticosteroid combination therapy for vitiligo. Pediatr Dermatol. 2004;21:495-8.
11. Sun MC, Xu XL, Lou XF, Du YZ. Recent progress and future directions: The nano-drug delivery system for the treatment of vitiligo. Int J Nanomedicine. 2020;15:3267-79.
12. Li X, Sun Y, Du J, Wang F, Ding X. Excellent repigmentation of generalized vitiligo with oral baricitinib combined with NB-UVB phototherapy. Clin Cosmet Investig Dermatol. 2023;16:635-8.
13. Su X, Luo R, Ruan S, Zhong Q, Zhuang Z, Xiao Z, et al. Efficacy and tolerability of oral upadacitinib monotherapy in patients with recalcitrant vitiligo. J. Am. Acad. Dermatol. 2023; 89(6):1257-9.
14. Pan T, Mu Y, Shi X, Chen L. Concurrent vitiligo and atopic dermatitis successfully treated with upadacitinib: A case report. J. Dermatol. Treat. 2023;34:2200873.
15. Cavalié M, Ezzedine K, Fontas E, Montaudié H, Castela E, Bahadoran P, et al. Maintenance therapy of adult vitiligo with 0.1% tacrolimus ointment: a randomized, double blind, placebo-controlled study. J Invest Dermatol. 2015;135:970-4.

CHAPTER 6A

Systemic Treatments in Vitiligo: Immunosuppressants—Oral Mini Pulse, Methotrexate, Cyclosporine, and Others

Narayanan Baskaran, Muthu Sendhil Kumaran

INTRODUCTION

Vitiligo is an acquired pigmentary condition and is the most common cause of depigmentation, with an estimated worldwide prevalence of 1%.[1] In India, its prevalence is found to be 0.25–8.8% in various studies.[2,3]

Vitiligo is a chronic pigmentary disorder of the skin caused by targeted destruction of melanocytes. The understanding of the disease pathogenesis has led to several causative hypotheses—autoimmune theory (circulating autoantibodies, T-cell dysregulation, and histopathology), neural theory (raised serum catecholamines and neuropeptide Y), oxidative stress theory (raised oxidant and decreased antioxidant levels), and melanocytorrhagy theory (ultrastructural changes in melanocytes).[4]

According to the revised classification and nomenclature of vitiligo as outlined by the Vitiligo Global Issues Consensus Conference,[5] vitiligo is classified into nonsegmental type [including acrofacial, mucosal, generalized, universal, and mixed (associated with segmental)], segmental type (uni-segmental, bi-segmental, or pluri-segmental), and unclassified/indeterminate type (focal, mucosal).

Treatment of vitiligo is aimed at two outcomes which include stopping disease progression and achieving repigmentation. Early and aggressive treatment of vitiligo is necessary to achieve these outcomes. Treatment of vitiligo is decided based on multiple factors which majorly include extent of disease and disease activity. Systemic treatments become necessary in patients with extensive nonsegmental vitiligo and those with active disease. Repeated courses may also be required, owing to the unpredictable nature of the disease. Systemic treatments in vitiligo include immunosuppressants, small molecules, antioxidants, and hormone analogues **(Table 1)**; with recent advances providing hope in the treatment of this challenging condition.

TABLE 1: Systemic treatments for vitiligo.

Study	Study design	Number of patients	Treatment	Duration	Results
Systemic corticosteroids					
Pasricha et al.[8] 1993	Case series	40	• Oral mini pulse • Betamethasone 5 mg once daily for two consecutive days a week	4 months	• Disease progression arrest in 89% • Repigmentation in 80%
Kanwar et al.[9] 2013	Case series	444	• Low-dose oral mini pulse • Dexamethasone 2.5 mg once daily for two consecutive days a week	Until disease activity arrest or 6 months, whichever was earlier	• Disease progression arrest in 91.8% • Good repigmentation in 68.3% • Relapse rate 12.25%
Radakovic-Fijan et al.[33] 2001	Case series	29	• Oral mini pulse • Dexamethasone 10 mg for two consecutive days a week	6 months	• Disease progression arrest in 88% • Marked repigmentation in 6.9% and moderate repigmentation in 10.3%
Banerjee et al.[7] 2003	Case series	100	Oral prednisolone 0.3 mg/kg/day for 2 months, tapered over next 2 months	4 months	• Disease progression arrest in 90% • Repigmentation in 76%
Azathioprine					
Patra et al.[12] 2021	Randomized controlled trial	55	• Oral azathioprine 50 mg twice daily for 6 months tapered over next 4 months vs. • Oral mini pulse • Betamethasone 5 mg once daily for two consecutive days a week tapered over next 4 months	10 months	• Disease progression arrest 2 months: 18.2% (vs. 82.6% in OMP), 6 months: 77.8% (vs. 89.5% in OMP) • Repigmentation >10% at 6 months: 11.1% (vs. 21% in OMP)

Continued

Continued

Study	Study design	Number of patients	Treatment	Duration	Results
Methotrexate					
Singh et al.[15] 2015	Randomized open label study	52	• Oral methotrexate 10 mg/week vs. • Low-dose oral mini pulse • Dexamethasone 2.5 mg once daily for two consecutive days a week	6 months	• Disease progression arrest in 76% (vs. 72% in OMP) • Repigmentation in 44% (vs. 60% in OMP)
Cyclosporine					
Taneja et al.[17] 2019	Case series	18	Oral cyclosporine 3 mg/kg	3 months	• Disease progression arrest in 61% • Mean VASI improvement: 0.43
Mutalik et al.[19] 2017	Observational pilot study	50	• All patients had autologous melanocyte keratinocyte grafting • Cyclosporine 3 mg/kg for 3 weeks followed by 1.5 mg/kg for 6 weeks vs. • No postoperative treatment	6 months	Repigmentation >75% in 100% (vs. 28% in control group)
Mehta et al.[18] 2021	Randomized controlled trial	50	• Oral cyclosporine 3 mg/kg vs. • Low-dose oral mini pulse • Dexamethasone 2.5 mg once daily for two consecutive days a week	4 months	• Disease progression arrest in 88% (vs. 84% in OMP) • Repigmentation comparable in both groups

Continued

Study	Study design	Number of patients	Treatment	Duration	Results
Mycophenolate mofetil					
Bishnoi et al.[34] 2021	Randomized pilot study	50	• Oral mycophenolate (up to 2 g) vs. • Low-dose oral mini pulse • Dexamethasone 2.5 mg once daily for two consecutive days a week	6 months	Significant comparable reduction in VIDA and number of new lesions in both groups
Tofacitinib					
Liu et al.[20] 2017	Case series	10	Oral tofacitinib 5–10 mg once or twice daily	9.9 months mean	Repigmentation in 50% (site of sun exposure or suction blister graft)
Minocycline					
Parsad et al.[25] 2010	Case series	32	Oral minocycline 100 mg daily	3 months	• Disease progression arrest in 90% • Moderate to marked repigmentation in 21.9%
Singh et al.[26] 2014	Randomized controlled trial	50	• Oral minocycline 100 mg daily vs. • Low-dose oral mini pulse • Dexamethasone 2.5 mg once daily for two consecutive days a week	6 months	Significant decrease in VIDA and VASI in both groups
Siadat et al.[35] 2014	Prospective comparative trial	42	• Oral minocycline 100 mg daily vs. • Phototherapy twice weekly	3 months	• Disease progression arrest in 33.3% (vs. 76.1% with NB-UVB) • Repigmentation significantly better with NB-UVB

Continued

Continued

Study	Study design	Number of patients	Treatment	Duration	Results
Antioxidants					
Parsad et al.[27] 2003	Double-blind placebo-controlled trial	52	• Oral Gingko biloba extract 40 mg three times daily vs. • Placebo	6 months	• Disease progression arrest in 80% (vs. 36% with placebo) • Marked to complete repigmentation in 40% (vs. 11.1% with placebo)
Middelkamp-Hup et al.[36] 2007	Randomized double-blind placebo-controlled trial	50	• Oral Polypodium leucotomos 250 mg three times daily vs. • Placebo • Both in combination with NB-UVB weekly	6 months	Repigmentation in 44% in the head and neck area (vs. 27% with placebo)
Afamelanotide					
Lim et al.[28] 2015	Randomized trial	55	• Afamelanotide plus NB-UVB vs. • NB-UVB monotherapy	5 months	Repigmentation in 48.64% (vs. 33.26% with NB-UVB monotherapy)

(NB-UVB: narrowband ultraviolet B; OMP: oral mini pulse; VASI: Vitiligo Area Scoring Index; VIDA: Vitiligo Disease Activity Score)

IMMUNOSUPPRESSANTS

Systemic Corticosteroids

Systemic corticosteroids are primarily aimed at the autoimmune hypothesis of vitiligo, thereby stopping disease progression, achieving stability, and promoting repigmentation. They are the first-choice drugs for rapidly progressive vitiligo.

Systemic corticosteroids can be administered as daily therapy or as a mini-pulse therapy. Oral prednisolone is the choice for daily therapy, started at a dose of 0.3–0.5 mg/kg, tapered over a period of 4–6 months. Kim et al. demonstrated that oral prednisolone, starting at 0.3 mg/kg and tapered over 4 months, halted vitiligo progression in 87.7% of cases. Additionally, 70.4% of patients showed visible repigmentation.[6] A study on 100 vitiligo patients treated with low-dose oral prednisolone (0.3 mg/kg) showed halted progression in 90% of cases and repigmentation in 76%. Younger patients (<15 years) and males had significantly better repigmentation outcomes, with minimal side effects reported.[7]

Pulse therapy [oral mini pulse (OMP)] refers to the administration of a long-acting steroid such as dexamethasone or betamethasone at weekly intervals, which is aimed at reducing the long-term adverse effects of corticosteroids. Pasricha and Khaitan used oral pulses of betamethasone or dexamethasone (5 mg) for two consecutive days weekly, continuing up to 4 months. Disease progression ceased in 89% within 1–3 months, and 80% showed repigmentation, though only three patients achieved >90% pigment restoration.[8] Lower doses of pulse therapy have also shown to be effective in achieving stability vitiligo. Kanwar et al. conducted a retrospective study on 444 vitiligo patients treated with low-dose oral mini-pulse therapy (2.5 mg/day for two consecutive days weekly). Disease progression stopped in 91.8%, with a 12.25% relapse rate, while 68.3% achieved good repigmentation and 17.9% showed minimal improvement.[9]

The choice of daily versus pulse therapy can be decided on a case-to-case basis, as comparative studies have shown equal efficacy of both in terms of halting progression or achieving repigmentation.[10] Pulse therapy can also be safely administered in children, with closer monitoring.[11] Systemic corticosteroids can be combined with other immunosuppressants, antioxidants and phototherapy; especially during the tapering phase.

Possible side effects include weight gain, hypothalamic-pituitary-adrenal (HPA) suppression, acne, hypertrichosis, menstrual irregularities, growth retardation, and immune suppression. Patients should be monitored for weight, height (especially in children approaching growth spurt), body mass index, and blood pressure during every visit. Laboratory investigations are not generally required, however, measurement of blood glucose, fasting lipid levels, and bone densitometry could be performed in patients on long-term therapy.

Azathioprine

Azathioprine acts by suppressing nucleic acid (DNA and RNA) synthesis, thereby inhibiting T- and B-lymphocyte activity. It primarily acts on the autoimmune component of vitiligo pathogenesis, inducing stability and promoting repigmentation.

Azathioprine can be administered at a dose of 2–2.5 mg/kg, up to a period of 6–12 months. It can be used for patients for progressive vitiligo, either alone or in combination with corticosteroids or phototherapy.

Azathioprine has shown comparable efficacy to pulse therapy in treatment of vitiligo. Pulse therapy however halts progression faster at 2 months (82.3% vs. 18.2%), but stabilization rates are similar at 6 months. Repigmentation with good color match is higher in the pulse group (84.2% vs. 61.1%).[12] A study on 60 vitiligo patients compared oral psoralen plus ultraviolet-A (PUVA) alone to a combination of azathioprine (0.6–0.75 mg/kg/day) and twice-weekly PUVA over 4 months. The combination group achieved earlier repigmentation (5.4 sessions vs. 8 sessions) and higher repigmentation rates (58.4% vs. 24.8%), with 30% showing excellent results compared to none in the monotherapy group.[13]

Possible adverse effects include myelosuppression, liver toxicity, gastric intolerance, and increased chance of infections.

Methotrexate

Methotrexate inhibits DNA synthesis and leads to apoptosis in active CD4+ T cells. It decreases pro-inflammatory cytokines (IL-1, IL-6, TNF-α), suppresses IL-2 and IFN-γ expression, and boosts anti-inflammatory cytokines (IL-4, IL-10), targeting cytokine dysfunction seen in vitiligo.

Methotrexate can be administered at weekly doses of 7.5–20 mg, for a period of 6–12 months, and can be combined with phototherapy.

Methotrexate leads to arrest of disease progression and activates repigmentation, as shown by Nageswaramma et al. where weekly methotrexate 15 mg in 20 cases of unstable vitiligo resulted in moderate repigmentation in 70% of patients and halted disease progression in 90% of cases.[14]

Methotrexate is an effective alternate to corticosteroids when the latter is contraindicated, with comparable efficacy. A study comparing methotrexate (10 mg/week) with OMP corticosteroid therapy (dexamethasone 2.5 mg on two consecutive days weekly) in unstable vitiligo found that 76% of patients on methotrexate stabilized, with 44% showing variable repigmentation. In the corticosteroid group, 72% stabilized and 60% achieved repigmentation.[15]

Possible adverse effects include transaminitis, hepatotoxicity, cytopenias, and gastric intolerance.

Cyclosporine

Cyclosporine works by binding with cyclophilin to inhibit calcineurin, which in turn suppresses the nuclear factor of activated T cells (NFAT) and IL-2 expression. This action reduces lymphocytes and macrophages in the skin, particularly inhibiting T-helper lymphocytes. In vitiligo lesions, there are elevated levels of CD4+ and CD8+ lymphocytes, as well as increased type-1 cytokines, TNF-α, IL-8, IFN-γ, and specific dendritic cells and Langerhans cells, all of which cyclosporine downregulates.[16]

Cyclosporine is administered at doses of 3–5 mg/kg, for a period of 4–6 months, mostly as monotherapy.

Cyclosporine can be used as alternative to systemic corticosteroids for halting disease progression and inducing repigmentation. Cyclosporine (3 mg/kg/day) caused cessation of vitiligo progression in 61% of patients (11 out of 18), and nine of these patients exhibited repigmentation.[17] Cyclosporine has also shown to induce stability more rapidly as compared to pulse steroids. Mehta et al. compared dexamethasone mini-pulse therapy (2.5 mg twice weekly) with cyclosporine (3 mg/kg/day) in active vitiligo. Disease stabilization was faster with dexamethasone (10.92 weeks vs. 13.90 weeks).[18]

Cyclosporine can also be used perioperatively to maintain stability, prevent postsurgery perilesional loss of pigment, and induce better repigmentation in patients undergoing cellular grafting for vitiligo. Cyclosporine postoperatively (3 mg/kg/day for 3 weeks, followed by 1.5 mg/kg/day for 6 weeks) in patients who underwent autologous nonculture melanocyte–keratinocyte cell transplant resulted in 100% of patients achieving over 75% repigmentation as compared to only 28% in the untreated group, where most patients achieved 25–50% repigmentation.[19]

Possible adverse effects include hypertension, hyperglycemia, renal toxicity, electrolyte imbalances, gingival hyperplasia, gastric intolerance, and increased risk of malignancy.

SMALL MOLECULES

Janus Kinase Inhibitors

Vitiligo is driven by interferon (IFN)-γ. IFN-γ binds to the receptor and activates the Janus kinase (JAK)-STAT pathway, resulting in the secretion of CXCL10 (C-X-C motif chemokine 10) in the skin. JAK inhibitors act on this pathway, which explains its efficacy in vitiligo.

Tofacitinib acts by causing inhibition of JAK1/3. The dose administered varies from 5 to 20 mg per day. In a case series involving 10 patients treated with oral tofacitinib, five patients showed a mean 5.4% decrease in vitiligo body surface area (BSA) over 9.9 months.[20] JAK inhibitors have demonstrated better repigmentation on facial lesions and when combined with phototherapy.

Possible adverse effects include reactivation of herpes zoster, lipid derangements, transaminitis, acne, nausea, and nasopharyngitis.

The other selective JAK inhibitors found efficacious in vitiligo include ritlecitinib (selective JAK 3 inhibitor) and upadacitinib (selective JAK1 inhibitor).[21,22]

Apremilast

Apremilast is a phosphodiesterase 4 (PDE4) inhibitor that acts by increasing intracellular cyclic adenosine monophosphate (cAMP) levels, which reduces the production of proinflammatory mediators such as IL-23, IL-17, TNF-α, and IFN-γ and increases the levels of anti-inflammatory mediators such as IL-10.

It is given at a dose of 30 mg twice daily for 3–6 months. It can be used in patients with slowly progressive disease as an adjuvant to or as alternative to corticosteroids and immunosuppressants. Majid et al. conducted a pilot study involving 13 patients with rapidly progressing nonsegmental vitiligo. Topical tacrolimus was allowed on exposed body parts. The results showed disease stabilization in all, with partial repigmentation observed in 61.5% of cases.[23]

Possible adverse effects include nausea, vomiting, diarrhea, headache, weight loss, and depression.

ANTIBIOTICS

Minocycline

Minocycline, an antibiotic with antioxidant properties, has demonstrated reduced hydrogen peroxide (H_2O_2)-induced melanocytes apoptosis in vitro.[24]

The prescribed dose is 100 g once daily for a period of 3 months. Minocycline is generally preferred in patients with slowly progressive disease, especially when immunosuppressants are contraindicated.

Out of 32 patients with slowly progressive vitiligo treated using 100 mg of minocycline daily for 3 months, 29 patients experienced disease stability, while three showed progression. 10 patients achieved arrest disease activity after 4 weeks, and seven patients demonstrated good repigmentation.[25] Minocycline has also shown comparable results to low-dose pulse therapy in halting disease progression.[26]

ANTIOXIDANTS

Alpha-lipoic acid is a scavenger for fatty-acid peroxyl and hydroxyl radicals, inhibits lipoxygenase, promotes glutathione synthesis, and recycles vitamins C and E. Ginkgo biloba extracts (GBEs) have antioxidant and anti-inflammatory properties, reducing oxidative stress in inflammatory cells, neutralizing superoxide free radicals, and offering protection against ultraviolet B (UVB)-induced cytotoxicity.

Antioxidants are usually combined with topical treatments, other systemic treatments, and phototherapy. By reducing oxidative stress, they aid in enhancing repigmentation induced by other therapies. It can also help in halting disease progression in slowly spreading vitiligo.[27]

HORMONE ANALOGUES

Afamelanotide

Afamelanotide is an analog of alpha-melanocyte-stimulating hormone (α-MSH) that stimulates proliferation of melanocytes and melanogenesis.

Afamelanotide can be used in combination with phototherapy to enhance repigmentation. Combination of afamelanotide with phototherapy has shown to induce superior repigmentation [48.64% reduction in Vitiligo Area Scoring Index (VASI)] and faster repigmentation compared to the monotherapy group, especially in patients with Fitzpatrick skin phototypes IV–VI.[28]

TREATMENT PROTOCOLS[29-32]

There are significant variations in definitions of unstable disease, progressive disease, and stability in vitiligo. However, the following cutoffs can be taken as a guide in deciding treatment protocols.

Unstable disease is characterized by the emergence or expansion of lesions within 6–12 weeks. Slowly progressive disease involves fewer than three new patches, each <2 cm, appearing in proximity. Rapidly progressive disease is defined by three or more new patches, or patches exceeding 2 cm in size or occurring in multiple anatomical regions. Treatment of stable disease shows no new or expanding lesions in the past 6 months.

Oral mini pulse therapy is indicated for patients with rapidly progressive vitiligo. OMP can be combined with whole-body phototherapy for patients with >5% BSA involvement, and widespread lesions across multiple regions. OMP is tapered over 12–16 weeks after achieving stability. If disease activity returns, OMP is restarted, and steroid-sparing immunosuppressive agents such as methotrexate, azathioprine, mycophenolate mofetil, or cyclosporine are introduced to maintain stability for 6 months, with necessary monitoring. Alternatively, steroid-sparing immunosuppressive agents or tofacitinib can be used as monotherapy for achieving disease stability when corticosteroids are contraindicated.

Antioxidants, apremilast, and minocycline can be considered in patients with slowly progressive disease. If inadequate control is noticed after adequate therapy, low-dose OMP, immunosuppressants such as azathioprine and methotrexate, or tofacitinib can be added.

CONCLUSION

Vitiligo is a complex disorder with a varying course, and its management requires a personalized approach based on disease activity and extent. Early intervention is essential for halting disease progression and promoting repigmentation. Systemic treatments, including corticosteroids, immunosuppressants, and small molecules, are central to managing active and extensive disease. OMP, alone or combined with phototherapy, has shown significant efficacy in stabilizing vitiligo. As research advances, newer therapies such as JAK inhibitors and afamelanotide offer promising alternatives. Overall, a combination of therapies tailored to individual patients' needs is key to achieving optimal treatment outcomes in vitiligo management.

REFERENCES

1. Ezzedine K, Eleftheriadou V, Whitton M, van Geel N. Vitiligo. Lancet. 2015;386:74-84.
2. Vora R, Patel B, Chaudhary A, Mehta M, Pilani A. A clinical study of vitiligo in a rural set up of Gujarat. Indian J Community Med. 2014;39:143-6.
3. Mahajan V, Vashist S, Chauhan P, Mehta KS, Sharma V, Sharma A. Clinico-epidemiological profile of patients with vitiligo: A retrospective study from a tertiary care center of North India. Indian Dermatol Online J. 2019;10:38-44.
4. Parsad D, Sahni K. Stability in vitiligo: Is there a perfect way to predict it? J Cutan Aesthet Surg. 2013;6:75-82.

5. Ezzedine K, Lim HW, Suzuki T, Katayama I, Hamzavi I, Lan CC, et al. Revised classification/nomenclature of vitiligo and related issues: the Vitiligo Global Issues Consensus Conference. Pigment Cell Melanoma Res. 2012;25:E1-13.
6. Kim SM, Lee HS, Hann SK. The efficacy of low-dose oral corticosteroids in the treatment of vitiligo patients. Int J Dermatol. 1999;38:546-50.
7. Banerjee K, Barbhuiya JN, Ghosh AP, Dey SK, Karmakar PR. The efficacy of low-dose oral corticosteroids in the treatment of vitiligo patients. Indian J Dermatol Venereol Leprol. 2003;69:135-7.
8. Pasricha JS, Khaitan BK. Oral mini-pulse therapy with betamethasone in vitiligo patients having extensive or fast-spreading disease. Int J Dermatol. 1993;32:753-7.
9. Kanwar AJ, Mahajan R, Parsad D. Low-dose oral mini-pulse dexamethasone therapy in progressive unstable vitiligo. J Cutan Med Surg. 2013;17:259-68.
10. Khan MS. Comparative efficacy of low-dose oral corticosteroids and oral mini pulse dexamethasone in patients of vitiligo. J Armed Forces Med Coll Bangladesh. 2015;11:54-8.
11. Majid I, Masood Q, Hassan I, Khan D, Chisti M. Childhood vitiligo: response to methylprednisolone oral minipulse therapy and topical fluticasone combination. Indian J Dermatol. 2009;54:124-7.
12. Patra S, Khaitan BK, Sharma VK, Khanna N. A randomized comparative study of the effect of betamethasone oral mini-pulse therapy versus oral azathioprine in progressive nonsegmental vitiligo. J Am Acad Dermatol. 2021;85:728-9.
13. Radmanesh M, Saedi K. The efficacy of combined PUVA and low-dose azathioprine for early and enhanced repigmentation in vitiligo patients. J Dermatolog Treat. 2006;17:151-3.
14. Nageswaramma S, Vani T, Indira N. Efficacy of methotrexate in vitiligo. IOSR J Dental Med Sci. 2018;17:16-9.
15. Singh H, Kumaran MS, Bains A, Parsad D. A Randomized Comparative Study of Oral Corticosteroid Minipulse and Low-Dose Oral Methotrexate in the Treatment of Unstable Vitiligo. Dermatology. 2015;231:286-90.
16. Tarlé RG, Nascimento LM, Mira MT, Castro CC. Vitiligo—part 1. An Bras Dermatol. 2014;89:461-70.
17. Taneja A, Kumari A, Vyas K, Khare AK, Gupta LK, Mittal AK. Cyclosporine in treatment of progressive vitiligo: an open-label, single-arm interventional study. Indian J Dermatol Venereol Leprol. 2019;85:528-31.
18. Mehta H, Kumar S, Parsad D, Bishnoi A, Vinay K, Kumaran MS. Oral cyclosporine is effective in stabilizing active vitiligo: results of a randomized controlled trial. Dermatol Ther. 2021;34:e15033.
19. Mutalik S, Shah S, Sidwadkar V, Khoja M. Efficacy of cyclosporine after autologous noncultured melanocyte transplantation in localized stable vitiligo—a pilot, open label, comparative study. Dermatol Surg. 2017;43:1339-47.
20. Liu LY, Strassner JP, Refat MA, Harris JE, King BA. Repigmentation in vitiligo using the Janus kinase inhibitor tofacitinib may require concomitant light exposure. J Am Acad Dermatol. 2017;77:675-82.
21. Ezzedine K, Peeva E, Yamaguchi Y, Cox LA, Banerjee A, Han G, et al. Efficacy and safety of oral ritlecitinib for the treatment of active nonsegmental vitiligo: a randomized phase 2b clinical trial. J Am Acad Dermatol. 2023;88:395-403.
22. Passeron T, Ezzedine K, Hamzavi I, van Geel N, Schlosser BJ, Wu X, et al. Once-daily upadacitinib versus placebo in adults with extensive non-segmental vitiligo: a phase 2, multicenter, randomized, double-blind, placebo-controlled, dose-ranging study. EClinicalMedicine. 2024;73:102655.
23. Majid I, Imran S, Batool S. Apremilast is effective in controlling the progression of adult vitiligo: a case series. Dermatol Ther. 2019;32:e12923.
24. Song X, Xu A, Pan W, Wallin B, Kivlin R, Lu S, et al. Minocycline protects melanocytes against H_2O_2-induced cell death via JNK and p38 MAPK pathways. Int J Mol Med. 2008;22:9-16.
25. Parsad D, Kanwar A. Oral minocycline in the treatment of vitiligo—a preliminary study. Dermatol Ther. 2010;23:305-7.

26. Singh A, Kanwar AJ, Parsad D, Mahajan R. Randomized controlled study to evaluate the effectiveness of dexamethasone oral minipulse therapy versus oral minocycline in patients with active vitiligo vulgaris. Indian J Dermatol Venereol Leprol. 2014;80:29-35.
27. Parsad D, Pandhi R, Juneja A. Effectiveness of oral Ginkgo biloba in treating limited, slowly spreading vitiligo. Clin Exp Dermatol. 2003;28:285-7.
28. Lim HW, Grimes PE, Agbai O, Hamzavi I, Henderson M, Haddican M, et al. Afamelanotide and narrowband UV-B phototherapy for the treatment of vitiligo: a randomized multicenter trial. JAMA Dermatol. 2015;151:42-50.
29. Bishnoi A, Meghana KB, Parsad D. Medical treatment of vitiligo: a narrative review. Pigment Int 2024;11:167-80.
30. Fatima S, Abbas T, Refat MA, Harris JE, Lim HW, Hamzavi IH, et al. Systemic therapies in vitiligo: a review. Int J Dermatol. 2023;62:279-89.
31. Searle T, Al-Niaimi F, Ali FR. Vitiligo: an update on systemic treatments. Clin Exp Dermatol. 2021;46:248-58.
32. Seneschal J, Speeckaert R, Taïeb A, Wolkerstorfer A, Passeron T, Pandya AG, et al. Worldwide expert recommendations for the diagnosis and management of vitiligo: position statement from the International Vitiligo Task Force—Part 2: specific treatment recommendations. J Eur Acad Dermatol Venereol. 2023;37:2185-95.
33. Radakovic-Fijan S, Fürnsinn-Friedl AM, Hönigsmann H, Tanew A. Oral dexamethasone pulse treatment for vitiligo. J Am Acad Dermatol. 2001;44:814-7.
34. Bishnoi A, Vinay K, Kumaran MS, Parsad D. Oral mycophenolate mofetil as a stabilizing treatment for progressive non-segmental vitiligo: results from a prospective, randomized, investigator-blinded pilot study. Arch Dermatol Res. 2021;313:357-65.
35. Siadat AH, Zeinali N, Iraji F, Abtahi-Naeini B, Nilforoushzadeh MA, Jamshidi K, et al. Narrow-Band Ultraviolet B versus Oral Minocycline in Treatment of Unstable Vitiligo: A Prospective Comparative Trial. Dermatol Res Pract. 2014;2014:240856.
36. Middelkamp-Hup MA, Bos JD, Rius-Diaz F, Gonzalez S, Westerhof W. Treatment of vitiligo vulgaris with narrow-band UVB and oral Polypodium leucotomos extract: a randomized double-blind placebo-controlled study. J Eur Acad Dermatol Venereol. 2007;21:942-50.

6B CHAPTER

Systemic Treatments in Vitiligo: Emerging Biologics and Systemic Janus Kinase Inhibitors

Priyansh Gupta, Davinder Parsad

INTRODUCTION

Vitiligo is a complex autoimmune disorder characterized by the progressive loss of skin pigmentation, resulting in white patches on the skin. It arises from the selective destruction of melanocytes, the cells responsible for producing melanin. Affecting about 0.5–2% of the global population, vitiligo has a profound psychosocial impact due to its visible nature and unpredictable progression.[1-3] Despite its prevalence, the treatment of vitiligo has historically been challenging, relying on conventional approaches such as topical corticosteroids, calcineurin inhibitors, systemic corticosteroids, adjuvants, and phototherapy. These therapies are often inconsistent and fail to address the underlying autoimmune mechanism.

In recent years, advancements in immunology have shed light on the molecular and cellular processes driving vitiligo, leading to the development of targeted therapies. Biologics and systemic Janus kinase (JAK) inhibitors are at the forefront of this therapeutic revolution, offering hope for more effective and durable outcomes. This chapter explores the role of emerging biologics and systemic JAK inhibitors in vitiligo, providing insights into their mechanisms, clinical trials, benefits, and limitations.

PATHOGENESIS OF VITILIGO

Understanding vitiligo's pathogenesis is essential for developing effective targeted therapies. At its core, vitiligo is an autoimmune disorder involving a complex interplay of genetic predisposition, environmental factors, and immune dysregulation, as summarized in **Figure 1**.

Role of Autoimmune T Cells

Cytotoxic CD8+ T cells are central to the autoimmune destruction of melanocytes. These T cells are attracted to the skin by the chemokine CXCL10, which is induced by interferon-gamma (IFN-γ) signaling.[4,5] Once in the skin, they release granzyme B and perforin, leading to melanocyte apoptosis.

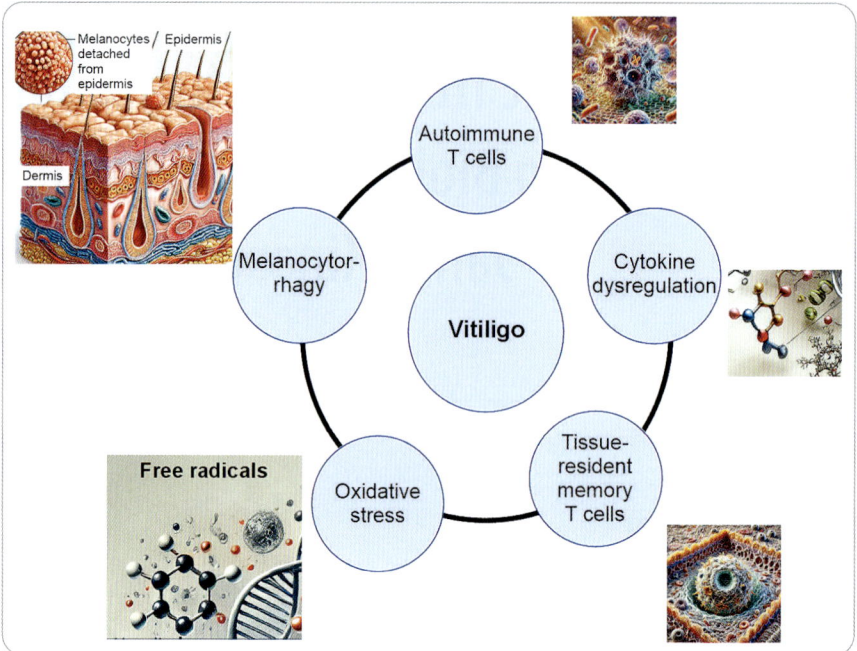

FIG. 1: Schematic representation of various pathogenic mechanisms implicated in vitiligo.

Cytokine Dysregulation

Pro-inflammatory cytokines, particularly IFN-γ, drive vitiligo progression. IFN-γ activates the Janus kinase-signal transducer and activator of transcription (JAK-STAT) pathway, which amplifies the inflammatory response and recruits additional T cells to the affected areas.[6]

Tissue-resident Memory T Cells

Tissue-resident memory T (TRM) cells are a subset of T cells that reside in the skin and persist even after active inflammation subsides. These cells maintain a "memory" of the autoimmune response, contributing to disease recurrence and resistance to treatment.[7]

Oxidative Stress

Oxidative stress is a significant contributor to melanocyte damage in vitiligo. Excessive production of reactive oxygen species (ROS) not only injures melanocytes but also enhances their immunogenicity, making them more susceptible to autoimmune attack.[8]

Melanocytorrhagy

The pathogenic mechanism of melanocytorrhagy in vitiligo involves the chronic detachment and loss of melanocytes from the basal layer of the epidermis, often triggered by mechanical stress, oxidative damage, impaired adhesion, and autoimmune targeting. Detached melanocytes may become immunogenic, provoking an autoimmune response that accelerates their destruction by cytotoxic T cells.[9]

This interplay between mechanical, oxidative, and immune factors perpetuates melanocyte depletion, contributing to the progression of vitiligo.

This multifaceted pathogenesis has driven the development of therapies that target specific immune pathways, particularly cytokines and signaling cascades such as the JAK-STAT pathway.

SYSTEMIC JANUS KINASE INHIBITORS IN VITILIGO

The JAK-STAT pathway is a critical signaling mechanism in vitiligo, mediating the effects of cytokines such as IFN-γ and IL-15. Systemic JAK inhibitors are small molecules that block the activity of JAK enzymes, offering a targeted approach to disrupt autoimmune signaling. They prevent the phosphorylation and activation of STAT proteins, which are transcription factors that regulate the expression of pro-inflammatory cytokines and chemokines. By inhibiting this pathway, JAK inhibitors reduce inflammation, T-cell recruitment, and melanocyte destruction.

Approved and Investigational Janus Kinase Inhibitors (Fig. 2)

Ruxolitinib

Ruxolitinib, a JAK1/2 inhibitor, has shown remarkable efficacy in vitiligo.[10] Phase 3 trials (TRuE-V1 and TRuE-V2) demonstrated the efficacy of ruxolitinib cream 1.5% for facial and body repigmentation.[11] The trials showed that over 50% of participants achieved ≥75% facial repigmentation within 52 weeks, making it a landmark therapy for localized vitiligo which paved the way for its Food and Drug Administration (FDA) approval for vitiligo in 2022. Initially developed as a topical formulation, systemic ruxolitinib has shown improvement in case reports

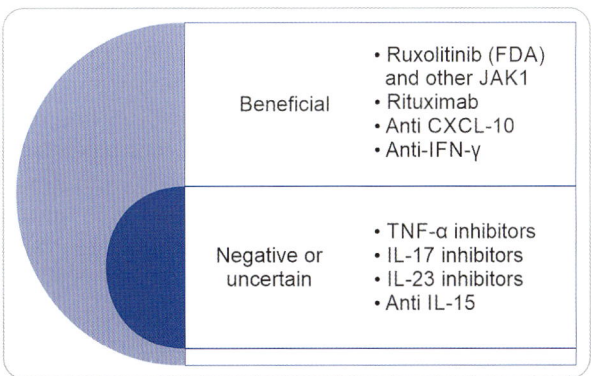

FIG. 2: Representation of Janus kinase (JAK) inhibitors and biologics in relation to their beneficial or negative effect in vitiligo.

when given for coexistent alopecia areata.[12] However, the pigmentation achieved did not last after 12 weeks of treatment discontinuation.[12] Comprehensive clinical trials evaluating the efficacy and safety of oral ruxolitinib specifically for vitiligo are lacking. When it comes to safety only adverse effects observed with topical ruxolitinib in TRuE-V1 and TRuE-V2 trials were local site pruritus, acne, and nasopharyngitis.[11] Ruxolitinib has been seen to be more effective on lesions located on face possibly due to thinner epidermis and greater sun exposure. In addition, repigmentation is more pronounced when used in combination with NB-UVB.[13] Long-term efficacy and safety of topical as well as oral ruxolitinib needs evaluation.

Tofacitinib

Tofacitinib, a JAK1/3 inhibitor, has been studied in small-scale trials and case reports.[10] A recent open label study of topical tofacitinib 2% cream on 16 patients showed significant improvement in 13 patients, with four patients experiencing >90% repigmentation; five patients experiencing 25–75% repigmentation; and four patients experiencing 5–15% repigmentation.[14] Only adverse effect noted was application site acne. Even oral tofacitinib alongside narrowband ultraviolet B (NB-UVB) phototherapy has been tried in vitiligo with almost 50% patients showing decrease in body surface area amounting to 5%.[15] Likewise, combination with micro-phototherapy or excimer laser showed better response than phototherapy alone.[16,17] Tofacitinib in vitiligo can be used as both stabilizing agent as well as repigmenting agent as was seen in a retrospective study of 25 patients.[18] However, variable responses were observed in previous studies, highlighting the need for further long-term studies with larger sample size. Oral tofacitinib is not devoid of adverse effects with a study on 42 patients showed mild pain, derangement of lipid profile and uric acid levels as well as coagulation dysfunction.[19] Recommended dosing is 5 mg once daily which can be escalated to twice daily in case of less than expected response.

Baricitinib

Baricitinib, a JAK1/2 inhibitor approved for rheumatoid arthritis, is being explored for its potential in vitiligo. Preliminary studies suggest that at a dose of 4 mg daily it reduces inflammation and promotes melanocyte regeneration.[20] Baricitinib could promote tyrosinase activity, melanin content and TYR, *TRP1* gene expression of MC-Ds in vitro.[21] The positive in vitro results were also replicated in vivo by clinical improvement seen in four patients.[21] Combination of baricitinib has been utilized for refractory vitiligo with good tolerability.[22] A phase 2 trial named comparing baricitinib and phototherapy in adult patients with progressive vitiligo (BARVIT) is underway.[23]

Upadacitinib, Delgocitinib (Topical), and Filgotinib[24-26]

These next-generation JAK inhibitors are more selective for JAK1, potentially offering improved safety profiles. Upadacitinib is used in treatment refractory vitiligo at a dose of 15 mg daily and showed better response in lesions over face. While their role in vitiligo is still under investigation, they hold promise for future treatment.

Safety Profile of Systemic Janus Kinase Inhibitors

Common side effects include gastrointestinal symptoms, fatigue, and laboratory abnormalities (e.g., elevated liver enzymes, changes in lipid profiles). Long-term use has been associated with an increased risk of thrombosis, malignancy, and cardiovascular events, necessitating regular monitoring. The safety profiles of these therapies are under continuous evaluation, with efforts to develop more selective agents to minimize adverse effects.

EMERGING BIOLOGICS IN VITILIGO (FIG. 2)

Biologics are engineered molecules, such as monoclonal antibodies, designed to target specific immune components. While biologics have revolutionized the management of other autoimmune diseases, their application in vitiligo is relatively new.

- *Tumor necrosis factor-alpha (TNF-α) inhibitors:* Tumor necrosis factor-alpha is a pro-inflammatory cytokine implicated in various autoimmune diseases. TNF-α inhibitors, such as etanercept and infliximab, have been evaluated in vitiligo with mixed results. While they reduce inflammation, their direct impact on melanocyte repigmentation has been limited. The lack of efficacy is reported in many studies while few authors showed beneficial effect in treatment refractory vitiligo.[27-29] Hence, their potential use in vitiligo should be apprehended with caution as studies have also shown onset of vitiligo in patients on TNF-α inhibitors.[30]
- *Anti-interferon-gamma and CXCL10 pathway blockade*[31,32]: Given the pivotal role of IFN-γ in vitiligo pathogenesis, biologics targeting this cytokine or its downstream mediators are under investigation in animal models. These therapies aim to disrupt the JAK-STAT signaling cascade and reduce T-cell recruitment to the skin.
- *Anti-CXCL10 Antibodies*[32]: Blocking CXCL10 may prevent CD8+ T-cell infiltration into vitiligo lesions, thereby halting disease progression. Early studies have shown promising results, though more research is needed.
- *Interleukin-17 inhibitors: Secukinumab:* Controversial results were reported with secukinumab, an interleukin-17 (IL-17) inhibitor when used for vitiligo. Adalimumab-induced vitiligo showed response to secukinumab.[33,34] However larger trial on eight patients showed worsening of depigmentation.[35] Newer data suggests against the use of IL-17 inhibitors in vitiligo.
- *Dupilumab: Targeting type 2 inflammation:* Dupilumab, an IL-4 receptor antagonist approved for atopic dermatitis, has shown anecdotal evidence of repigmentation in vitiligo patients. While IL-4 and IL-13 are traditionally associated with type 2 inflammation, their interplay with IFN-γ in vitiligo

suggests a broader role for these cytokines. Nevertheless, dupilumab has also been implicated in the causation of vitiligo.[36-38]
- *Monoclonal antibodies against CD-20 (rituximab) and interleukin-23 (tildrakizumab)*[39,40]: Studies have shown mixed results with a 6-month follow-up showing improvement in four out of five patients. In contrast, an elderly male showed 90% repigmentation after 1 year treatment with tildrakizumab.
- *Interleukin-15 and tissue-resident memory T Cells:*
  - Interleukin-15 (IL-15) is a cytokine critical for the survival and activation of TRM cells, which are implicated in vitiligo persistence. Blocking IL-15 or its receptor offers a promising strategy for long-term disease control.
  - Bimagrumab is a monoclonal antibody targeting the IL-15 receptor. Preclinical studies suggest that it reduces TRM activity, leading to decreased inflammation and potential repigmentation.[41]

Safety and Tolerability of Biologics

While biologics are generally well-tolerated, their use is not without risks. Adverse effects are typically mild and include injection site reactions and hypersensitivity. Rarely, patients may experience infections or reactivation of latent infections (e.g., tuberculosis). However, in absence of robust efficacy trials, use of biologics requires further study in treatment of vitiligo.

COMBINATION THERAPIES

Combining JAK inhibitors with NB-UVB or topical agents has shown synergistic effects, promoting faster, and more extensive repigmentation. This approach addresses both immune dysregulation and melanocyte regeneration. This will also deter the requirement of higher doses of JAK inhibitors thus preventing dose-related adverse effects. Integrating biologics or JAK inhibitors with established therapies, such as phototherapy and topical agents, may optimize outcomes. Future studies should focus on refining these combinations. The combination of JAK inhibitors with biologics and other adjuvant immunosuppressants has not been studied and is better avoided till robust data is available.

CHALLENGES AND FUTURE DIRECTIONS

Despite their promise, biologics and JAK inhibitors face several challenges in clinical practice.

Heterogeneous Response

Not all patients respond equally to treatment. Biomarkers to predict therapeutic response are needed to personalize therapy.

Tissue-resident Memory T Cells and Disease Chronicity

Tissue-resident memory T cells pose a significant barrier to durable remission. Future therapies must target these cells to achieve long-lasting results.

Cost and Accessibility

The high cost of biologics and JAK inhibitors limits their accessibility, particularly in resource-limited settings. Biosimilars and generic formulations could address this issue.

Pediatric and Long-term Use

The safety of these therapies in children and their long-term effects remain areas of active investigation.

CONCLUSION

The emergence of biologics and systemic JAK inhibitors marks a new era in the management of vitiligo. By targeting the immune mechanisms at the heart of the disease, these therapies offer the potential for more effective and sustained repigmentation. Since JAK inhibitors have role in active disease also, they reduce the requirement of systemic corticosteroids as bridge therapy during progressive stage and hence the side effects. While challenges remain, ongoing research and clinical trials are paving the way for precision medicine in vitiligo, offering hope to millions of patients worldwide. With further advancements in understanding the disease's pathogenesis and optimizing treatment strategies, the goal of achieving complete and lasting repigmentation is becoming increasingly attainable.

REFERENCES

1. Bergqvist C, Ezzedine K. Vitiligo: A Review. Dermatology. 2020;236(6):571-92.
2. Ezzedine K, Eleftheriadou V, Whitton M, van Geel N. Vitiligo. Lancet. 2015;386(9988):74-84.
3. Parsad D, Dogra S, Kanwar AJ. Quality of life in patients with vitiligo. Health Qual Life Outcomes. 2003;1:58.
4. Iannella G, Greco A, Didona D, Didona B, Granata G, Manno A, et al. Vitiligo: Pathogenesis, clinical variants and treatment approaches. Autoimmun Rev. 2016;15(4):335-43.
5. Rodrigues M, Ezzedine K, Hamzavi I, Pandya AG, Harris JE. New discoveries in the pathogenesis and classification of vitiligo. J Am Acad Dermatol. 2017;77(1):1-13.
6. Samaka RM, Basha MA, Menesy D. Role of Janus kinase 1 and signal transducer and activator of transcription 3 in vitiligo. Clin Cosmet Investig Dermatol. 2019;12:469.
7. Frączek A, Owczarczyk-Saczonek A, Placek W. The Role of TRM Cells in the Pathogenesis of Vitiligo-A Review of the Current State-Of-The-Art. Int J Mol Sci. 2020;21(10).
8. Xuan Y, Yang Y, Xiang L, Zhang C. The Role of Oxidative Stress in the Pathogenesis of Vitiligo: A Culprit for Melanocyte Death. Oxid Med Cell Longev. 2022;2022:8498472.
9. Kumar R, Parsad D. Melanocytorrhagy and apoptosis in vitiligo: connecting jigsaw pieces. Indian J Dermatol Venereol Leprol. 2012;78(1):19-23.
10. Pala V, Ribero S, Quaglino P, Mastorino L. Updates on Potential Therapeutic Approaches for Vitiligo: Janus Kinase Inhibitors and Biologics. J Clin Med. 2023;12(23):7486.
11. Rosmarin D, Passeron T, Pandya AG, Grimes P, Harris JE, Desai SR, et al. Two Phase 3, Randomized, Controlled Trials of Ruxolitinib Cream for Vitiligo. N Engl J Med. 2022;387(16):1445-55.
12. Harris JE, Rashighi M, Nguyen N, Jabbari A, Ulerio G, Clynes R, et al. Rapid skin repigmentation on oral ruxolitinib in a patient with coexistent vitiligo and alopecia areata (AA). J Am Acad Dermatol. 2016;74(2):370-1.

13. Rothstein B, Joshipura D, Saraiya A, Abdat R, Ashkar H, Turkowski Y, et al. Treatment of vitiligo with the topical Janus kinase inhibitor ruxolitinib. J Am Acad Dermatol. 2017;76(6):1054-1060.e1.
14. Mobasher P, Guerra R, Li SJ, Frangos J, Ganesan AK, Huang V. Open Label Pilot Study of 2% Tofacitinib for the Treatment of Refractory Vitiligo. Br J Dermatol. 2019;182(4):1047.
15. Liu LY, Strassner JP, Refat MA, Harris JE, King BA. Repigmentation in vitiligo using the Janus kinase inhibitor, tofacitinib, may require concomitant light exposure. J Am Acad Dermatol. 2017;77(4):675.
16. Gianfaldoni S, Tchernev G, Wollina U, Roccia MG, Fioranelli M, Lotti J, et al. Micro-Focused Phototherapy Associated to Janus Kinase Inhibitor: A Promising Valid Therapeutic Option for Patients with Localized Vitiligo. Open Access Maced J Med Sci. 2018;6(1):46-8.
17. Fang WC, Lin SY, Huang SM, Lan CCE. Low-dose tofacitinib with 308-nm excimer therapy successfully induced repigmentation in patients with refractory vitiligo. Clin Exp Dermatol. 2022;47(4):782-3.
18. Sun XK, Sheng AQ, Xu AE. Tofacitinib for the Treatment of Refractory Progressive Vitiligo: A Retrospective Case Series. Dermatol Ther. 2024;2024(1):9944826.
19. Song H, Hu Z, Zhang S, Yang L, Liu Y, Wang T. Effectiveness and safety of tofacitinib combined with narrowband ultraviolet B phototherapy for patients with refractory vitiligo in real-world clinical practice. Dermatol Ther. 2022;35(11).
20. Mumford BP, Gibson A, Chong AH. Repigmentation of vitiligo with oral baricitinib. Australas J Dermatol. 2020;61(4):374-6.
21. Dong J, Huang X, Ma LP, Qi F, Wang SN, Zhang ZQ, et al. Baricitinib is Effective in Treating Progressing Vitiligo in vivo and in vitro. Dose Response. 2022;20(2):15593258221105370.
22. Li X, Sun Y, Du J, Wang F, Ding X. Excellent Repigmentation of Generalized Vitiligo with Oral Baricitinib Combined with NB-UVB Phototherapy. Clin Cosmet Investig Dermatol. 2023;16:635-8.
23. University Hospital Bordeaux. Evaluation of Effect and Tolerance of the Association of Baricitinib and Phototherapy Versus Phototherapy in Adults with Progressive Vitiligo (BARVIT). Bethesda, MD: U.S. National Library of Medicine; 2023.
24. Su X, Luo R, Ruan S, Zhong Q, Zhuang Z, Xiao Z, et al. Efficacy and tolerability of oral upadacitinib monotherapy in patients with recalcitrant vitiligo. J Am Acad Dermatol. 2023;89(6):1257-9.
25. Dhillon S. Delgocitinib: First Approval. Drugs. 2020;80(6):609-15.
26. Yagi K, Ishida Y, Otsuka A, Kabashima K. Two cases of vitiligo vulgaris treated with topical Janus kinase inhibitor delgocitinib. Australas J Dermatol. 2021;62(3):433-4.
27. Kim NH, Torchia D, Rouhani P, Roberts B, Romanelli P. Tumor necrosis factor-α in vitiligo: direct correlation between tissue levels and clinical parameters. Cutan Ocul Toxicol. 2011;30(3):225-7.
28. Rigopoulos D, Gregoriou S, Larios G, Moustou E, Belayeva-Karatza E, Kalogeromitros D. Etanercept in the treatment of vitiligo. Dermatology. 2007;215(1):84-5.
29. AlGhamdi KM, Khurrum H, Rikabi A. Worsening of vitiligo and onset of new psoriasiform dermatitis following treatment with infliximab. J Cutan Med Surg. 2011;15(5):280-4.
30. Sachdeva M, Mufti A, Kashetsky N, Georgakopoulos JR, Naderi-Azad S, Salsberg J, et al. A systematic review of vitiligo onset and exacerbation in patients receiving biologic therapy. JAAD Int. 2020;2:37.
31. Liu H, Wang Y, Le Q, Tong J, Wang H. The IFN-γ-CXCL9/CXCL10-CXCR3 axis in vitiligo: pathological mechanism and treatment. Eur J Immunol. 2024;54(4):2250281.
32. Rashighi M, Harris JE. Interfering with the IFN-γ/CXCL10 pathway to develop new targeted treatments for vitiligo. Ann Transl Med. 2015;3(21):343.
33. Yang Y, Xu Q, Zhang Z, Yao Z. Segmental vitiligo following acitretin treatment for infantile generalized pustular psoriasis resulting in repigmentation under secukinumab therapy. Dermatol Ther. 2022;35(4).
34. Palazzo G. Resolution of post-adalimumab vitiligo with secukinumab in a patient with psoriasis vulgaris. Oxf Med Case Reports. 2020;2020(1):omz134.

35. Speeckaert R, Mylle S, van Geel N. IL-17A is not a treatment target in progressive vitiligo. Pigment Cell Melanoma Res. 2019;32(6):842-7.
36. Picone V, Napolitano M, Torta G, Fabbrocini G, Patruno C. Vitiligo during dupilumab therapy. JAAD Case Rep. 2023;36:51.
37. Shao X, Chen T, Pan X, Chen S, Chen Y, Chen J. Biologic drugs induced vitiligo: case reports and review of literature. Front Immunol 2024;15:1455050.
38. Takeoka S, Kamata M, Yokoi I, Takehara A, Tada Y. Rapid Enlargement of Vitiligo Vulgaris after Initiation of Dupilumab for Atopic Dermatitis: A Case Report. Acta Derm Venereol. 2021;101(10):545.
39. Ruiz-Argüelles A, García-Carrasco M, Jimenez-Brito G, Sánchez-Sosa S, Pérez-Romano B, Garcés-Eisele J, et al. Treatment of vitiligo with a chimeric monoclonal antibody to CD20: a pilot study. Clin Exp Immunol 2013;174(2):229-36.
40. Jerjen R, Moodley A, Sinclair R. Repigmentation of acrofacial vitiligo with subcutaneous tildrakizumab. Australas J Dermatol. 2020;61(4):e446-8.
41. Kaur M, Misra S. Bimagrumab: an investigational human monoclonal antibody against activin type II receptors for treating obesity. J Basic Clin Physiol Pharmacol. 2024;35(6):325-34.

CHAPTER 7A

Tissue Grafting Techniques in Vitiligo

Imran Majid, Seerat Fatima, Aaqib Aslam

INTRODUCTION

Vitiligo is an acquired depigmenting disorder characterized by the loss of melanocytes, leading to white patches on the skin. It affects approximately 0.5–2% of the global population and can significantly impact quality of life[1] due to its cosmetic appearance and social stigma associated with it, especially in skin of color. Various medical and surgical treatments have been developed, with different grafting techniques emerging as viable options for patients with disease resistant to medical therapy. The success of medical treatments for vitiligo largely hinges on the availability of a melanocyte reservoir.[2] Certain lesions, particularly those of late-stage segmental vitiligo, those with leukotrichia (hair that has turned white or gray), and lesions found on hairless skin tend to show inadequate responses to medical therapies. When such lesions stabilize, a viable approach is to surgically introduce new melanocytes to promote effective repigmentation.[3,4]

Tissue grafting in vitiligo involves the transplantation of melanocytes, either from unaffected skin or cultured in vitro, into the depigmented areas to achieve repigmentation. It is typically considered when vitiligo is stable, meaning no new lesions have appeared, and existing ones have not expanded for at least 6–12 months. This chapter explores the various tissue grafting techniques used in the treatment of vitiligo, their mechanisms, indications, advantages, limitations, and outcomes.

HISTORY OF TISSUE GRAFTING IN VITILIGO

Tissue grafting in the treatment of vitiligo has evolved significantly over the years, adapting principles from general surgical grafting and integrating novel dermatological insights. The various contributions and developments in grafting techniques over the years are described in **Table 1**.

TABLE 1: The contributions and developments in grafting techniques over the years.		
Contributors	Year	Description
Ollier	1872	First introduced thin split-thickness grafting
Thiersch	1874	Introduced thin split-thickness grafting
Brown	1944	Developed an electric dermatome to harvest thin and homogenous grafts
Haxthausen	1947	Transplanted thin split-thickness skin grafts from normal to vitiliginous skin in three cases
Behl	1964	First described the surgical treatment of vitiligo in a large series of 107 patients
Falabella	1971	Described the suction blister technique for repigmentation of vitiligo
Falabella	1978	Described the miniature punch grafting technique
Falabella et al.	1989	Described the use of in vitro cultures of melanocyte-bearing epidermis for the treatment of vitiligo
Gauthier and Surleve-Bazeille	1992	Described the use of epidermal suspensions obtained by trypsinization
Kahn et al.	1996	Reported the use of a short-pulse carbon dioxide laser to dermabrade the recipient area
Olsson and Juhlin	1997	Modified the Surleve–Bazeille technique by adding a melanocyte culture medium
Kahn and Cohen	1998	Utilized the motorized dermatome to obtain ultrathin grafts

FUNDAMENTALS OF STABILITY AND TISSUE GRAFTING IN VITILIGO

Achieving stability in vitiligo is crucial for the success of surgical interventions. Stability is typically defined as the absence of new lesions or no progression of existing lesions over a given time period. However, opinions differ on the exact duration required to define stability, ranging from 4 months to 2 years, depending on various studies.[5-8] Recent guidelines recommend a 1-year period of stability, defined by no new lesions, no spread of existing lesions, and no occurrence of the Koebner phenomenon over the preceding year.[9]

Falabella and colleagues introduced the test graft method, in which several punch grafts are placed within a vitiligo lesion, and the extent of repigmentation is observed over the next 12 weeks. Repigmentation extending >1 mm from the graft indicates stability. However, some researchers question its reliability, as it has been observed that the test may yield positive results even in cases where the disease is not entirely stable. Moreover, the test only confirms the stability of the specific lesion tested, not necessarily the overall disease.

Njoo et al.[10] proposed the vitiligo disease activity score (VIDA) scoring system, a six-point scale used to assess disease activity by tracking the appearance of new lesions or the growth of existing ones over periods ranging from <6 weeks to 1 year.

Surgical interventions are typically recommended for patients with VIDA scores of −1 or 0, indicating stability.

Another important question in the field of stability is the relative importance of lesional versus overall disease stability. One multicentric study has looked at this aspect and concluded that lesional stability is as important as overall disease stability in vitiligo grafting. Any patient with lesional stability of >1 year with just six months of overall disease stability can also be considered for vitiligo grafting.[11]

Various types of tissue grafting techniques are available, and the selection of the appropriate technique depends on factors, such as the type of vitiligo, the size and location of the lesions, and the equipment and expertise of the surgeon performing the procedure.

TYPES OF GRAFTING TECHNIQUES (BOX 1)

Mini-punch Grafting

Principle

Mini-punch grafting (MPG) is one of the oldest and simplest grafting techniques in vitiligo surgery, first described in the early 1970s. The basic principle involves transferring healthy and pigmented skin-containing melanocytes (the cells responsible for skin pigmentation) from a donor site to depigmented areas (recipient sites). Small circular grafts, typically 1 mm in diameter, are taken from the donor site and implanted into corresponding sites in the vitiliginous areas to encourage repigmentation through melanocyte migration.

Technique

Mini-punch grafting involves the use of a punch biopsy instrument to harvest small skin grafts from normally pigmented areas and implant them into depigmented areas. Each graft is typically 1 mm in size. The procedure is particularly suitable for small and localized patches of stable vitiligo and is performed under local anesthesia. This technique is often selected for its simplicity, ease of execution, and minimal requirement for specialized equipment.

BOX 1 Tissue grafting techniques can be broadly classified into the following categories.

Grafting techniques:
- Mini-punch grafting (MPG)
- Suction blister epidermal grafting (SBEG)
- Ultrathin skin grafting (UTSG)
- Hair follicle grafts
- Mesh grafts
- Smash grafting
- Flip-top pigment transplantation

Harvesting of Grafts

The donor skin is usually taken from a well-pigmented area of the patient's body, such as the thighs, buttocks, inner arms or other inconspicuous areas. A punch biopsy tool is used to extract multiple small grafts (typically 1 mm in diameter) from the donor site. The punch biopsy instrument is pressed onto the skin and rotated until the graft is cut free. The extracted grafts are carefully stored in saline solution to prevent drying until they are ready to be transplanted. Nowadays, one can use motorized punches to harvest these grafts of 0.8–1.0 mm in diameter.

Preparation of Donor Site

Before harvesting the grafts, the donor site is cleansed with an antiseptic solution, such as povidone-iodine or chlorhexidine, to minimize the risk of infection. Local anesthesia is administered intradermally to separate the deep dermis and ensure patient's comfort during the procedure. After harvesting the grafts, the small donor site wounds are typically left to heal by secondary intention. Healing of these small wounds is usually rapid and leaves minimal scarring.

Procedure and Transfer of Grafts

Once the grafts have been harvested, the recipient site is prepared. The depigmented skin is punctured with the same punch biopsy tool to create tiny holes for graft placement. The holes must be shallow, typically just deep enough to accommodate the grafts. The harvested punch grafts are then carefully inserted into these holes, with the epidermal surface of each graft facing outward. Each graft is gently pressed into place, and once the grafting is complete, a sterile dressing is applied over the area.

Postoperative Care

After the procedure, the recipient site is dressed with sterile gauze, which may be secured with tape or a bandage. The dressing typically remains in place for about 5–7 days to protect the grafts and ensure they adhere properly. Patients are advised to avoid washing or disturbing the grafted area during this time. Mild analgesics can be prescribed to manage any postoperative discomfort, and antibiotics may be prescribed to reduce the risk of infection. Patients should avoid sun exposure and strenuous activities that could affect healing.

Follow-up

Patients are usually asked to return for a follow-up visit about a week after the procedure to remove the dressing and assess the success of the grafts. Subsequent follow-ups are scheduled at intervals to monitor repigmentation and ensure the grafts have taken properly. Repigmentation typically begins within 3-4 weeks and may continue to improve for several months. Patients may also be advised to undergo phototherapy [such as narrowband ultraviolet B (NB-UVB)] to enhance repigmentation and maintain long-term results.

Outcomes and Efficacy

Mini-punch grafting is highly effective for small and stable patches of vitiligo, with reported success rates ranging from 60 to 80%.[12] Repigmentation usually begins within a few weeks to a few months, depending on factors, such as lesion location, graft size, and postoperative care. Patients with facial vitiligo tend to experience the best outcomes, while those with lesions on acral areas (such as hands and feet) may have less predictable results.[12,13] Long-term maintenance of repigmentation varies, but it is generally favorable if the disease remains stable **(Fig. 1)**.

Complications

Though MPG is generally considered a safe procedure, it can carry some risks and complications as described in **Table 2 (Fig. 2)**.

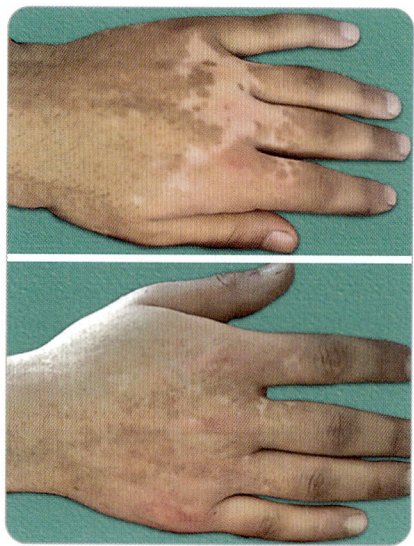

FIG. 1: Miniature-punch grafting with good result on left hand.

TABLE 2: Complications.	
Complications	**Description**
Cobblestoning	Raised, uneven areas of skin at the graft site
Depression at the graft site	Sunken areas where the grafts were placed
Mismatched pigmentation	A slight difference in color between the grafted and surrounding skin
Infection	Rare, but possible if postoperative care guidelines are not followed
Scarring	Small scars may occur at both the donor and recipient sites
Failure of grafts	In some cases, the grafts may not "take" or survive, leading to incomplete or no repigmentation

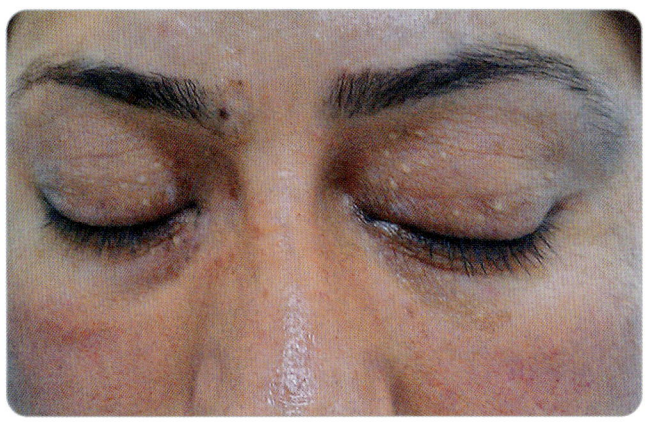

FIG. 2: Cobblestoning after mini-punch grafting (MPG).

TABLE 3: Advantages and description.	
Advantages	Description
Simplicity	The procedure is relatively simple and can be performed with minimal equipment
Minimal invasiveness	The small size of the grafts reduces the risk of scarring and complications
Cost-effective	Compared to more advanced surgical techniques, mini-punch grafting is affordable and accessible
Favorable cosmetic results	In some areas, such as acral areas, areolae, mini-punch grafting can provide good cosmetic outcomes

TABLE 4: Limitations/Disadvantages.	
Disadvantages	Description
Cobblestoning and depigmentation	Uneven skin texture and color mismatch may occur, especially in highly visible areas
Limited to small areas	Mini-punch grafting is not suitable for large areas of vitiligo or rapidly progressing cases
Variable success rates	The outcome may depend on lesion location
Time-consuming for large lesions	Since the grafts are small, covering larger areas requires many grafts, which can be time-consuming and labor-intensive
Risk of graft failure	Some grafts may not take, leading to incomplete repigmentation

Advantages

Refer **Table 3**.

Limitations/Disadvantages (Table 4)

In summary, MPG is a valuable option for treating small, stable vitiligo lesions that have not responded to medical treatments. While it offers simplicity and relatively good cosmetic outcomes, its limitations must be considered, especially in cases involving large or difficult-to-treat areas.

Suction Blister Epidermal Grafting

Principle
The fundamental principle behind suction blister grafting is to create blisters on the donor site through negative pressure, which causes the epidermis to separate from the dermis. The epidermal layer, which contains melanocytes (the pigment-producing cells), is then harvested and transplanted onto the depigmented areas. This method capitalizes on the body's natural healing processes, aiming to promote repigmentation in the affected areas by supplying viable melanocytes.

Technique
The technique of suction blister grafting involves creating controlled blisters using a suction device. A suction blister apparatus is applied to a donor site, often on areas like the thigh or abdomen, where the skin is normally pigmented.[14] The suction creates negative pressure that results in fluid accumulation beneath the epidermis, leading to the formation of blisters within 1–3 hours. Once the blisters have formed, the epidermal roof is removed to obtain a graft. The harvested epidermal grafts are then placed onto the prepared recipient sites, ensuring good contact for optimal adherence and repigmentation.

Harvesting of Grafts
Harvesting in suction blister grafting involves careful management of the created blisters. After allowing sufficient time for blister formation, the epidermis is then separated from the underlying dermis using sterile instruments. The harvested grafts, typically measuring 1–3 cm in diameter, are meticulously handled to maintain their viability. Care must be taken to avoid damaging the melanocyte-rich epidermis during this process.

Preparation of Donor Site
Before commencing the procedure, the donor site is thoroughly cleaned with an antiseptic solution to reduce the risk of infection. Local anesthesia may be administered to minimize discomfort. It is essential to select a donor site with healthy, pigmented skin, as the success of the graft relies on the viability of the melanocytes present in the epidermis. After the blister roofs are harvested, the donor site may be left to heal by secondary intention, as the small wounds typically heal quickly and with minimal scarring.

Procedure and Transfer of Grafts
Once the grafts have been harvested, the recipient area is prepared by cleansing it with antiseptic solution and suitable anesthesia either with topical anesthetic creams or infiltration anesthesia is obtained. The area is then dermabraded, ensuring that any crusts or debris are removed. The harvested epidermal grafts are carefully placed onto the dermabraded depigmented areas, ensuring that they cover the entire affected surface[15,16] and are in direct contact with the underlying dermis. Gentle pressure is applied to secure the grafts, and a sterile dressing is applied to protect the area and maintain moisture.

Postoperative Care

After the procedure, the grafted areas are covered with sterile dressings, which should remain in place for about 5-7 days to protect the grafts and allow for proper adhesion. Patients are advised to avoid excessive moisture, sun exposure, and trauma to the grafted area during the initial healing phase. Monitoring for any signs of complications, such as infection or graft failure, is essential.

Follow-up

Patients typically return for follow-up visits approximately one week after the procedure to assess graft take and the healing process. During these visits, the dressing is removed, and the area is inspected for signs of repigmentation. Regular follow-ups may continue for several months to monitor ongoing repigmentation and to evaluate the long-term success of the grafts. If necessary, adjunctive treatments, such as phototherapy may be considered to enhance and sustain pigmentation.

Outcomes and Efficacy

Suction blister grafting is known to be an effective treatment for stable vitiligo, with reported success rates ranging from 60 to 90%,[12] depending on factors, such as the size and location of the grafts, the stability of the vitiligo, and the patient's skin type. Facial vitiligo tends to respond particularly well to this technique, with patients often achieving satisfactory cosmetic outcomes. Repigmentation typically begins within 4-6 weeks postsurgery and can continue to improve over the following months.

Complications (Table 5)

Although suction blister grafting is generally safe, some potential complications may arise,[14] including:

Advantages

Refer **Table 6**.

Limitations/Disadvantages (Table 7)

In summary, suction blister grafting is a valuable surgical option for treating stable vitiligo, particularly for small-depigmented areas. Its efficacy, combined

TABLE 5: Complications.

Complications	Description
Graft failure	The grafts may not adhere properly or survive, leading to incomplete or no repigmentation
Infection	If postoperative care is not adhered to, there is a risk of infection at the donor or recipient sites
Scarring	While scarring is usually minimal, there is a potential for some scarring at both the donor and recipient sites
Mismatched pigmentation	Grafted areas may not blend seamlessly with surrounding skin, leading to visible differences in skin tone

TABLE 6: Advantages.

Advantages	Description
Minimal invasiveness	The procedure is less invasive compared to full-thickness grafting or other surgical techniques[9]
Good cosmetic results	Patients often achieve satisfactory repigmentation with minimal scarring

TABLE 7: Limitations/Disadvantages.

Limitations/Disadvantages	Description
Limited to small lesions	Suction-blister grafting is best suited for small, stable patches of vitiligo and may not be effective for larger areas
Potential for graft failure	Some grafts may not take, leading to variable outcomes in repigmentation
Requires specialized equipment	Access to suction devices is necessary, which may limit its availability in some clinical settings
Time-consuming procedure	Blister formation takes a long time and is inconvenient and painful for the patient

with minimal invasiveness and good cosmetic outcomes, makes it a preferred choice for many patients. However, careful consideration of its limitations and complications is essential for optimal results.

Split-thickness Skin Grafting

Principle

Split-thickness skin grafting (STSG) is a surgical technique used to treat stable vitiligo by transferring a portion of the patient's own pigmented skin (autograft) to areas of depigmentation.[16] The basic principle is to transplant the epidermis and part of the dermis, which includes melanocytes, from a donor site (usually an inconspicuous, normally pigmented area) to a depigmented recipient site. This method allows melanocytes to repopulate the depigmented skin, leading to repigmentation over time. Unlike full-thickness grafts, STSGs involve only partial dermis transfer, which facilitates faster healing and less donor-site morbidity.

Types of Split-thickness Skin Grafts

Split-thickness skin graftings can be categorized based on the thickness of the graft harvested:
- Thin split-thickness grafts (0.08–0.20 mm)
- Intermediate split-thickness grafts (0.20–0.35 mm)
- Thick split-thickness grafts (0.35–0.50 mm)
- Ultrathin skin grafts (0.05–0.1 mm)

Ultrathin Skin Grafting

Ultrathin skin grafting (UTSG) is practically the only type of STSG used in today's era and time. UTSG is a surgical method used in stable vitiligo to achieve even repigmentation by transferring melanocytes from pigmented donor skin to depigmented areas. This technique has gained popularity due to its minimally invasive nature, reduced scarring, and excellent color matching. One of the early reports of the use of UTSG followed by NB-UVB therapy showcased that the procedure leads to an excellent cosmetic outcome with faster onset of repigmentation in resistant stable vitiligo.[17]

Principle: The principle of UTSG is to harvest a very thin layer of skin, typically <0.1 mm thick, that contains melanocytes, keratinocytes, and the basal membrane. The graft here differs from a STSG in that it does not remain in the recipient area and is shed after 7–10 days. The graft just donates viable melanocytes into vitiligo-affected areas and thus restores pigmentation.

Technique: Ultrathin skin grafting utilizes thin grafts, approximately 0.05–0.1 mm, which is finer than conventional STSG. This minimal thickness ensures that only the epidermal layer, containing melanocytes and keratinocytes, is harvested. The characteristics of an UTSG are that the graft is translucent without any whitish dermal tissue and floats on the normal saline or Ringer's lactate (RL) solution. It is very difficult to ascertain the epidermal and dermal surfaces of the graft as there is essentially no dermal tissue. Only the skin markings on the epidermal surface help is delineating the dermal from the epidermal surfaces of the graft **(Figs. 3A and B)**.

Harvesting of graft: To harvest the graft, a suitable donor area, such as the thigh, buttocks, or upper arm, is selected and cleaned thoroughly. The graft harvesting is typically done under topical anesthesia by utilizing an eutectic mixture of lignocaine and prilocaine in a cream form. The topical anesthetic cream is applied for about 60 minutes both at the donor and the recipient sites before the procedure is done. After attaining a good anesthetic effect, the graft is harvested using a Silver's knife, a specialized dermatome blade or even a simple blade in a hemostatic forceps. Maintaining skin tension is essential during harvesting to achieve a uniform graft thickness, ensuring effective results without risking donor site morbidity.

Preparation of donor site: The donor site is cleaned, sterilized, and treated with a topical anesthetic. A dermatome blade is calibrated to ensure precise and controlled removal of an ultrathin layer of skin. Proper skin tension is applied during harvesting to avoid uneven graft thickness.

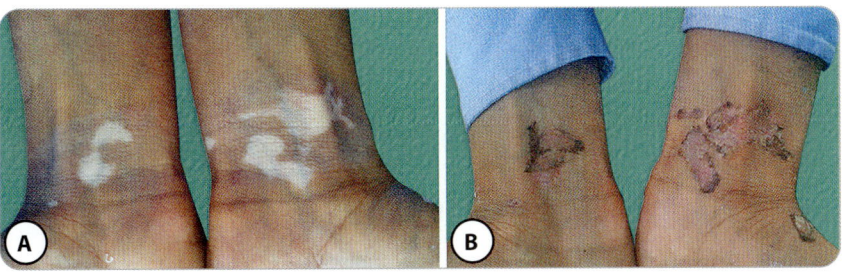

FIGS. 3A AND B: Ultrathin skin grafting after 7 days—the graft will fall off in few days.

Procedure and transfer of grafts: The depigmented area is cleansed and prepared with dermabrasion or a fractional CO_2 laser, which creates a superficial wound bed to improve graft adherence and facilitate melanocyte migration. One can use either manual dermabraders or motorized ones to achieve a uniform superficial dermabrasion. Once prepared, the ultrathin graft is carefully placed onto the recipient's site, ensuring there are no air pockets or wrinkles, which could cause graft failure or irregular repigmentation. The graft is then covered with a nonstick gauze and a pressure dressing to enhance adherence and prevent displacement during the initial healing phase.

Postoperative care: Postoperative care is essential to support graft survival and proper healing. The dressing is typically left undisturbed for 5–7 days to avoid displacement. Following this period, mild topical antibiotics may be applied for a few days followed by topical tacrolimus ointment or any other suitable topical agent to enhance the repigmentation.

Follow-up: Regular follow-up is critical to monitor healing and pigmentation. Typically, the repigmentation starts after 2–3 weeks and complete repigmentation may take 2–3 months. In some cases, phototherapy, such as NB-UVB or excimer laser, may be added to encourage melanocyte migration and enhance repigmentation.

Outcome and efficacy: Ultrathin skin grafting has shown promising outcomes, with studies indicating 70–90% repigmentation in patients with stable vitiligo. The thin graft allows for excellent color blending with the surrounding skin, leading to a natural appearance, and the achieved repigmentation is typically long-lasting if the vitiligo remains stable. However, complications, though rare, may include graft rejection, perigraft halo, and color irregularities, such as hypo- or hyperpigmentation. Minimal scarring may also occur at the donor or recipient site, particularly if the graft was thicker than intended or improperly handled **(Figs. 4 and 5)**.

Complications: Refer **Table 8**.

Advantages: Refer **Table 9**.

Limitations/Disadvantages: Refer **Table 10**.

In summary, UTSG is a refined and effective approach for treating stable and localized vitiligo. By addressing key aspects of donor site preparation, meticulous

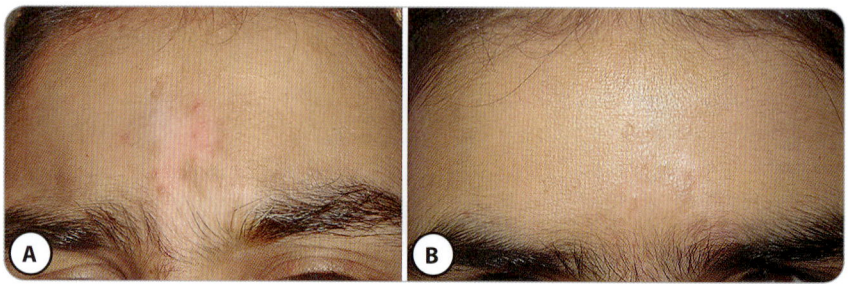

FIGS. 4A AND B: Excellent response to ultrathin skin grafting (UTSG) in segmental vitiligo.

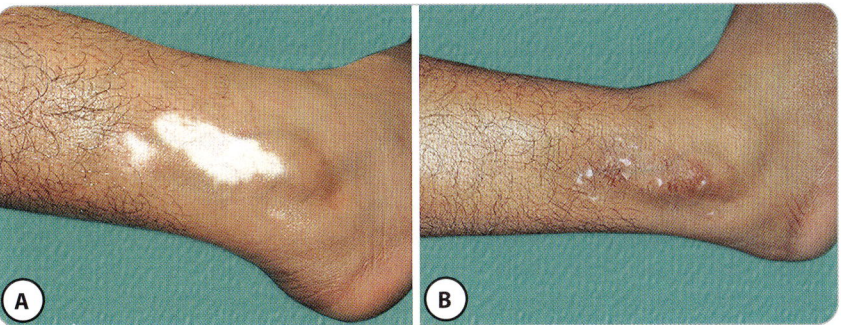

FIGS. 5A AND B: Response to ultrathin skin grafting (UTSG) on the leg.

TABLE 8: Complications.	
Complications	**Description**
Graft rejection	In some cases, the graft may not adhere properly, leading to partial or complete failure
Infection	Postoperative infections can occur but are typically manageable with antibiotics
Hypopigmentation/ Hyperpigmentation	Uneven color changes may occur, particularly in areas with high ultraviolet (UV) exposure or friction
Scarring	Although rare, minimal scarring can develop at the donor or recipient site, especially if the graft is too thick or improperly handled

TABLE 9: Advantages.	
Advantages	**Description**
Cosmetic outcomes	Ultrathin grafts provide excellent color matching, minimal scarring, and a natural appearance
Minimal donor site morbidity	The thinness of the graft minimizes trauma to the donor site, reducing pain, scarring, and risk of secondary infections. Grafts can be taken again from the same site at multiple times
Efficient melanocyte migration	Ultrathin grafts allow melanocytes to migrate effectively across the depigmented area, ensuring even pigmentation

TABLE 10: Limitations/Disadvantages.	
Disadvantages	**Description**
Limited coverage for large lesions	This technique is best suited for small-to-medium areas of vitiligo, as extensive depigmentation may require alternative or multiple grafts
Technical skill requirement	Achieving consistent ultrathin graft thickness requires precision and expertise, making the procedure more technically demanding
Risk of graft loss	Due to the delicate nature of the graft, there is a risk of graft failure if postoperative care is not followed strictly

graft placement, and close follow-up, this technique offers promising repigmentation results with minimal side effects. However, as with any surgical procedure, patient's selection and surgical expertise are crucial to maximizing outcomes and minimizing complications.

Hair Follicle Grafts in Vitiligo

Principle

The principle behind hair follicle grafting in vitiligo is based on the presence of melanocyte reservoirs in the hair follicles. These melanocytes can be used to repigment vitiliginous skin when transferred to depigmented areas.[14] The hair follicle is harvested from areas like the scalp or beard area and grafted onto depigmented patches. Over time, the melanocytes within the follicles migrate into the surrounding skin, promoting repigmentation.

This method is particularly beneficial for patients with lesions in areas where traditional skin grafts may not work effectively, such as glabrous skin (hairless skin) and areas resistant to medical therapy, like lesions with leukotrichia (white hair).

Outcomes and Efficacy

Hair follicle grafting has shown high efficacy, particularly in treating smaller areas of stable vitiligo or lesions in cosmetically sensitive locations, such as the face and neck.[18] Studies report a repigmentation success rate ranging from 60 to 90%, especially when combined with adjuvant therapies, such as NB-UVB. The long-term outcomes are positive, with grafted follicles continuing to provide a melanocyte reservoir for years after the procedure, allowing for sustained repigmentation.

One of the major advantages of hair follicle grafting is its ability to induce melanocyte migration from the follicle into surrounding skin,[16] leading to broader repigmentation than the size of the graft itself. This makes the technique particularly useful for small and resistant lesions or areas, such as the lips and eyelids, where traditional grafting methods may be less effective.

Mesh Grafting in Vitiligo

Principle

The principle of mesh grafting lies in expanding the surface area of a STSG by creating small slits or holes in a grid-like pattern, which allows the graft to stretch and cover a larger area.[14] The mesh pattern also provides drainage for fluids that might accumulate under the graft, promoting better adherence to the recipient site.[13] The transplanted graft brings melanocytes from the donor area, which then migrate to the depigmented region, leading to repigmentation.

Outcomes and Efficacy

Mesh grafting has proven to be effective in achieving repigmentation in large and stable vitiligo patches. Studies have shown success rates ranging from 60 to 80%, depending on the location of the lesion, the patient's skin type, and adherence to postoperative care protocols.

The cosmetic outcomes of mesh grafting are generally good, especially when the graft takes well and repigmentation is uniform. When combined with postoperative NB-UVB phototherapy, the likelihood of successful repigmentation is further increased.

Smash Graft Technique in Vitiligo

Principle

The principle behind the smash graft technique is to transplant melanocyte-rich tissue into depigmented areas.[14] By finely mincing the skin into small pieces, the surface area of the grafts increases, allowing for more widespread application over vitiliginous regions.[13] The melanocytes from these grafts can then migrate and repopulate the recipient site, leading to repigmentation. Unlike other techniques, smash grafting covers a relatively large surface area with minimal donor skin, making it cost-effective and straightforward.

Outcomes and Efficacy

The smash graft technique is effective in causing repigmentation in stable vitiligo patches, especially in cases where other treatment options are not feasible. Studies suggest that success rates range from 60 to 90%, depending on the patient's skin type, lesion location, and adherence to postoperative care.

One of the key benefits of the smash graft technique is that it can cover a large-depigmented area with a small amount of donor skin, making it both cost-effective and minimally invasive. The cosmetic results are generally good, although the final outcome may take several months to fully develop. When combined with postoperative phototherapy, such as NB-UVB, the likelihood of successful and even repigmentation is further enhanced. Smash grafting can serve as a cost-effective technique in resource-poor settings to treat larger areas of vitiligo **(Figs. 6A and B)**.

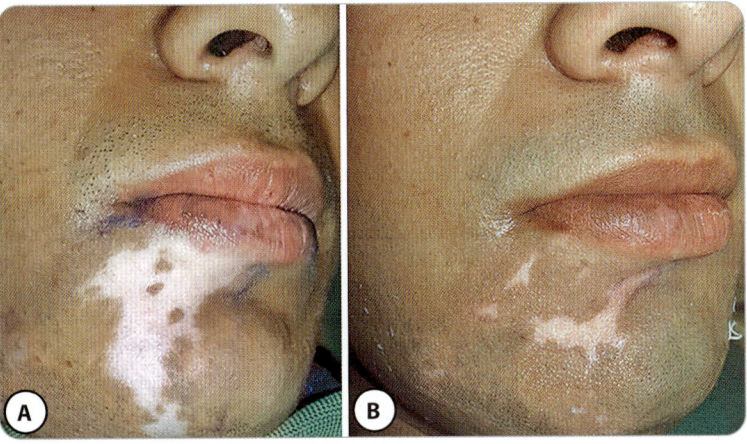

FIGS. 6A AND B: Smash grafting in beard area.

Flip-top Pigment Transplantation Technique in Vitiligo

Principle

The principle of the flip-top pigment transplantation (FTPT) technique is to transfer melanocytes from normally pigmented skin to vitiliginous areas through the application of a skin flap.[19,20] This flap remains partially attached to the donor site (allowing vascular connections to remain intact), which helps to ensure graft survival and enhances melanocyte migration.[21] Unlike other grafting methods, where skin grafts are completely detached, this "flip-top" method reduces the risk of graft failure by maintaining a partial blood supply. The technique is particularly suited for localized and stable vitiligo and provides a novel alternative when other grafting methods are not feasible.

Conclusion

Tissue-grafting techniques represent a crucial advancement in the treatment of stable vitiligo, offering a chance for significant repigmentation where medical therapy has failed. Each technique has its own set of advantages, limitations, and indications, and the choice of method should be individualized based on lesion characteristics, patient's preference, and available expertise. With continued advancements in cellular biology and grafting technologies, the success and accessibility of these techniques are expected to improve **(Table 11)**.

RECENT ADVANCES

Robotic-assisted Skin Grafting[22]

Robotic-assisted grafting systems are being developed to automate the harvesting and transplantation process, ensuring more precise and consistent outcomes. These systems are designed to:
- *Improve precision*: Robots can remove and transplant extremely thin layers of skin with more accuracy than manual techniques, reducing donor site morbidity and improving cosmetic results.
- *Speed up procedures*: Automation reduces the time required for skin harvesting and grafting, making procedures more efficient for both patients and clinicians.

Phototherapy and Laser-assisted Grafting[22,23]

The combination of tissue-grafting techniques with advanced phototherapy and laser treatments has improved outcomes by enhancing melanocyte survival and repigmentation postgrafting:
- *Excimer laser*: Using the excimer laser postgrafting can target specific areas to stimulate melanocyte activity and enhance repigmentation in a focused manner. This laser is also used pregrafting to prepare the recipient site, leading to better graft acceptance.

CHAPTER 7A: Tissue Grafting Techniques in Vitiligo

TABLE 11: This table provides an overview of the various grafting techniques used in vitiligo treatment. Each method has its specific use case, advantages, and disadvantages, which help to determine the most suitable option depending on the patient's condition, location, and extent of vitiligo.

Technique	Principle	Donor site preparation	Procedure	Postoperative care	Advantages	Limitations/Disadvantages
Mini-punch grafting	Transplanting small, circular grafts (usually 1 mm) of pigmented skin into depigmented areas	Donor skin (often from thigh or gluteal area) is prepared and local anesthesia is applied	Punch grafts are harvested and implanted into prepared depigmented areas using corresponding punch tools	Immobilize grafts with pressure dressings for 5–7 days. Avoid trauma to the area	Simple technique, minimal donor skin needed, useful for stable lesions	Cobblestone appearance, risk of poor cosmetic outcome, limited to small areas
Suction blister grafting	Harvesting a thin graft from the epidermis using suction blisters and transferring it to the depigmented areas	Suction cups create blisters at the donor site, which is often on the thigh	Blister roofs are transferred to dermabraded recipient sites	Dressings kept in place for 5–7 days. Patient advised to avoid movement or trauma to the treated areas	Minimal scarring, ideal for cosmetically sensitive areas, such as the face, good aesthetic results	Labor-intensive, time-consuming blister formation, suitable only for small lesions
Ultrathin split skin grafting	Similar to split-thickness grafting, but with a thinner graft that includes only the epidermis	Similar to split-thickness grafting; a very thin sheet is harvested from the thigh	Graft is placed onto the recipient area	Dressings and immobilization required as in split-thickness grafting	Less scarring compared to thicker grafts, better cosmetic outcomes	Thin grafts are delicate and have a higher chance of failure or sloughing off
Hair follicle grafting	Transplanting hair follicles from pigmented areas (since melanocytes reside in hair follicles) to depigmented skin	Follicles are harvested using a punch tool from areas like the scalp	Individual hair follicles are transplanted into the depigmented area via small incisions	Area should remain undisturbed postoperatively. Instruct patients to avoid direct sun exposure	Minimal donor site trauma, potential for hair-bearing areas, and long-lasting pigmentation	Limited use to areas where hair presence is acceptable, can result in patchy appearance

Continued

Continued

Technique	Principle	Donor site preparation	Procedure	Postoperative care	Advantages	Limitations/Disadvantages
Mesh grafting	Uses a split-thickness skin graft, which is expanded into a mesh to cover a larger area	Same as split-thickness grafting; the skin is prepared and harvested with a dermatome	The graft is meshed and stretched to cover more extensive depigmented areas	Dressings applied, area immobilized for 7–10 days	Can cover large vitiligo patches with minimal donor skin	Mesh pattern may remain visible, particularly in cosmetically sensitive areas
Smash grafting	Tiny pieces of minced epidermis or dermal tissue are spread over a dermabraded depigmented area, allowing for spontaneous repigmentation	Harvested from pigmented areas using a razor or surgical blade	Small pieces of skin are minced into tiny bits and spread evenly over the dermabraded recipient site	Pressure dressings applied. Monitor for signs of graft failure or infection	Quick procedure, covers irregular-shaped lesions effectively, no need for exact graft matching	Results may vary, pigmentary irregularities are common, and limited use for large lesions
Flip-top pigment transplantation	A partial-thickness skin flap remains attached to its donor site on one end while the free end is transferred to the depigmented area, keeping blood supply intact	The donor site is adjacent to the vitiligo lesion; a partial-thickness skin flap is harvested with one side remaining attached to the donor site	The attached side provides blood supply, and the free end is flipped over the recipient area. Secured with sutures and left to heal in place	Graft immobilized for 1 week; patient advised to avoid any activity that could displace the graft	Maintains blood supply, higher graft survival rate, good cosmetic outcome, especially in small and localized vitiligo	Limited to small and localized areas, requires adequate donor skin nearby, technically demanding

- *Fractional CO_2 laser*: Fractional lasers are now used to create microwounds on the recipient's site, promoting graft adherence, and stimulating the migration of melanocytes. This combination treatment enhances the success rate of grafting techniques.

CONCLUSION

Recent advances in tissue-grafting techniques for vitiligo have revolutionized the approach to repigmentation, offering better cosmetic outcomes, higher success rates, and more efficient procedures. The combination of innovations in cell biology, tissue engineering, and immunology holds promise for even more effective treatments in the future. While some of these techniques are still experimental, their potential to transform vitiligo treatment is significant, providing new hope for patients with this challenging condition.

REFERENCES

1. Parsad D, Dogra S, Kanwar AJ. Quality of life in patients with vitiligo. Health Quality Life Outcomes. 2003;1:58.
2. Maleki M, Banihashemi M, Sanjari V. Efficacy of suction blister epidermal graft without phototherapy for locally stable and resistant vitiligo. Indian J Dermatol. 2012;57:282-4.
3. Mulekar SV. Melanocyte-keratinocyte cell transplantation for stable vitiligo. Int J Dermatol. 2003;42:132-6.
4. VanGeel NA, Ongenae K, Vander Haeghen YM, Naeyaert JM. Autologous transplantation techniques for vitiligo: how to evaluate treatment outcome? Eur J Dermatol. 2004;14:46-51.
5. Das SS, Pasricha JS. Punch grafting as a treatment for residual lesions in vitiligo. Indian J Dermatol Venereol Leprol. 1992;58:315-9.
6. Boersma BR, Westerhof W, Bos JD. Repigmentation in vitiligo vulgaris by autologous minigrafting: Results in nineteen patients. J Am Acad Dermatol. 1995;33:990-5.
7. Olsson M, Juhlin L. long-term follow-up of leukoderma patients treated with transplants of autologous cultured melanocytes, ultrathin epidermal sheets and basal cell layer suspension. Br J Dermatol. 2002;47:893-904.
8. Falabella R. Surgical treatment of vitiligo: Why, when and how. J Eur Acad Dermatol Venereol. 2003;17:518-20.
9. Parsad D, Gupta S. Standard guidelines of care for vitiligo surgery. Indian J Dermatol Venereol Leprol. 2008;74:37-45.
10. Njoo MD, Das PK, Bos JD, Westerhof W. Association of the Kobner phenomenon with disease activity and therapeutic responsiveness in vitiligo vulgaris. Arch Dermatol. 1999;135:407-13.
11. Majid I, Mysore V, Salim T, Lahiri K, Chatterji M, Khunger N, et al. Is lesional stability in vitiligo more important than disease stability for performing surgical interventions? Results from a multicentric study. J Cutan Aesthet Surg. 2016;9(1):13-9.
12. Njoo MD, Westerhof W, Bos JD, Bossuyt PM. A systemic review of autologous transplantation methods in vitiligo. Arch Dermatol. 1999;135(12):1532-9.
13. Gauthier Y, Benzekri L. Surgical management of vitiligo: An update. Dermatol Clin. 2012; 30(2):301-13.
14. Falabella R. Surgical approaches for stable vitiligo. Dermatol Surg. 2001;27(2):175-82.
15. Mulekar SV. Surgical interventions for vitiligo: What's new? J Cutan Aesthetic Surg. 2003; 1(1):13-7.
16. Olsson MJ, Juhlin L. Treatment of vitiligo by suction blister grafting: A retrospective study of 50 patients. J Am Acad Dermatol. 1998;38(5):761-4.

17. Majid I, Imran S. Ultrathin split-thickness skin grafting followed by narrowband UVB therapy for stable vitiligo: an effective and cosmetically satisfying treatment option. Indian J Dermatol Venereol Leprol. 2012;78(2):159-64.
18. Thakur P, Sacchidanand S, Nataraj HV, Savitha AS. A study of hair follicular transplantation as a treatment option for vitiligo. Journal of Cutaneous and Aesthetic Surgery. 2015;8(4):211-7.
19. Gupta S, Olsson MJ. Surgical intervention for stable vitiligo: Autologous non-cultured melanocyte transplantation versus suction blister epidermal grafting. J Cutan Aesthetic Surg. 2003;1(1):19-23.
20. Bergamaschi OM, Meneguin S. A novel approach to surgical treatment of vitiligo: Flip-top grafting technique. J Dermatol Surg. 2010;36(2):215-9.
21. McGovern TW, Bolognia J, Leffell DJ. Flip-top pigment transplantation: A novel transplantation procedure for the treatment of depigmentation. Archives of dermatology. 1999;135(11):1305-7.
22. Taneja A, Trehan M, Taylor CR. 308-nm excimer laser for the treatment of localized vitiligo. Int J Dermatol. 2003;42(8):658-62.
23. Wu CS, Lan CC. Enhancing repigmentation in vitiligo by fractional CO_2 laser treatment. J Cosmet Laser Ther. 2008;10(4):210-3.

7B CHAPTER

Surgical and Adjunctive Therapies: Cellular Grafting in Vitiligo

Salim Thurakkal, S Prasannakumar

INTRODUCTION

Surgical therapy of vitiligo is the gold standard in the management of resistant and residual lesions. Certain types of vitiligo, such as segmental, mucosal, acral, and leukotrichia commonly fail to respond well to medical therapies and in those cases that do respond, residual areas of depigmentation persist.

Cellular grafting methods constitute important advances in the surgical management of leukoderma. Different methods, such as noncultured epidermal suspensions (NCES), hair follicle cell suspension (HFCS), pure melanocyte cultures, and melanocyte-keratinocyte cultures have all been shown to be effective.[1,2] It is possible to treat very large areas using a small donor area. It yields faster, uniform, normal textured, and natural pigmentation.[1,3] This chapter deals with the "Cellular Grafting" techniques.

HISTORIC ASPECTS

In the early 1980s, researchers began to recognize that melanocytes could be cultured and isolated from the skin, opening the door for the development of cellular grafting techniques.[4] In the 1990s, the NCES technique emerged as a simpler and quicker alternative to cultured melanocyte transplantation.

The first noncultured epidermal cellular grafting was performed under experimental conditions on piebald guinea pig skin by Billingham and Medawar.[3] In 1992, Gauthier and Surleve–Bazeille used this technique for the treatment of stable vitiligo.[5] The donor sample was obtained from the scalp and treated with 0.25% trypsin solution for 18 hours. Liquid nitrogen was used to raise blisters at the recipient site into which the suspension was inoculated.

This technique was then modified by Olsson and Juhlin in 1998, where the donor skin was taken from the gluteal region and the trypsinization time was reduced to 60 minutes and the suspension was directly applied on to dermabraded vitiligo lesion.[6] A limiting factor to this technique was the fixation of the liquid suspension at the recipient area. To overcome this hurdle, further modification in the technique was introduced by Van Geel et al. in 2001 with the use of hyaluronic acid to increase the viscosity of the suspension and to prevent its run-off.[7]

PRINCIPLE OF CELLULAR GRAFTING

All grafting techniques rely on the basic principle of repopulating depigmented lesions with functional melanocytes arising from normal epidermis or outer root sheath (ORS) and bulge areas of the hair follicle. These cells are enzymatically separated, and then concentrated in suspending media. This can be either transplanted directly or cultured and transplanted after 3–4 weeks. The transplanted melanocyte will establish and function as an epidermal melanin unit and the cells will continue to survive and function if the disease remains stable.[5]

Noncultured epidermal suspension is based on extraction of basal cell layer followed by concentration of these cells by centrifugation. The basal cell extraction is carried out by enzymatic separation of the intercellular bridges and dermoepidermal junction using the proteolytic enzyme, trypsin. Trypsin separates the basal keratinocytes and melanocytes.[5] These separated cells are concentrated in suspending media and further transplanted over the recipient area **(Figs. 1A to F)**.

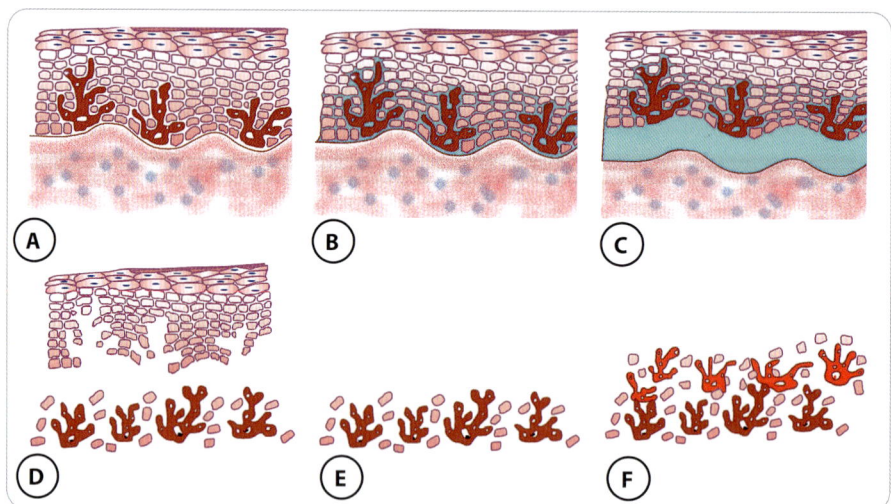

FIGS. 1A TO F: Principle of noncultured epidermal suspensions (NCES). (A) Cross-section of normal skin showing dermis, epidermis, and dermoepidermal junction with basal melanocytes and keratinocytes; (B) Trypsin entering through the intercellular bridges and dermoepidermal junction; (C) Cells getting separated due to the action of trypsin; (D) Basal melanocytes and keratinocytes separated; (E) Basal cells are concentrated in the suspending media and the epidermal and dermal components are discarded; and (F) New melanocytes after culture.

In culture techniques, the cells are cultured in flasks under anaerobic incubation and transplanted after 3–4 weeks.

INDICATIONS FOR CELLULAR GRAFTING TECHNIQUES AND PATIENT'S SELECTION

Proper case selection is of paramount importance for any surgical method to yield good results. Stability of vitiligo should be the primary consideration while opting for any transplantation methods. Proper counseling is essential; the nature of the disease, procedure, expected outcome, and possible complications should be clearly explained to the patient.[6]

Type of Vitiligo

Cellular grafting is indicated for all types of stable vitiligo including segmental, generalized, and acrofacial types that do not respond to medical treatment. However, the best of the result is obtained in segmental vitiligo. The chance of reactivation is much lower in segmental variants in comparison with other types of vitiligo. Moreover in segmental vitiligo accompanied by leukotrichia, it may be considered as a first-line of therapy as the reservoir of melanocyte is lacking.[6,7]

Other indications include piebaldism, postburn leukoderma, chemical leukoderma, nevus depigmentosus, and halo nevus.

Area of Involvement

Cellular grafting is useful in treating leukoderma of all anatomical areas including "the difficult to treat areas", such as hairy areas, and those areas with excessive movements, such as the joints, acral area, mucosa, angle of mouth, eyelids, and genital area. Nonhair bearing areas and mucosal surfaces are resistant to medical treatments. As the reservoir is lacking in these areas these techniques may be considered to replenish with melanocytes to regain pigment.[8]

Stability

Stability indicates absence of new lesions and arrest of spreading of the existing lesions. The stability status of vitiligo is the single most important prerequisite in case selection. Parameters for establishing stability of vitiligo include absence of new lesions, or extension of old lesions, no Koebner phenomenon, and a successful test grafting.[7,8] The recent consensus recommendations by most of the Task Forces regarding stability is that, vitiligo can be considered as being stable if a patient is presenting with no new lesions, no progression of existing lesions, and absence of Koebner phenomenon during the past 1 year.[7,8] Spontaneous repigmentation, presence of well-defined borders, and spotty pigmentation are considered as favorable signs for vitiligo surgery.

Age of the Patient

There is no uniformly accepted opinion concerning the minimum age for surgery. Even though the progress of the disease is difficult to predict in children, studies have suggested that results of transplantation procedures were better in younger individuals than in older ones.[8] The author is of the opinion that surgeries can be of great help in pediatric population with stable segmental vitiligo unresponsive to medical treatments. The dermatosurgeon should exercise judgment after taking all aspects of the individual patient into consideration.

Contraindications

Bleeding disorders, active vitiligo, and keloidal tendency are the absolute contraindications for "Cellular Grafting" techniques.

NONCULTURED EPIDERMAL SUSPENSION

This technique has revolutionized the scenario of the surgical therapy of vitiligo helping to treat very large area utilizing a donor skin of one-tenth area of recipient site. NCES yields cosmetically acceptable results in a short period of time. More recently NCES have come out of tissue culture laboratory to operating theater settings. These techniques have become more practitioner friendly, more widely used, and almost an office procedure now.

Instruments and Consumables

Skin-grafting knife in the form of Humby's knife, Silver's knife, straight artery forceps with razor blade or Padget's, and Zimmer's or Davol's dermatome can be used for harvesting. **(Box 1 and Fig. 2)**.

BOX 1 **Consumables and equipment for noncultured epidermal suspensions (NCES).**

Consumables:
- 0.25% trypsin—0.8% ethylenediaminetetraacetic acid (EDTA) solution
- Trypsin inhibitor, to neutralize excess trypsin
- Dulbecco's Modified Eagle's Medium (DMEM)

Equipment:
- Centrifuge
- Aerobic incubator
- Micromotor diamond-fraise dermabrader or a CO_2 laser
- A manual or electric dermatome
- Two pairs of fine pointed nontoothed forceps
- Pasture pipette or calibrated micropipette
- Centrifuge tubes, petridishes

Dressings:
- Collagen dressings
- Tulle dressings

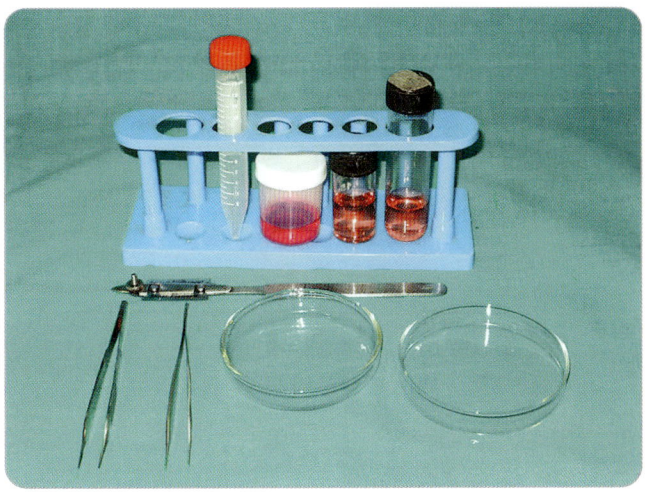

FIG. 2: Reagents and instruments required for noncultured epidermal suspensions (NCES).

Technique

The technique involves three steps:
1. Harvesting of donor skin
2. Preparation of melanocyte rich basal layer cell suspension
3. Dermabrasion followed by application of the cells over the recipient area

Harvesting of donor skin: Usually one-fifth to one-tenth the size of the recipient area is harvested from the lateral aspect of the gluteal region. After cleaning with povidone iodine and alcohol, a superficial skin sample is obtained using a skin grafting knife under local anesthesia or topical anesthesia. The donor site is then covered with nonadherent tulle dressing **(Figs. 3A to E)**.

Preparation of Cell Suspension

The skin sample is immediately transferred into a petridish containing 8 mL of 0.25% trypsin—0.8% ethylenediaminetetraacetic acid (EDTA) solution (Sigma, St. Louis, Mo, USA). Complete contact of the graft with the solution should be ensured by turning the sample back and forth. It is finally placed epidermis facing upward. The sample is then incubated in an ordinary aerobic incubator at 37°C for 50 minutes. After incubation excess of trypsin, EDTA solution is removed and about 5 mL of trypsin inhibitor (Sigma, St. Louis, Mo, USA) is added to stop further action of trypsin. Further cell separation is done in Dulbecco's Modified Eagle's Medium (DMEM) with F-12 nutrient mixture, 1:1 v/v, and a 15-mmole/L HEPES Buffer system (Sigma, St. Louis, Mo, USA) **(Figs. 4A to H)**.

The epidermis and the dermis are separated with the help of a pair of nontoothed forceps in the petridish-containing DMEM with F-12 nutrient mixture, 1:1 v/v and a 15-mmole/L HEPES Buffer system (Sigma, St. Louis, Mo, USA). The cells adherent to the dermis are also separated. Dermal tissue is then discarded. Simple phosphate buffer saline can also be used in place of DMEM.

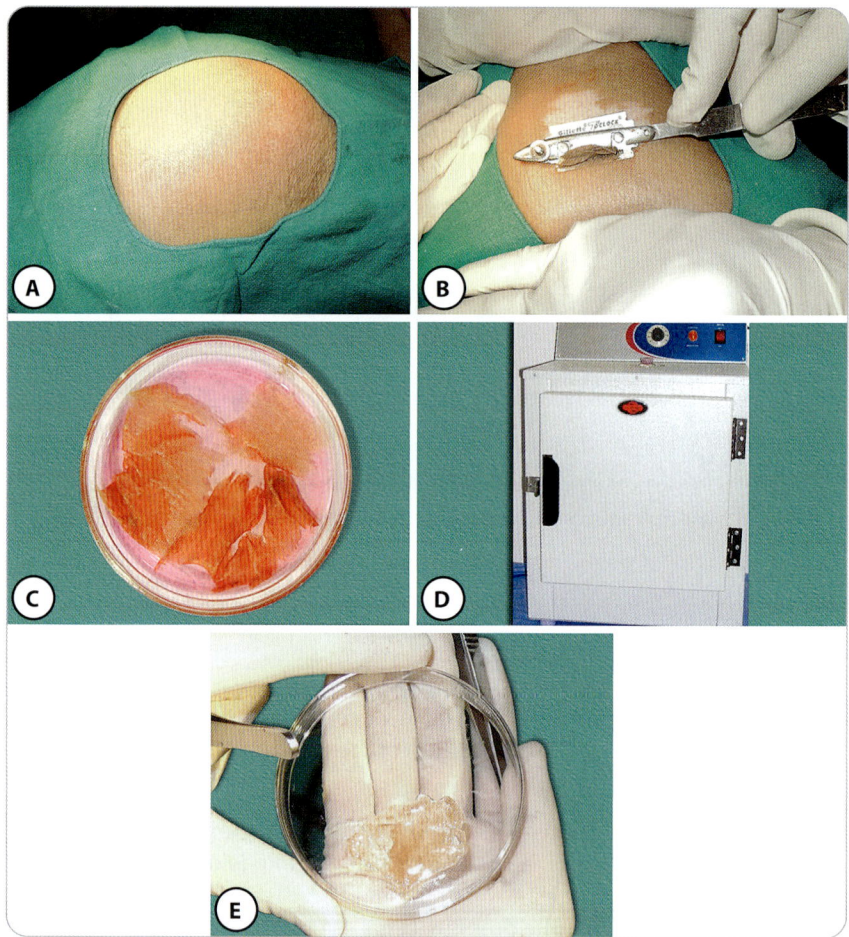

FIGS. 3A TO E: Procedure. (A) Donor site prepared for harvesting split thickness skin; (B) Harvesting donor skin with modified silver's knife; (C) Skin sample transferred to petridish-containing trypsin—ethylenediaminetetraacetic acid (EDTA) solution and kept epidermal surface facing upward; (D) The sample is incubated in aerobic incubator at 37°C for 50 minutes; and (E) Skin sample after trypsinization. You can notice the separated cells here.

The epidermis is washed in the media and the basal cells are separated. The epidermal pieces are then discarded. The media along with the cells is centrifuged at 2,000 rpm for 10 minutes. A cell pellet rich in melanocyte and basal keratinocytes is formed at the bottom of the tube. The supernatant is discarded, and the pellet is resuspended in a total volume of 0.8 mL of fresh medium in a 1-mL syringe **(Figs. 5A to C)**.

Transplantation

The recipient area is surgically cleaned with povidone iodine and alcohol. Under local anesthesia, using a high-speed diamond-fraise dermabrader or carbon-dioxide laser, the recipient area is abraded down to the dermoepidermal junction.

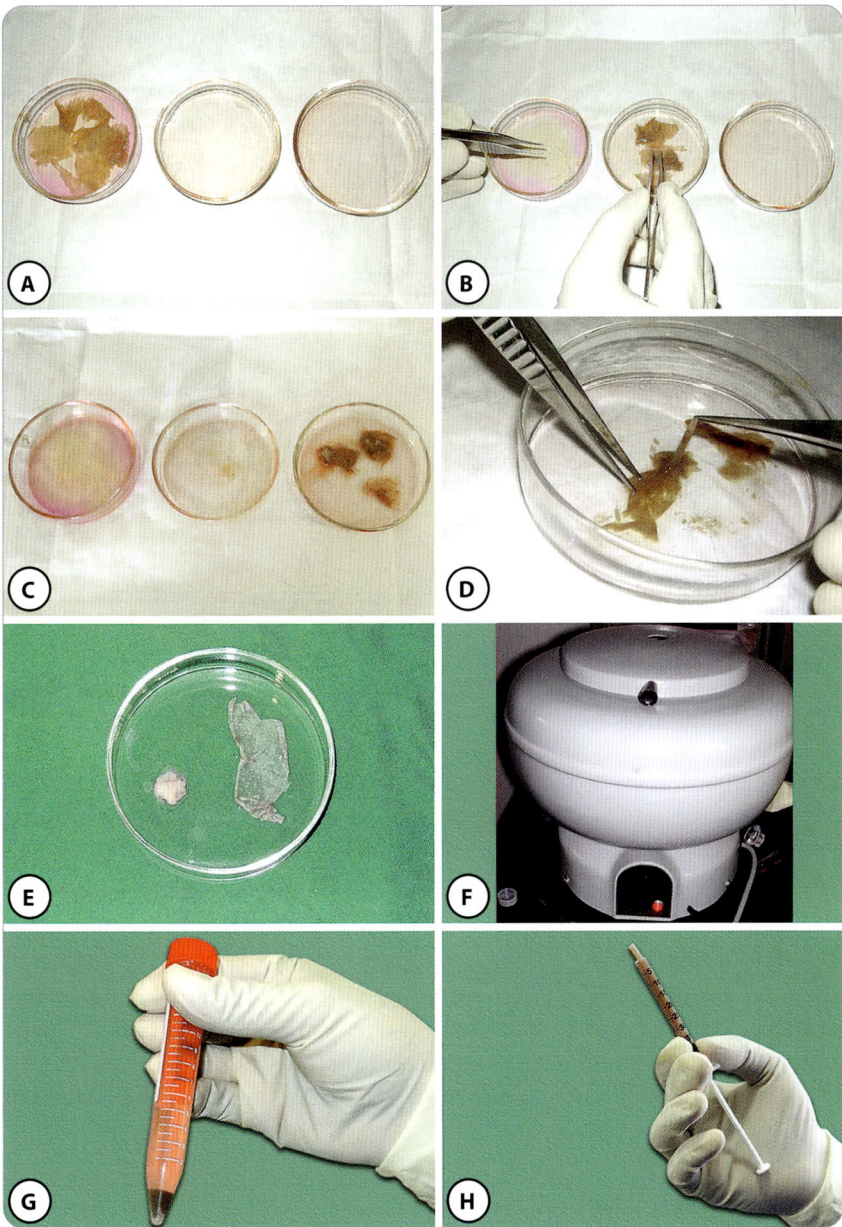

FIGS. 4A TO H: (A) Three petridishes with reagents. First one with trypsin and grafts, second one with trypsin inhibitor, and third one with Dulbecco's Modified Eagle's Medium (DMEM) suspending medium; (B) Grafts transferred to second petridish with trypsin inhibitor to stop further action of trypsin; (C) Grafts transferred from second petridish to the third containing DMEM for cell separation; (D) Cell separation done with nontoothed forceps; (E) Dermis and epidermal component after separating the basal cells; (F) The separated basal cells along with DMEM are centrifuged for concentrating the cells; (G) Cell pellet of basal cells obtained after centrifugation; and (H) Basal cell rich suspension reconstituted in fresh DMEM ready for transplantation.

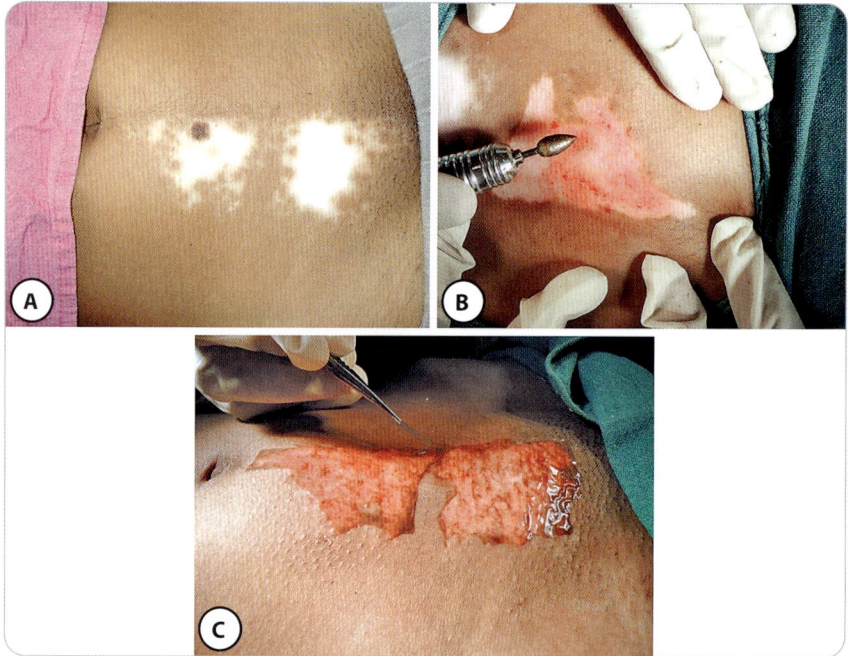

FIGS. 5A TO C: (A) Recipient area prepared; (B) Dermabrasion done using diamond fraise dermabrader; and (C) Application of cellular suspension followed by collagen sheets.

The cell suspension is evenly applied with the syringe and spread out with its tip over the recipient area. Cells are covered with a thin-transparent collagen film. This is then covered with a sterile pad and finally with tegaderm (3 M) dressing **(Figs. 6A to C)**.

Postoperative Care

All patients are advised to take complete rest and avoid vigorous physical activities. All cases with area treated <150 cm^2 can be managed as daycare. The patient is sent home under antibiotic coverage and the dressings are removed after a week. Anti-inflammatory medicines are prescribed to manage the postoperative pain.

Surgical Outcome

The onset of pigmentation usually occurs in 3–6 weeks and it is complete in 2–6 months' time **(Figs. 7 to 11)**. The pigmentation is uniform with good textural and cosmetic color match. This method is much simpler than culture-based techniques and less time-consuming. It does not require expensive culturing conditions and high-tech laboratories; but still requires trained personnel familiar with cell separation to get an optimal survival rate of cells. Cell separation can be done under sterile conditions in the operating room itself. Key features of NECS are given in **Box 2**.

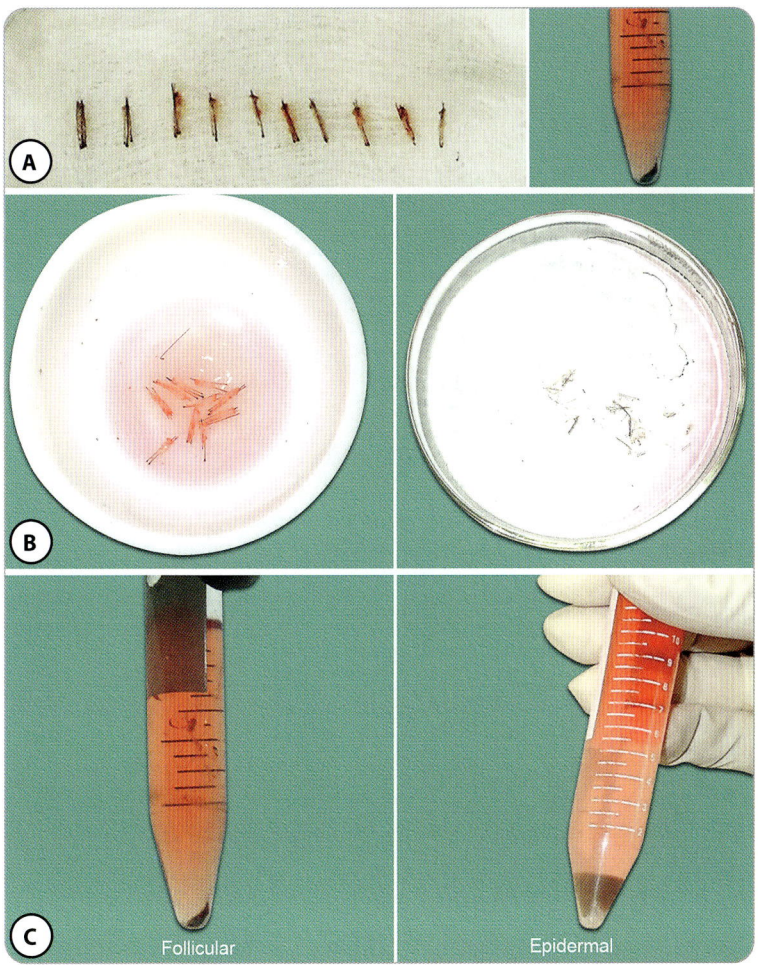

FIGS. 6A TO C: Hair follicle cell suspension (HFCS). (A) Extracted hair follicles and HFCS; (B) HFCS before and after trypsinization; and (C) Follicular and epidermal suspension.

HAIR FOLLICLE CELL SUSPENSION

Autologous noncultured ORS-HFCS is a new novel cellular grafting technique for the treatment of vitiligo. This is a recently described novel cellular graft technique for the surgical treatment of stable vitiligo. Hair-follicle melanocytes have some unique characteristics that make them an attractive source of melanocytes than epidermis for cell-based therapies in vitiligo.

Inactive melanocytes or melanocyte stem cells are found to reside in the ORS and bulge areas of the hair follicle. These melanocytes did not produce melanin under normal conditions but became active to produce melanin when stimulated either by ultraviolet radiation or dermabrasion.[2,9] Cui et al. proposed the hair follicle to be the reservoir of "inactive" melanocytes (melanocyte stem cells).[9,10] It was also observed that in vitiliginous lesions, there was destruction of only the

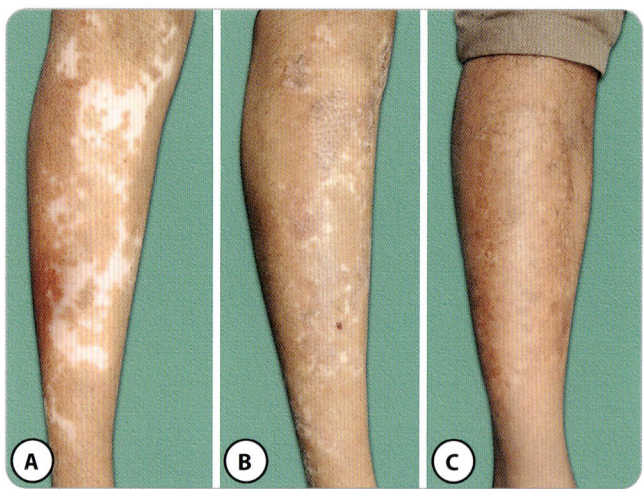

FIGS. 7A TO C: (A) Vitiligo vulgaris before noncultured epidermal suspensions (NCES); (B) Early repigmentation at three weeks; and (C) Repigmentation after six months.

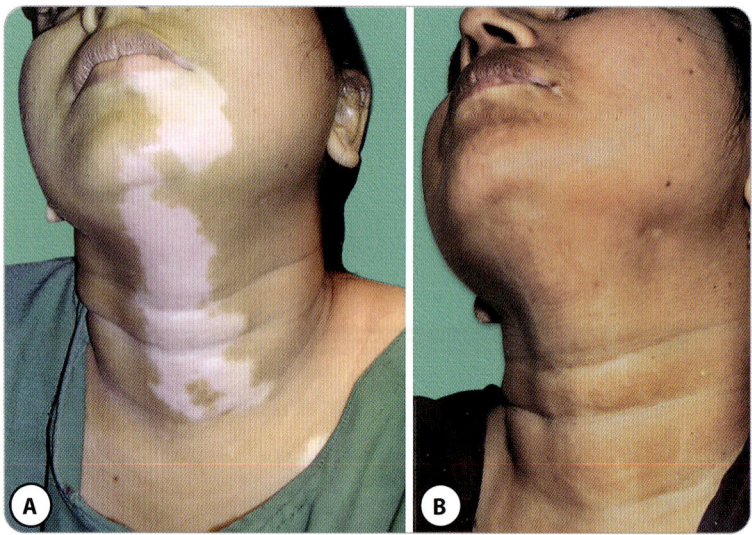

FIGS. 8A AND B: (A) Segmental vitiligo before noncultured epidermal suspensions (NCES) and (B) After three months.

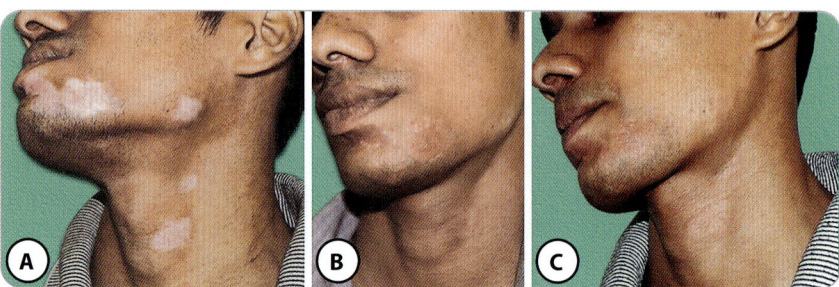

FIGS. 9A TO C: Cellular grafting with hair melanocytes before and after.

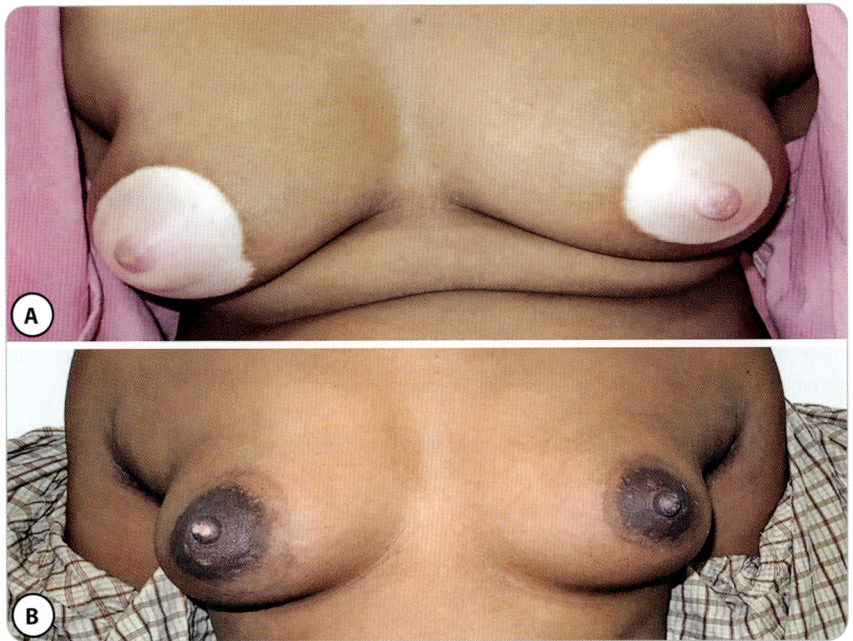

FIGS. 10A AND B: (A) Before noncultured epidermal suspensions (NCES) and (B) After 6 months. Note the recipient predominance pattern here.

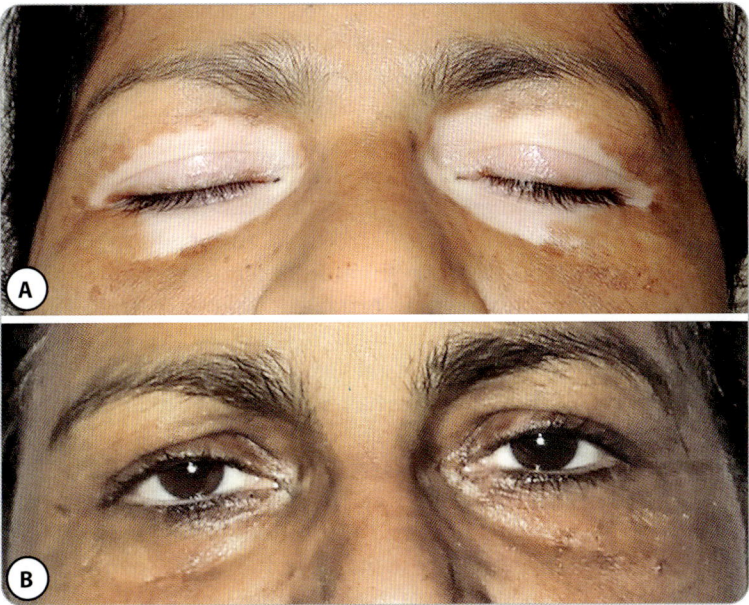

FIGS. 11A AND B: Periorbital area. (A) Before and (B) After.

> **BOX 2: Advantages and disadvantages of noncultured epidermal suspensions (NCES).**
>
> *Advantages:*
> - Large area can be treated using a small skin sample. Donor recipient ratio 1:10
> - It can be used in difficult areas, such as joints, pressure sites, mucosa, etc.
> - Faster, uniform pigmentation matching with adjoining skin
> - It does not need laboratory as the cell separation can be done in operating room itself
> - Daycare procedure
> - Donor site pigments with minimal scaring
>
> *Disadvantages:*
> - Requires specific cell culture grade biochemicals and media
> - The operating room has to be equipped with incubator, centrifuge, and equipment for preparation of cell suspension
> - Surgical skill required to harvest adequate sized, thin grafts
> - Perilesional Halo seen in few cases

TABLE 1: Comparison of noncultured epidermal suspensions (NCES) and HFCS.

Noncultured epidermal cell suspension (NCES)	Hair follicle outer root sheath cell suspension (HFCS)
• Easy to perform • Single Incubation required • Melanocyte keratinocyte ratio 1:36 • Load of melanocyte is less in comparison with HFCS • Skin melanocytes are less influenced by age	• Follicular unit extraction and cellular suspension preparation are time consuming • Three incubations are required • Melanocyte keratinocyte ratios 1:1 to 1:6 • Load of melanocyte is much higher than NECS. Few hairs can yield large quantity of melanocyte • Hair melanocyte undergo aging (graying)

active (DOPA-positive) melanocytes, whereas the inactive melanocytes in the ORS of the hair follicle were undamaged. These melanocytes were proposed to be responsible for repigmentation in vitiligo by dividing and migrating upward along the surface of hair follicle to the nearby epidermis and surrounding skin.

Follicular unit extraction is done from the scalp using follicular extraction device. About 15–25 hair follicles are extracted. These are then trimmed and transferred to a petridish containing 10 mL of 0.25% of trypsin EDTA solution. Three different incubations of 20 minutes at each at 37°C is required for cell separation. After each incubation, the hair is transferred to another pertridish-containing DMEM and the separated cells are scraped. The cells fall into the DMEM. The hair is again transferred to trypsin and incubated. The cells are then concentrated by centrifugation and the cell pellet formed is resuspended in fresh medium. The cell suspension is spread over dermabraded-recipient area and covered with collagen sheet as in case of epidermal cell suspension technique. The comparison of NCES and HFCS is given in **Table 1**.

Vanscheidt et al.,[10] in a small case series, have used single cell suspension of "plucked" hair follicles in the treatment of vitiligo. They found almost complete (>90%) repigmentation in three out of five patients with vitiligo, around 50% repigmentation in one patient and <10% repigmentation in one patient.

Mohanthy et al.[2] in their pioneering study reported follicular unit extraction followed by separation of melanocytes from ORS and transplantation in vitiligo patients with promising results.

Singh C et al.[11] compared the treatment outcome in patients of stable vitiligo treated with HFCS method and epidermal cell suspension method. Both epidermal cell suspension method and HFCS method were found to be of comparable efficacy in treating patients of stable vitiligo. But, the patient in NCES group was significantly more satisfied than the patients in HFCS group.

In a study published by Vinay et al., the mean number of melanocytes transplanted that was associated with optimum pigmentation was 1,187 cells/cm^2, which is much less than that described by earlier studies.[12] Hence, the requirement of melanocytes for optimal pigmentation is lesser than epidermal cell suspension technique. This is attributed to the different morphology and ultrastructural characteristics of hair follicle melanocytes, being larger, more dendritic, and a higher synthetic capacity. Cell suspension prepared from extracted hair follicles provides an excellent, relatively less invasive source for stem cells and/or melanocytes in the surgical management of vitiligo.

One concern about the follicular melanocyte transplantation is the influence of aging. Hair graying is noticed as an age-related phenomenon in melanocytes. The future of the transplanted hair melanocytes in the skin can be predicted only through long-term studies. Further studies are needed that suggest techniques to improve melanocytes survival, function, and multiplication to achieve optimal permanent pigmentation.

CULTURE TECHNIQUES

Melanocyte culture techniques are slowly moving out of vitiligo surgical scenario with the advent of less time-consuming nonculture techniques yielding freshly prepared melanocytes. Moreover, culture techniques employed for the expansion of the cell number are time consuming, expensive, and also require trained manpower and well-equipped tissue culture laboratory. In addition, there are concerns about the safety of the techniques owing to the xenobiotic properties of some of the additives in the culture medium.[13,14]

The techniques used are cultured melanocytes (CM) and cultured epidermis (CE).

Cultured Melanocytes

Melanocytes are cultured in vitro for 15–30 days by the addition of media and growth factors. Once sufficient numbers are present, melanocytes are detached from the culture plates and suspension is transplanted onto the denuded recipient area in a density of 1,000–2,000 melanocytes/mm^2. The vitiliginous patch is dermabraded or laser abraded, and cells' suspension is applied.[14]

Cultured Epidermis

Basal cells separated by trypsinization are seeded in a medium that allows cocultivation of keratinocytes and melanocytes. A few weeks later, a cultured epidermal sheet is obtained, released by dispase and attached to petrolatum gauze. This is applied on a dermabraded-recipient site.

Both the culture techniques are being replaced by nonculture techniques.

CONCLUSION

Vitiligo surgery has made major advances in techniques. Noncultured cellular grafting techniques, evolved from the culture techniques, have outgrown from the cell culture laboratories. It is now possible to treat very large areas of vitiliginous patches with excellent cosmetic results in operating theater settings. The improved techniques can encompass larger areas with better results at a substantially lower cost thus enabling us to reach a wider spectrum of the population.

REFERENCES

1. Olsson MJ, Juhlin L. Leukoderma treated by transplantation of basal cell layer enriched suspension. Br J Dermatol. 1998;138:644-8.
2. Mohanty S, Kumar A, Dhawan J, Sreenivas V, Gupta S. Non-cultured extracted hair follicle outer root sheath cell suspension for transplantation in vitiligo. Br J Dermatol. 2011;164(6):1241-6.
3. Salim T. Surgical Management of Vitiligo. In: Lahiri K, Chatterjee M, Sarkar R (Eds). Pigmentary Disorders: A Comprehensive Compendium. New Delhi: Jaypee Brothers Medical Publishers (P) Ltd; 2014. pp. 227-40.
4. Kaufmann R, Greiner D, Kippenberger S, Bernd A. Grafting of in vitro cultured melanocytes onto laser-ablated lesions in vitiligo. Acta Derm Venereol. 1998;78(2):136-8.
5. Falabella R. Surgical treatment of vitiligo: Why, when and how. J Eur Acad Dermatol Venereol. 2003;17:518-20.
6. Mysore V, Salim T. Cellular grafts in management of leucoderma. Indian J Dermatol. 2009;54:142-9.
7. Parsad D, Gupta S. Standard guidelines of care for vitiligo surgery. Indian J Dermatol Venereol Leprol. 2008;74:37-45.
8. Taieb A, Alomar A, Böhm M, Dell'anna ML, De Pase A, Eleftheriadou V, et al. Guidelines for the management of vitiligo: the European Dermatology Forum consensus. Br J Dermatol. 2013;168(1):5-19.
9. Cui J, Shen LY, Wang GC. Role of hair follicles in the repigmentation of vitiligo. J Invest Dermatol. 1991;97:410-6.
10. Vanscheidt W, Hunziker T. Repigmentation by outer-root-sheath-derived melanocytes: Proof of concept in vitiligo and leucoderma. Dermatology. 2009;218:342-3.
11. Singh C, Parsad D, Kanwar AJ, Dogra S, Kumar R. Comparison between autologous noncultured extracted hair follicle outer root sheath cell suspension and autologous noncultured epidermal cell suspension in the treatment of stable vitiligo: a randomized study. Br J Dermatol. 2013;169(2):287-93.
12. Vinay K, Dogra S. Stem cells in vitiligo: Current position and prospects. Pigment Int. 2014;1(1):8-12.
13. Verma R, Grewal RS, Chatterjee M, Pragasam V, Vasudevan B, Mitra D. A comparative study of efficacy of cultured versus non cultured melanocyte transfer in the management of stable vitiligo. Med J Armed Forces India. 2014;70(1):26-31.
14. Chen YF, Yang PY, Hu DN, Kuo FS, Hung CS, Hung CM. Treatment of vitiligo by transplantation of cultured pure melanocyte suspension: analysis of 120 cases. J Am Acad Dermatol. 2004;51(1):68-74.

CHAPTER 8

Role of Lasers and Medication in Depigmentation in Vitiligo

Munish Paul

INTRODUCTION

The aim of treatment in vitiligo is to produce a uniform skin color. In patients having limited disease, the aim of treatment is repigmentation through medical and or surgical methods, but patients who have more extensive disease, attaining a significant repigmentation and maintaining the repigmentation are quite difficult. It is very important that such cases are identified who are beyond repigmentation because even if repigmentation is achieved in such cases, it will be typically for a short duration, which does not make significance because it comes at a cost of possible numerous immediate or late side effects, because of the use of immune suppressive drugs, phototherapy, etc., hence these patients should be identified as candidates for active or induced depigmentation and managed accordingly.

The *indications* for depigmentations are patients of vitiligo having >50% area involved, unstable cases, patients with extensive diseases and multiple coexisting morbidities as old age, obesity, hypertension, diabetes, and cardiac, patients having acral vitiligo with extensively spreading disease, and patients having long-standing acral diseases and who have frequent relapses.

Detailed counseling is a very important aspect of depigmentation, the involves discussing in detail with the patient, the treatment time that will be required, the course of the treatment the role of medicines [monobenzyl ether of hydroquinone (MBEH)] and lasers, that is Q-switched neodymium-doped yttrium aluminum garnet (Nd:YAG) Laser. Patient should also be counseled that depigmentation process is irreversible. Also in counseling, the side effects like contact dermatitis, photosensitivity, have to be discussed and understand that they have to avoid direct exposure to sunlight forever.

Patient must be given enough time and assistance in making the decision and ideally family members should also be involved in the process of taking a decision about depigmentation.

MEDICAL DEPIGMENTATION

An ideal depigmenting agent would be that has a potent, rapid, and selective effect on destruction of melanocytes. It should lead to permanent removal of pigment. It should be nontoxic and has minimum side effects.[1]

The various options that are available are monobenzyl ether of hydroquinone also known as MBEH, monomethyl ether of hydroquinone, topical diphencyprone diphenylcyclopropenone (DPCP), imiquimod, phenol, cryotherapy, and lasers.

Amongst all of these, monobenzyl ether of hydroquinone is the one which is used most commonly and this is most readily available. So, the process of using, it is first an open use test which should be performed on the pigmented skin of the forearm on a small area and observe for any un-outward reactions.

The cream has to be applied at night on one area initially, there can be a reaction, i.e., itching, redness, and oozing. At this time, MBEH should be discontinued and the allergic reaction should be managed with a mild steroid and antihistamines. Once the reaction subsides lightening of the pigment can be noted and once the reaction has subsided the MBEH can be restarted. Patient is instructed to start treating sequentially moving from the highest to the lowest priority example, eventually a patient might want the face **(Figs. 1 and 2)** to be depigmented first, so we have to work on depigmenting the face and then we move to the hands, arms, and body.

With MBEH, there will be a gradual lightening of the skin over a period of 4–12 months[2] and the depigmentation that is usually irreversible and histologically associated with loss of melanosomes and melanocytes.[1] We can use different concentrations of MBEH. For example, for the face we use 10% or 20%, for the neck and eyelids, we can use 5%, 20% on the arms and legs and for the elbows and knees we can use 30 and 40%.

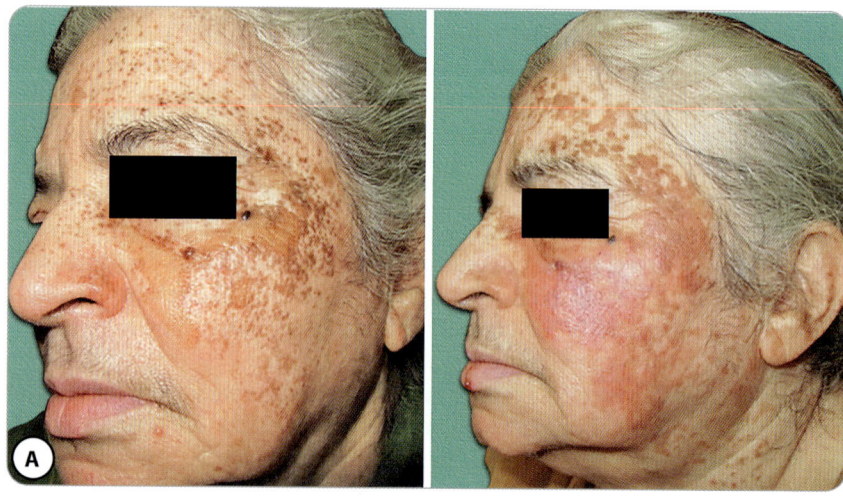

FIGS. 1A TO D: *Continued*

Continued

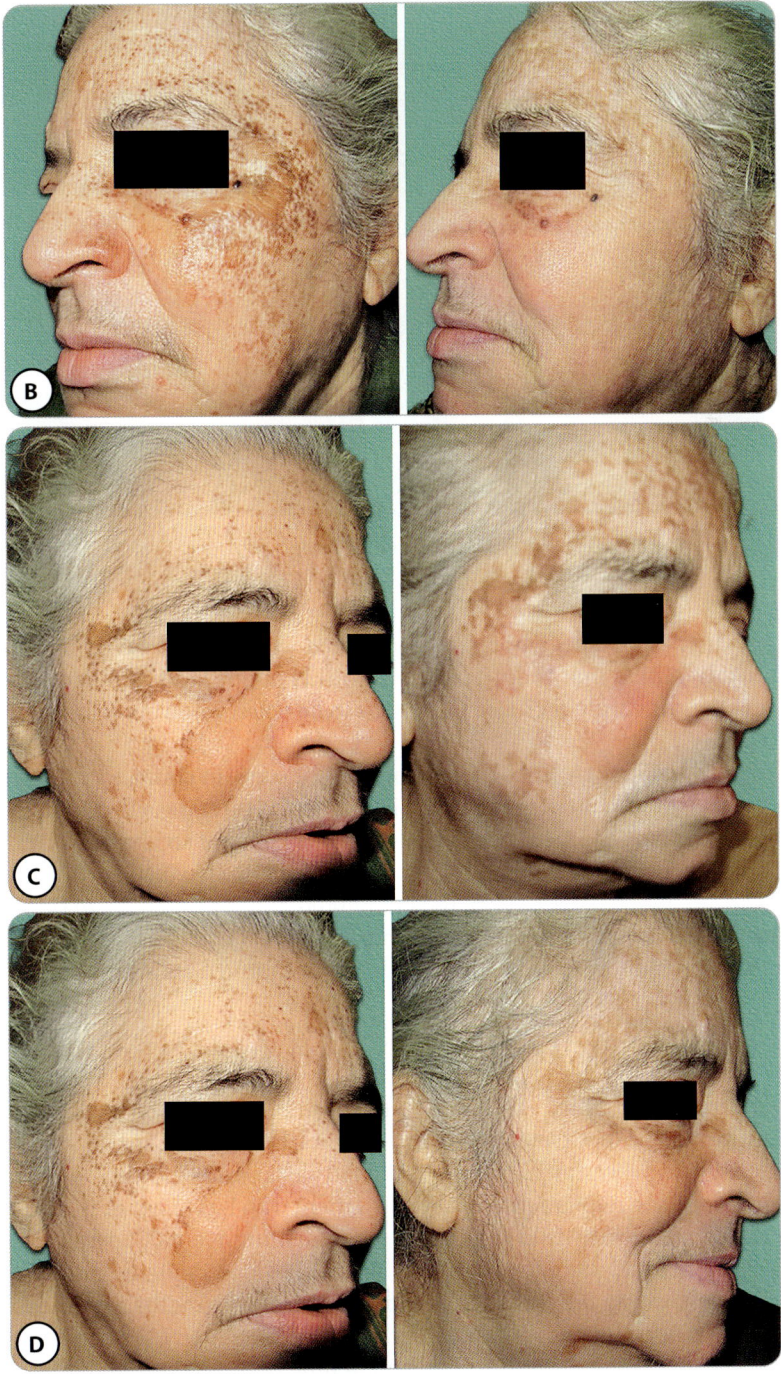

FIGS. 1A TO D: (A) Left: Pigmented left face; right: reaction to MBEH. (B) Left: Pigmented left face; right: complete depigmentation. (C) Left: Pigmented right face; right: reaction to MBEH. (D) Left: Pigmented right face; right: complete depigmentation.

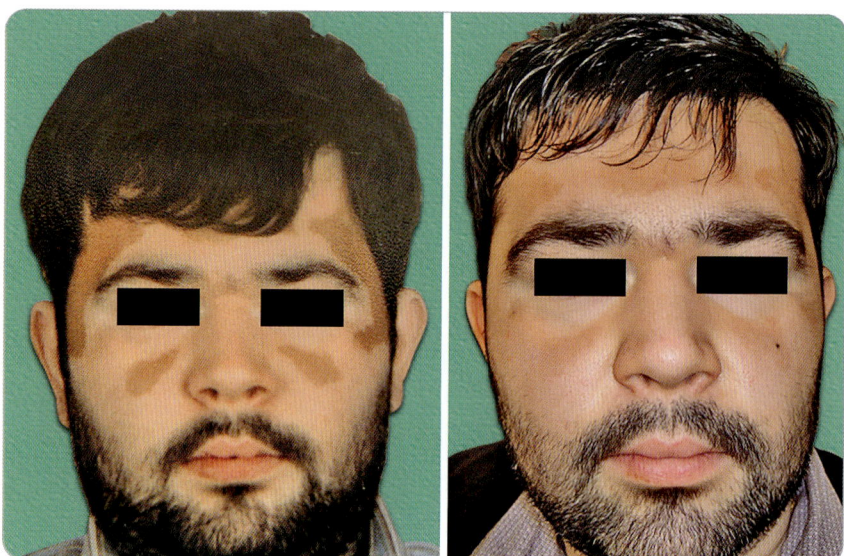

FIG. 2: Left: Pigmented face; right: Final depigmented face.

There are certain special precautions which we need to bear in mind when we are using MBEH that is application of MBEH at one side can lead to loss of pigment at distant body sites also.[3] Care has to be taken when applying very close to the eyes.

After application of MBEH, the person cannot come in contact with any other person because they can trigger a reduced pigmentation at the site of contact with the other person; all clothes beddings, etc., should be kept separate.

The side effects of MBEH will be contact dermatitis,[4] which is more irritant more than allergic and it is more in the pigmented skin than the vitiligo skin, and it can also lead to exogenous ochronosis unmasking of telangiectasias on the lower extremities, pruritus, xerosis, erythema, rash, edema, and distant depigmentation.

LASERS IN DEPIGMENTATION

The various lasers which are available for depigmentation are Q-switched Nd:YAG laser, 532-nm wavelength (most common laser used). The second laser is Q-switched ruby,[5] 694 nm. Third is Q-switched alexandrite, 755 nm.

Role of lasers in depigmentation is in a patient who has failed or is resistant to medical treatment with MBEH and other depigmenting agents. Second, areas like the face where faster depigmentation is desirable since depigmentation with a laser can occur over a few weeks as compared to several months with medicines. Lasers also overcome the disadvantages of topical therapy, i.e., local irritant reactions, contact dermatitis, burning, and itching.

Lastly, lasers are also useful in cases of patients who cannot use MBEH because of them coming in contact with other family members. With lasers, we can depigment larger areas faster as compared to that with the medical treatment.

The most common laser that is used is the Q-switched ND:YAG laser. The mechanism of action of Q-switched ND:YAG laser is that it induces selective photothermolysis of the pigmented lesion because the wavelength is absorbed by melanin. And the pulse duration of the Q-switched is shorter than the thermal relaxation time of the melanosomes so no energy or heat is going to the surrounding skin. So, there is no collateral damage.[1]

PROCEDURE

Considering the treatment is painful patient should be applied a thick layer of topical anesthesia (lidocaine and prilocaine mixture) 45 minutes to 1 hour before the procedure. Routinely, we can do roughly 100 cm^2 in one session. After 45 minutes, we remove the anesthesia cream, clean the area with betadine and spirit.

And then the Q-switched ND:YAG laser 532 nm is fired over the pigmented skin.

It is important that every person in the laser room is wearing the protective glasses which are specific to the 532 nm. Spot size is 8–10 mm. The frequency is between 5 and 10 Hz. Energy used will vary and has to be chosen according to the endpoint, which is the most important thing.

The endpoint with Q-switched Nd:YAG laser for depigmentation is the one that creates a minimum frost without any petechiae formation. Different lasers will have different parameters and the fluence, spot size, etc., can be variable but the endpoint is always the same laser will be same, i.e., minimum frost without any petechiaeor bleeding.

Once the appropriate energy has been decided, then the entire area is covered. With 10% overlap, single pass is required to cover the whole area. When doing the entire area, then we can increase the frequency to 5 or 10 Hz; the energy, spot size will still be the same depending on the laser operator.

Once the entire area has been covered, the area is cooled for half an hour to one hour with ice packs to tackle the burning sensation and reduce the pain.

Postlaser patient is given instructions to apply a topical antibiotic cream, containing fusidic acid and to avoid sun. They are given oral anti-inflammatory medication [nonsteroidal anti-inflammatory drugs (NSAIDS)].

The patient is counseled that the treated area will be inflamed and there will be swelling, crusting, scabbing for approximately 1 week. In 1 week that whole skin will peel off and there will be significant lightening. Once one area has lightened up, after 5–7 days, we can take up the second area. Since it is a painful procedure, we cannot do too much area at one session hence it has to be done in a very sequential pattern.

Secondly, the area that has been lasered once, there will be a loss of pigment or dilution of pigment. But it may require more than one session. On average, two to three sessions on the same area are required to depigment the pigment significantly. The interval between two laser sessions on the same area is roughly 1 month, postlaser patient has to strictly avoid sun exposure.

Following depigmentation, the patient becomes more photosensitive so they have to keep avoiding sunlight for the rest of the life and throughout the year to prevent sunburn and also to prevent some spotted repigmentation which may occur. If a person does not follow the sun avoidance, they can have recurrence of pigmentation especially in a follicular pattern which will require further depigmentation therapy to get loss of that pigment.

CONCLUSION

Depigmentation therapy, whether through MBEH or laser treatments, offers a viable option for patients with extensive vitiligo seeking a uniform skin appearance. Each method has its advantages and potential side effects, and the choice of treatment should be individualized based on patient preferences, medical history, and specific clinical considerations. Comprehensive patient counseling and involvement of family members in the decision-making process are crucial to ensure adherence and satisfaction with the treatment outcomes **(Figs. 3 to 13)**.

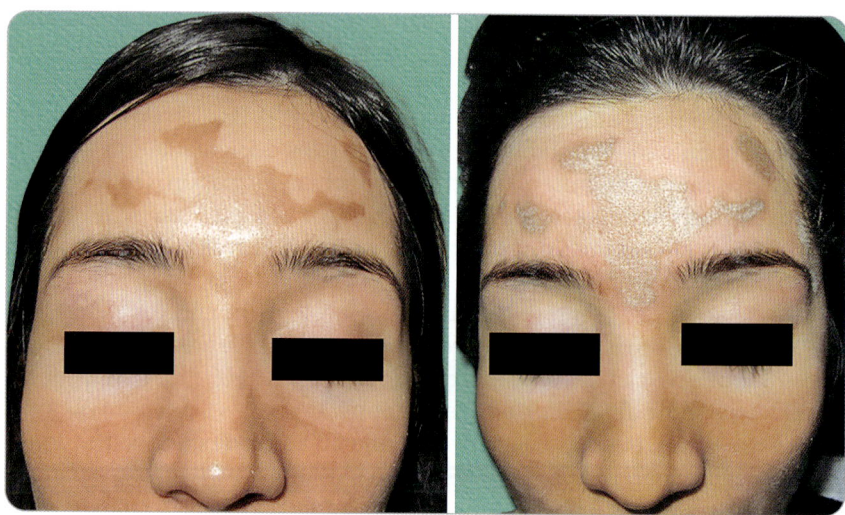

FIG. 3: Immediate frosting after laser irradiation.

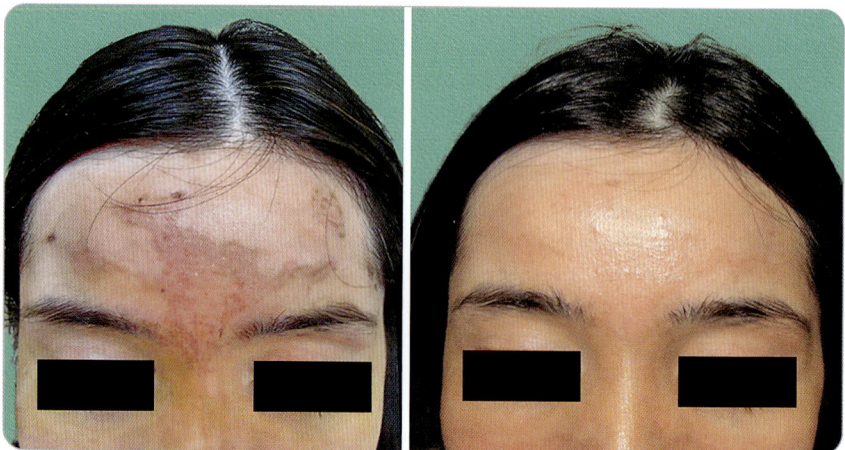

FIG. 4: Skin crust, peels in 7–10 days.

CHAPTER 8: Role of Lasers and Medication in Depigmentation in Vitiligo   111

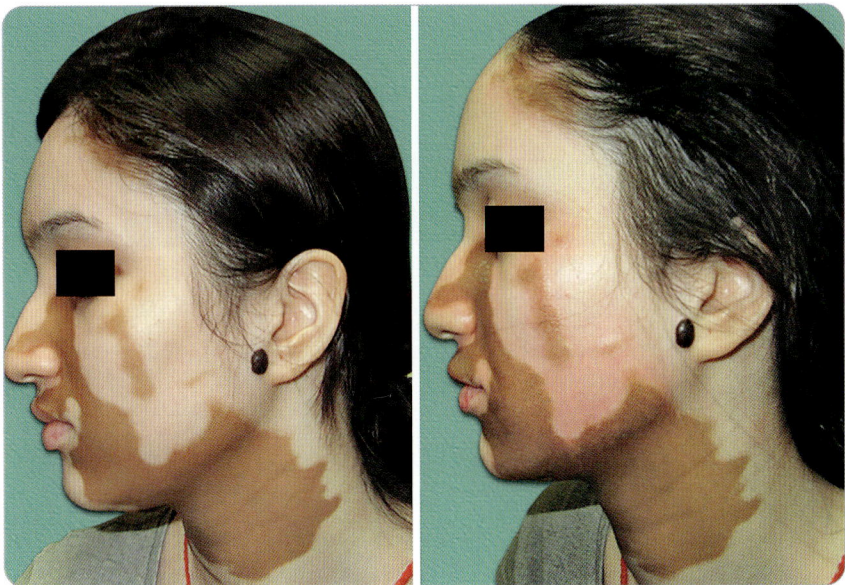

FIG. 5: Q-switched Nd:YAG laser immediate reaction.

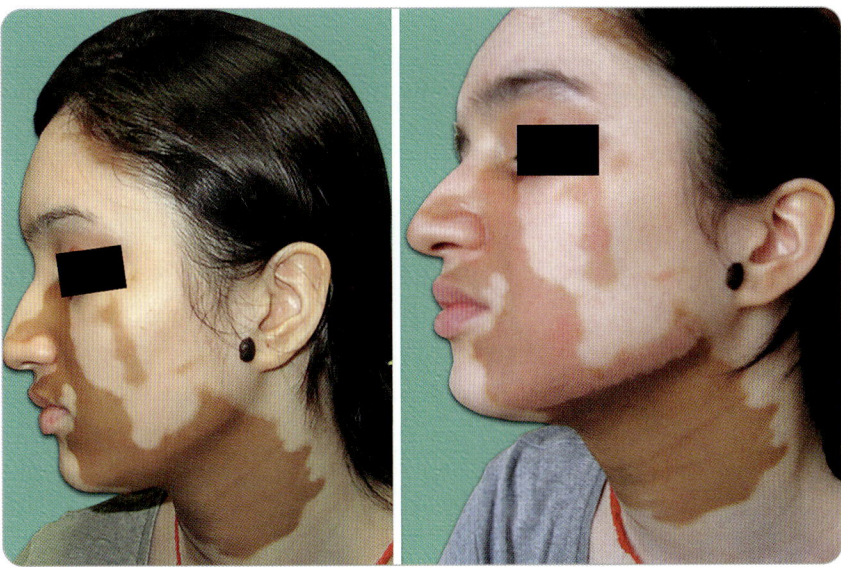

FIG. 6: Lightening after 10 days.

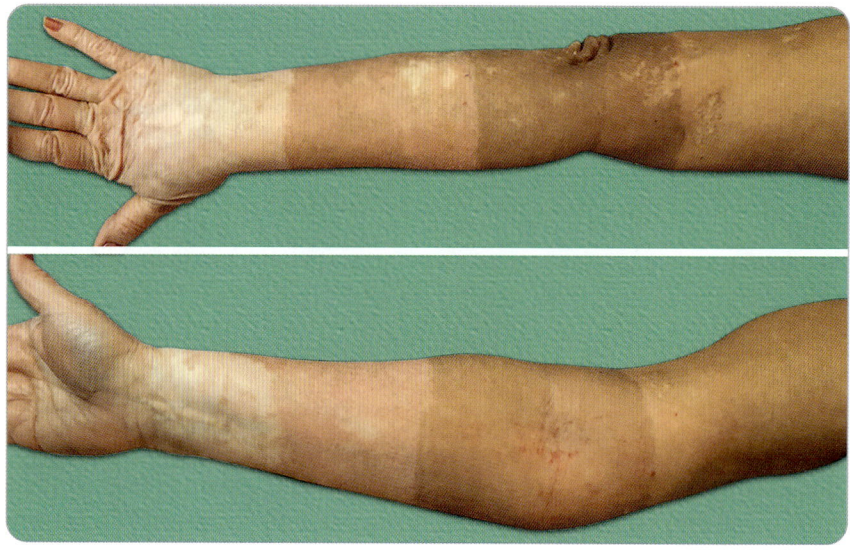

FIG. 7: Depigmentation over the arms done in a stage wise and sequential manner.

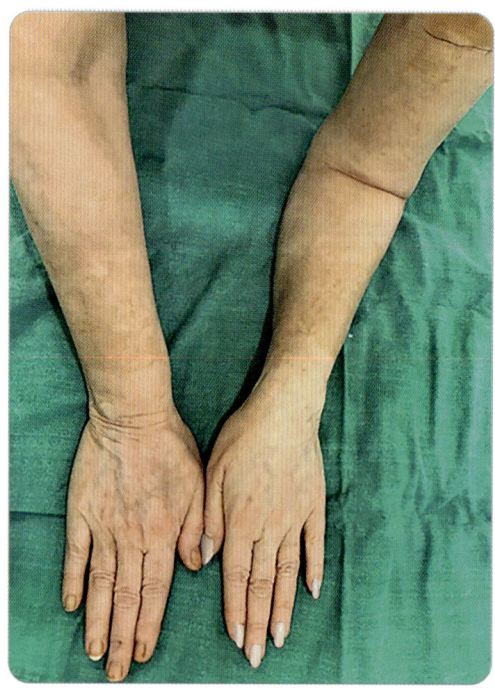

FIG. 8: Q-switched Nd:YAG laser induced full depigmentation of the arms.

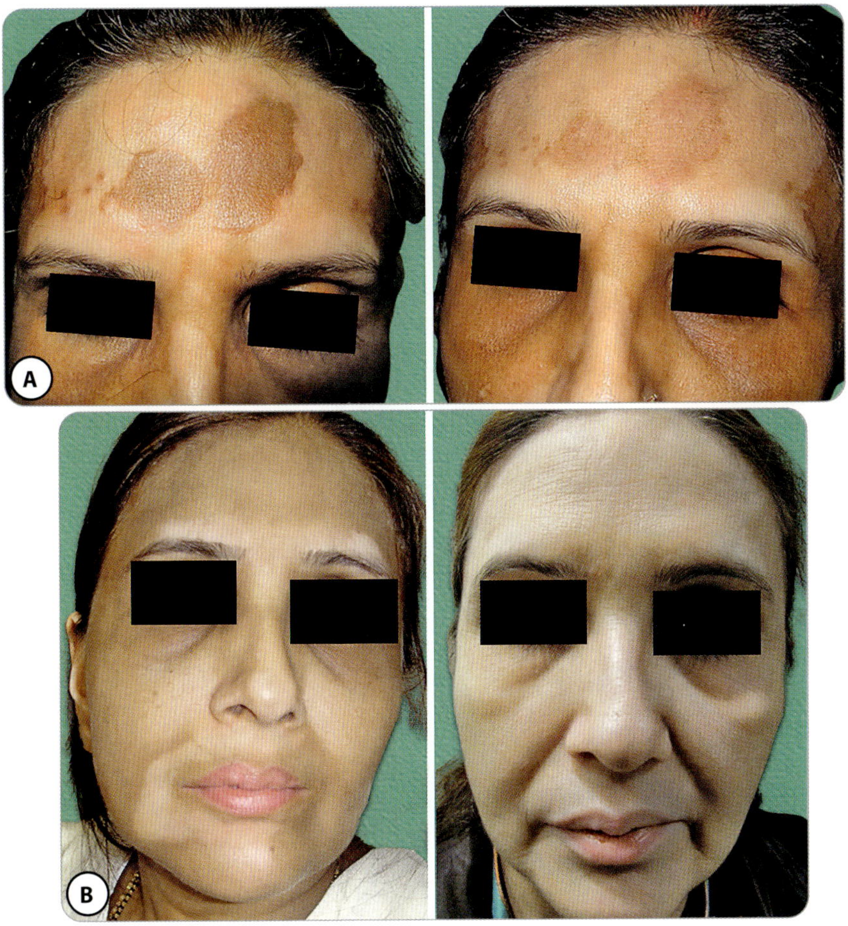

FIGS. 9A AND B: Q-switched Nd:YAG laser sequelae—frost–edema–crust–exfoliation–lightening.

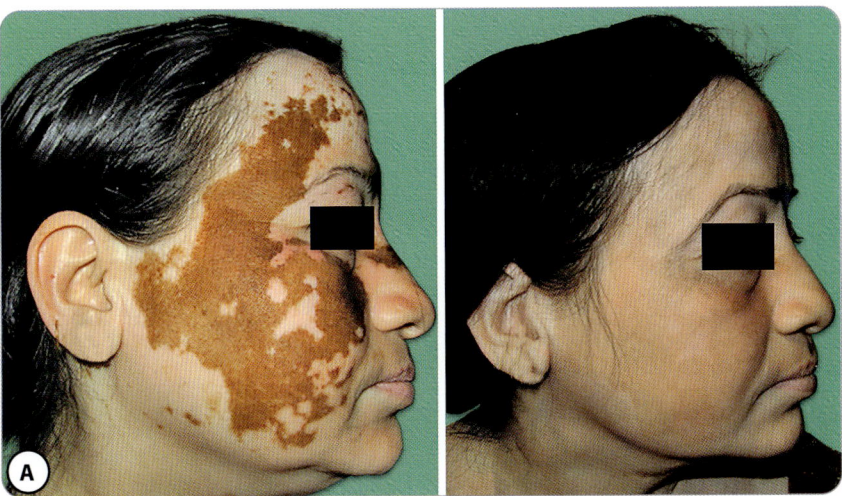

FIGS. 10A AND B: *Continued*

Continued

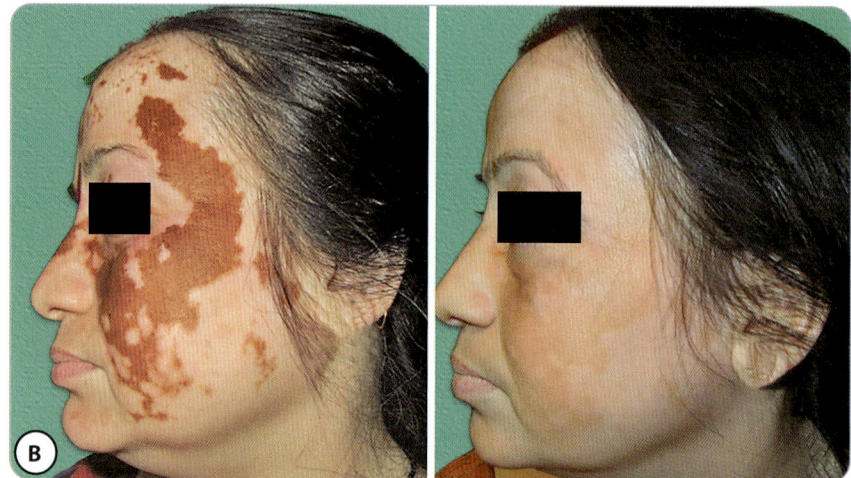

FIGS. 10A AND B: Q-switched Nd:YAG laser induced depigmentation.

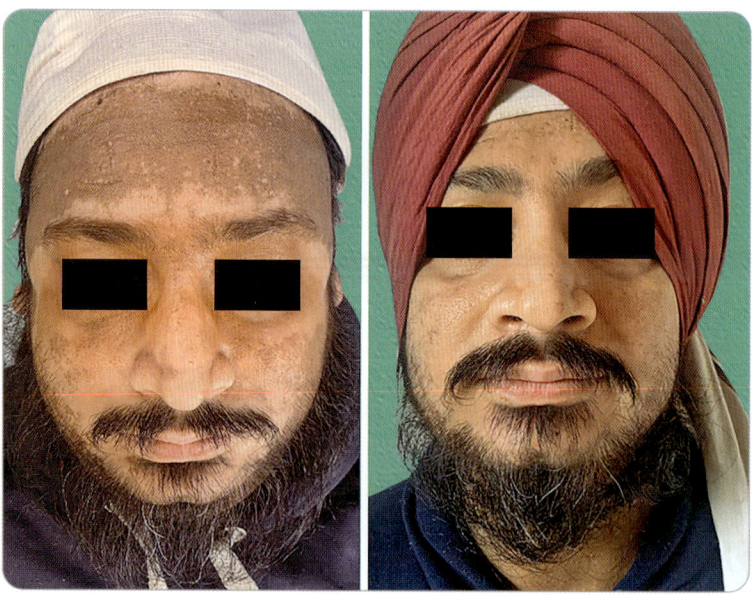

FIG. 11: Hair does not get white because of treatment. Important concern for Patients!!!

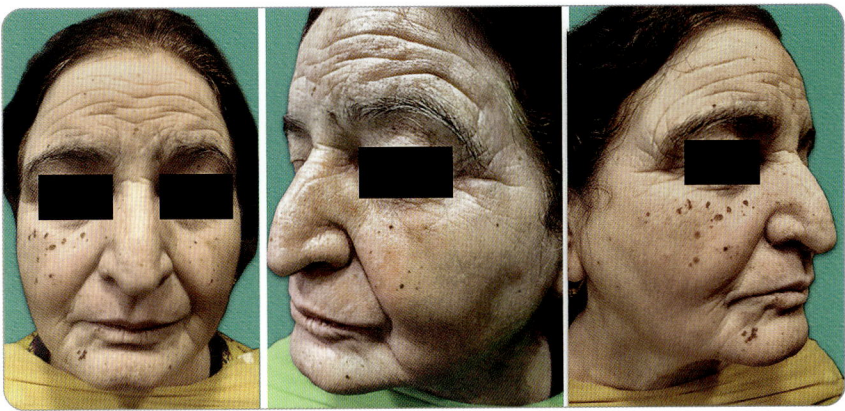

FIG. 12: Spotted repigmentation after sun exposure.

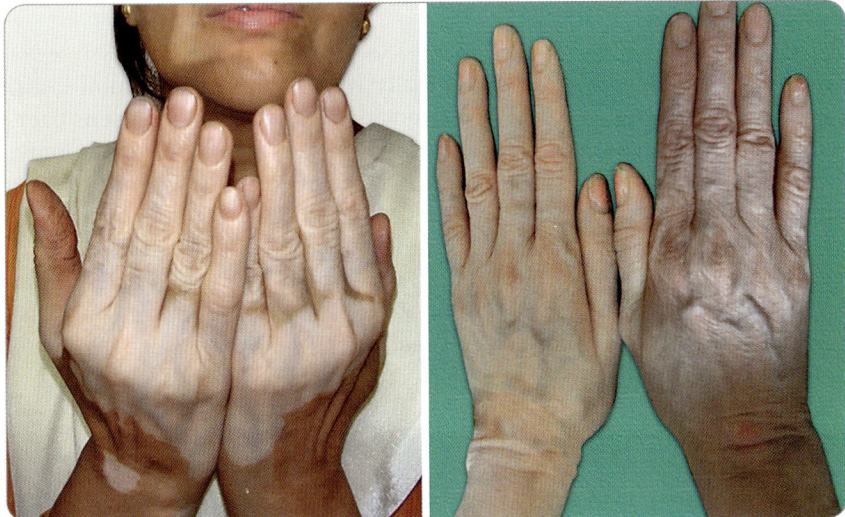

FIG. 13: Depigmentation: Hands.

REFERENCES

1. Alghamdi KM, Kumar A. Depigmentation therapies for normal skin in vitiligo universalis. J Eur Acad Dermatol Venereol. 2011;25:749-57.
2. Bolognia JL, Lapia BK, Somma S. Depigmentation therapy. Dermatol Ther 2001;14:29-34.
3. Drake LA, Dinehart SM, Farmer ER, Goltz RW, Graham GF, Hordinsky MK, et al. Guidelines of care for vitiligo. J Am Acad Dermatol. 1996;35:620-6.
4. Lyon CC, Beck MH. Contact hypersensitivity to monobenzyl ether of hydroquinone used to treat vitiligo. Contact Dermatitis. 1998;39:132-56
5. Njoo MD, Vodegel RM, Westerhof W. Depigmentation therapy in vitiligo universalis with topical 4-methoxyphenol and the Q-switched ruby laser. J Am Acad Dermatol. 2000;42:760-9.

CHAPTER 9

Light-based Therapy in Vitiligo

Deepti Ghia, Nidhi Pugalia

INTRODUCTION

Phototherapy or light therapy traditionally refers to the use of non-ionizing radiation in the absence of a photosensitizer. Use of a photosensitizer in combination with ultraviolet (UV) radiation is termed as photochemotherapy.

The ultraviolet B (UVB) (270–350 nm) and ultraviolet A (UVA) (320–400 nm) band from the light spectrum is utilized for phototherapy and photochemotherapy, respectively. The therapeutic range of UVB further can be divided as broadband (BB) UVB (280–320 nm), and narrowband (NB) UVB (311–313 nm). While narrowband ultraviolet B (NB-UVB) is the most effective range, broadband ultraviolet B (BB-UVB) is often seldom used. UVA photochemotherapy is usually combined with topical and oral photosensitizer called psoralens.

MECHANISM OF PHOTOTHERAPY

When light strikes the skin surface, it can be absorbed, scattered, or reflected. UVB, on account of its shorter wavelength, is primarily absorbed in the epidermis and upper dermis, whereas UVA, characterized by its longer wavelength, penetrates deeper into the dermis.

The radiation should be absorbed by target molecular components, such as deoxyribonucleic acid (DNA), nucleotides, porphyrins, amino acids, lipids, water, photosensitizing drugs, and tattoo pigments termed as "chromophores" that result in various photochemical reactions.

The keratinocyte-melanocyte loop works efficiently to protect the human integument from the harmful effects of the solar radiation **(Flowchart 1 and Fig. 1)**.[1]

HELIOTHERAPY

Heliotherapy (Helios = sun) is the utilization of sunlight as an age-old source for treatment of vitiligo in Greece, ancient Egypt, and Rome. Egyptians combined heliotherapy with plant extracts from the weed *Ammi majus* to treat vitiligo, as did ancient Indians who used sunlight and seeds from *Psoralea corylifolia*.

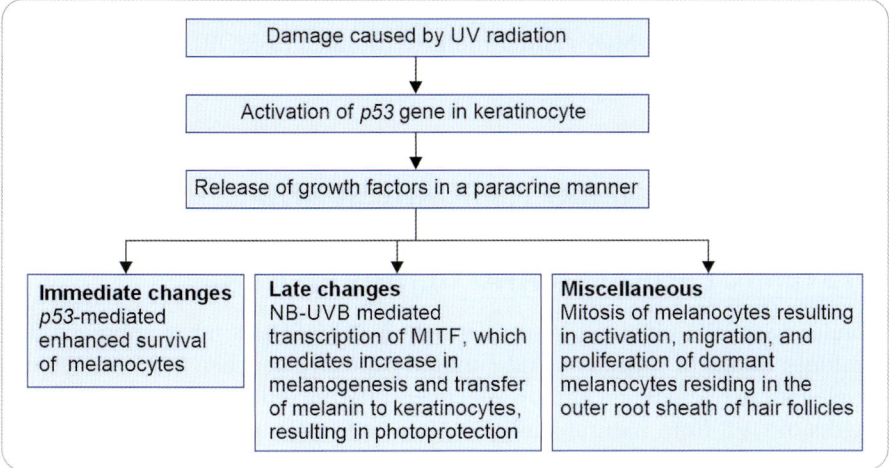

FLOWCHART 1: A photo-protective mechanism exerted by the interplay keratinocyte—melanocyte loop.
(MITF: microphthalmia-associated transcription factor; NB-UVB: narrowband ultraviolet B; UV: ultraviolet)

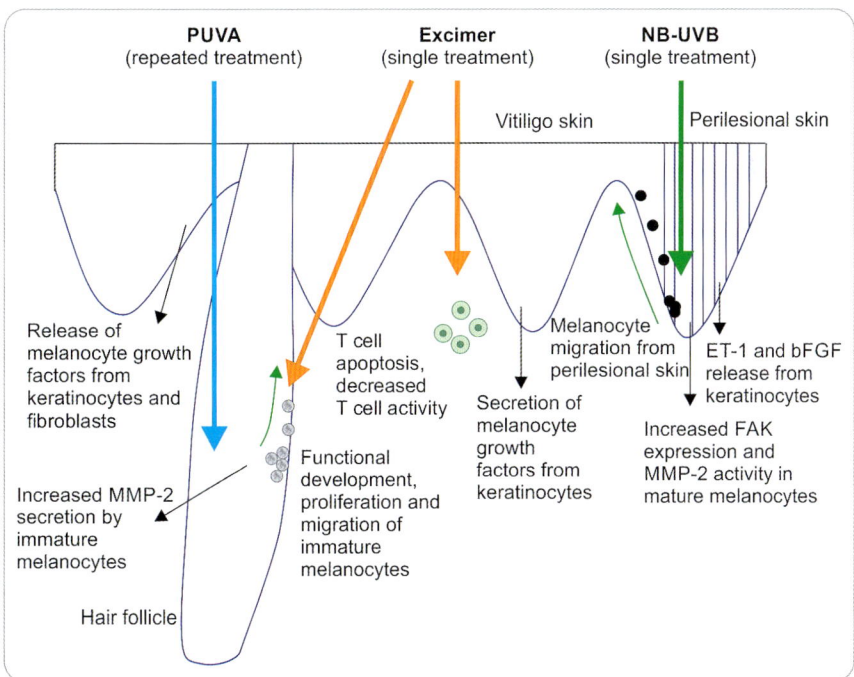

FIG. 1: Schematic diagram showing the proposed mechanisms of different forms of phototherapy [psoralen and ultraviolet A (PUVA), excimer laser/excimer light, narrowband ultraviolet B (NB-UVB)] inducing the repigmentation. The main proposed mechanism includes the induction of T-cell apoptosis, release of melanocyte growth factors, such as endothelin-1 and basic fibroblast growth factor from keratinocytes and fibroblasts, and increased matrix metalloproteinase-2 (MMP-2) secretion by melanocytes. This may lead to the proliferation and migration of functional melanocytes in the perilesional skin and immature melanocytes in hair follicle.[1]

Fahmy et al. isolated the active ingredients in these plant extracts in 1947 as 8-methoxypsoralen (8-MOP) and 5-methoxypsoralen (5-MOP) and Fahmy et al. and El-Mofty started treating patients of vitiligo with 8-MOP followed by sun exposure.[2]

PHOTOCHEMOTHERAPY: PSORALEN AND ULTRAVIOLET A OBTAINED BY SOLAR LIGHT (SYSTEMIC PSORALEN AND ULTRAVIOLET A)

Psoralen with UVA obtained from solar light is PUVASOL, a novel approach that combines intake of psoralens and sunlight exposure between 320 and 400 nm wavelength to treat vitiligo and by selectively filtering out non-therapeutic wavelengths of UVB from natural sunlight. After oral intake of 8-MOP, in a dose of 0.6 mg/kg body weight, UVA administration in the form of sunlight or UVA panel lights needs to be done within 1–2 hours after ingestion of psoralens with initial doses that range from 0.25 to 2 J/cm². Treatment is done two to three times a week, with increases of 0.2–0.5 J/cm² each session until erythema develops or a maximum dose is reached.[3,4]

Clinical studies indicate that PUVASOL can improve outcomes for patients with vitiligo, especially when combined with other therapies, such as topical calcipotriol and low-dose oral azathioprine.[5,6]

Types of Psoralen and Ultraviolet A Therapy (Table 1)[7]

Post-psoralen and Ultraviolet A Instructions
- If sunlight is used as the source of UVA, exposure starts with 5 minutes, increased by 1 minute with each exposure up to a maximum of 15–30 minutes. The treatment is given 3–4 times/week for 10–12 weeks.[7]
- The duration of sun exposure varies from place to place. The ideal time for sun exposure is 9:15–11:15 AM or 2:30–3:30 PM, when UVB and infrared radiation are minimum.[8]
- The eyes should be protected with UVA-protective goggles.
- Men need to cover their genitalia with dark undergarments.
- Post-treatment bathing is not required, but the exposed parts of the body should be protected from sunlight.[7]

Practice Point Highlights[9]
- As per the global consensus on vitiligo oral psoralen and ultraviolet A (PUVA) is no longer recommended for vitiligo and contraindicated in children and pregnancy.[9]
- *Psoralen and ultraviolet A side effects:*
    - Ocular and systemic toxicity
    - Increased risk of melanoma and non-melanoma skin cancer
    - Nausea and headache

TABLE 1: Administration of different types of psoralen and ultraviolet A (PUVA).[7]

	Method and concentration of 8–methoxy psoralen (8-MOP)	Time duration for soaking	Ultraviolet A (UVA) dose	Duration
Bath PUVA	• Bathtub filled with 100 L of warm water • 37.5 mL of 1% 8-MOP is added to obtain a concentration of 3.75 mg/L or 2.6 mg/L (lower concentration)	10 minutes in supine and 10 minutes in the prone position	1–2 J/cm^2 with increments of 0.5 J/cm^2	• 3 times a week × 1 month • Twice weekly maintenance
Soak PUVA	In a small plastic tub or a basin 3.75 mg/L solution of 8-MOP (prepared as above)	20 minutes	1–2 J/cm^2 with increments of 0.5 J/cm^2	3–4 times/week
Turban PUVA	An absorbent cotton cloth is soaked for 30 seconds in a 3.75 mg/L solution of 8-MOP, gently squeezed to remove excess water and wrapped around the head	5 minutes Repeat this four times (i.e., a total of 20 minutes)	1–2 J/cm^2 with increments of 0.5 J/cm^2	3–4 times/week for 10–12 weeks
Bath suit PUVA	2 L of water is taken in a bucket and 1 mL of 1% 8-MOP is added to obtain a concentration of 3.75 mg/L. A bathing suit of flannel material (stitched to suit the patient) is dipped in this solution for 5 minutes	Patient wears the suit for 15 minutes with a raincoat over it to prevent evaporation	1–2 J/cm^2 with increments of 0.5 J/cm^2	3–4 times/week

- *Topical psoralen and ultraviolet A:*
  - Requires fewer treatments and smaller cumulative dose of UVA
  - Safe for children
  - It can cause blistering and perilesional hyperpigmentation.
  - Less effective at arresting disease activity.
- Psoralen and UVA obtained by solar light uses sun light as a source of UVA is cost effective when machines are not available.[9]

NARROWBAND ULTRAVIOLET B

Narrowband ultraviolet B harnesses the most effective 311–313 nm wavelength of the UVB light spectrum. It is the preferred first-line therapy for widespread or rapidly progressive disease. Early initiation of NB-UVB is encouraged, because of its ability to halt disease activity and induce repigmentation.[10] This is especially important in segmental and acral vitiligo, where repigmentation is notoriously difficult in later stages. Limitations include resistant anatomical sites (e.g., fingers, toes, bony prominences) and areas lacking a melanocyte reservoir (e.g., lesions with leukotrichia).[10]

Rather than performing minimal erythema dose testing, experts propose to start at a fixed dose and use a recommended dosing schedule.[9,10]

Types of Narrowband Ultraviolet B Units

Full-body Units
These are large, specialized phototherapy cabinets that provide full-body exposure to NB-UVB light and are particularly beneficial for multiple vitiligo patches and patients with widespread depigmentation. They are typically found in dermatology clinics and are designed to treat extensive areas of skin affected by vitiligo **(Figs. 2A and B)**.

Handheld Units
Handheld NB-UVB devices are portable and designed for localized treatment. These units are suitable for both clinical and home use. They are particularly useful for small patches of vitiligo and can be easily maneuvered to treat hard-to-reach areas, such as the face, neck, and scalp. Handheld devices allow for greater precision and can be used in conjunction with topical medications to enhance therapeutic outcomes **(Figs. 3A and B)**.

Panel Units
Panel devices are smaller than full-body units and consist of multiple UVB lamps arranged in a panel format. These units are suitable for both clinical and home use and can be utilized for targeted treatment of specific areas, such as the arms or legs. They often feature adjustable height and angle settings to accommodate various body types and treatment needs **(Fig. 4)**.

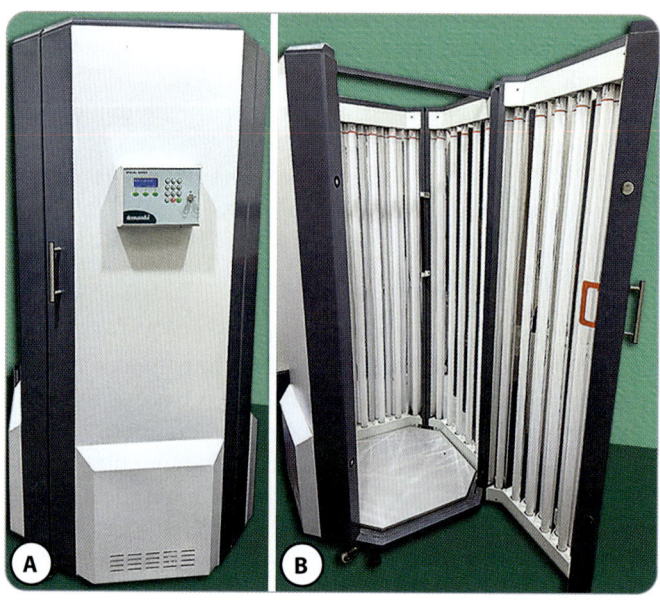

FIGS. 2A AND B: Narrowband ultraviolet B (NB-UVB) chamber.

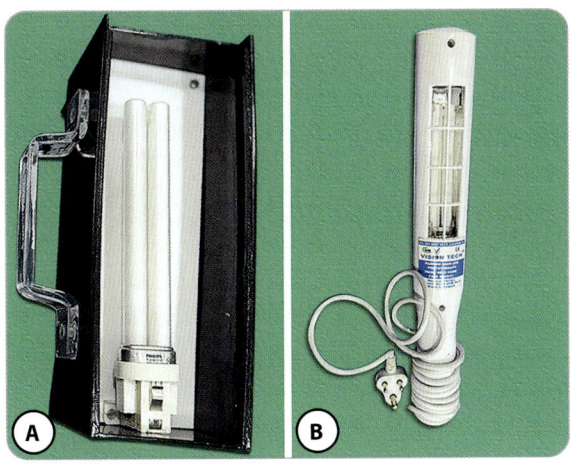

FIGS. 3A AND B: Handheld narrowband ultraviolet B (NB-UVB).

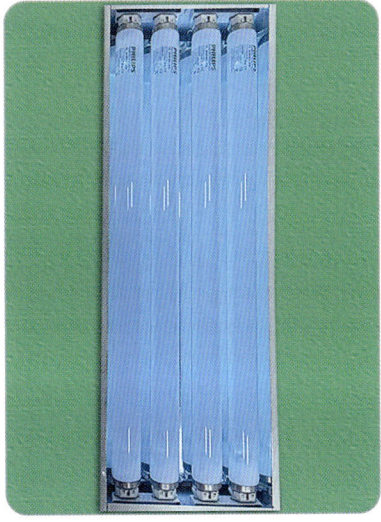

FIG. 4: Panel narrowband ultraviolet B (NB-UVB).

Administration of Narrowband Ultraviolet B Therapy

Table 2 highlights the Vitiligo Working Group phototherapy consensus recommendations for administration of NB-UVB therapy that involves specific protocols to maximize efficacy and minimize risks.[9]

Adverse Effects of Narrowband Ultraviolet B

The most common acute adverse effects of NB-UVB therapy are erythema and xerosis. Although a small increased risk of basal cell cancer (BCC) is observed with PUVA, there is no significant association of BCC, squamous cell cancer (SCC), melanoma with NB-UVB.[11] Actinic keratoses[12] and lichenoid papules[13] in vitiligo lesions were reported in individuals undergoing over 200 sessions **(Figs. 5A and B)**.

TABLE 2: The Vitiligo Working Group phototherapy consensus recommendations for administration of narrowband ultraviolet B (NB-UVB) therapy.[9]	
Weekly frequency of NB-UVB administration	• *Optimal:* Three times per week • *Acceptable:* Two times per week • Repigmentation is dependent on the total number of sessions • Earlier onset of pigmentation associated with thrice weekly dosing • Twice weekly regimen more convenient, less costly, and increases patient compliance
Initial dosing	• Initiate at—fixed dosing starting at 200 mJ/cm^2 (regardless of skin type, it is convenient and avoids phototoxic reactions) • Increase by 10–20% per treatment • For darker skin populations—higher starting doses 400–500 mJ/cm^2 are considered
Maximum acceptable dose per treatment	• 1,500 mJ/cm^2 for the face • 3,000 mJ/cm^2 for the body
Maximum number of acceptable exposures	• Skin phototypes (SPTs)[1] IV-VI—no upper limit • SPTs I-III, additional data needed
Course of therapy	• 18–36 sessions required for assessing response • Minimum 48 sessions required to determine lack of response
Dose adjustment based on degree of erythema	• *No erythema:* Increase next dose by 10–20% • *Pink asymptomatic erythema:* Hold at current dose until erythema disappears, then increase by 10–20% • *Bright red asymptomatic erythema:* Stop phototherapy until affected areas become light pink, then resume at last tolerated dose • *Symptomatic erythema (includes pain and blistering):* Stop phototherapy until the skin heals and erythema fades to a light pink, then resume at last tolerated dose
Tapering NB-UVB after complete repigmentation	• *First month:* Phototherapy twice week • *Second month:* Phototherapy once weekly • *Third and fourth months:* Phototherapy every other week. After 4 months, discontinue phototherapy
Dose adjustment following missed doses	• *4–7 days between treatments:* Hold dose constant • *8–14 days between treatments:* Decrease dose by 25% • *15–21 days between treatments:* Decrease dose by 50% • *>3 weeks between treatments:* Restart at initial dose
Pretreatment monitoring	Routine antinuclear antibody screening is not mandatory but may be recommended for non-photoadaptors
Response predictors	• *Before starting treatment:* Favorable response predictors include pediatric age, location on face and neck, and recent disease onset • In contrast, areas with white hair and large, longstanding-lesions, and acral areas are not expected to repigment readily • *During treatment:* The presence of perifollicular pigmentation on dermoscopy is predictive of a positive response to NB-UVB
Related medications	• No topicals are allowed before the session except for mineral oil to help UV penetration of xerotic skin • Non-steroidal anti-inflammatory drugs (NSAIDs), especially Ibuprofen helps achieving therapeutic doses for non-photoadaptors by minimizing burns and session interruption • Sun protection is recommended between the sessions to prevent phototoxicity from additional exposure to the sun

CHAPTER 9: Light-based Therapy in Vitiligo

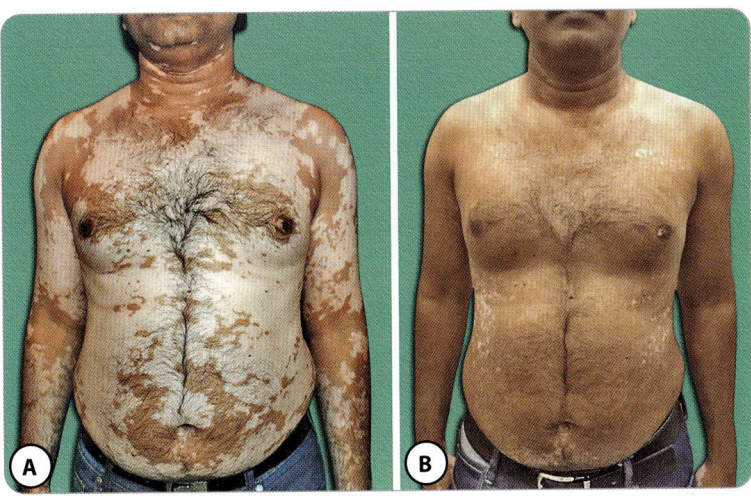

FIGS. 5A AND B: Patient of vitiligo vulgaris before and after narrowband ultraviolet B (NB-UVB) phototherapy.

TARGETED PHOTOTHERAPY: 308 NM EXCIMER LASER AND HANDHELD EXCIMER LAMP

Administration of Excimer Laser Therapy

Excimer laser therapy is particularly useful for patients with localized vitiligo or those who have not responded adequately to traditional NB-UVB therapy **(Fig. 6)**.
- *Mechanism of action:* The excimer laser emits UVB light at a wavelength of 308 nm, which is effective for stimulating melanocyte activity in targeted areas while minimizing the risk of exposure to surrounding skin.[14]

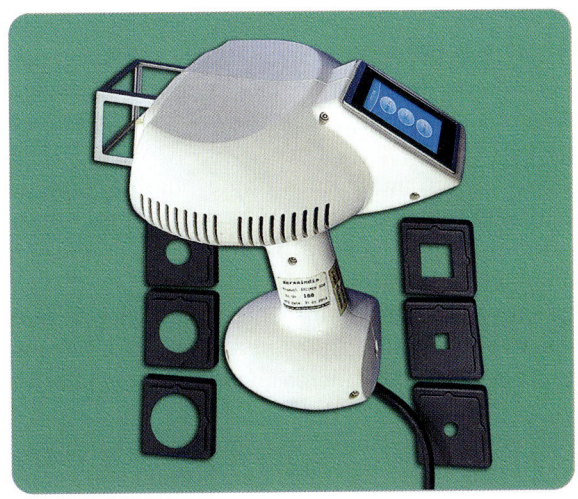

FIG. 6: Handheld excimer lamp.

TABLE 3: Treatment protocol of the 308-nm excimer laser for vitiligo.[16]	
Body site	**Initial dose**
Face and neck	150 mJ/cm²
Trunk and extremities	200 mJ/cm²
Hands and feet	300 mJ/cm²
Post-treatment	**Dose modification**
No erythema	Increase dose by 50 mJ/cm²
Transient asymptomatic erythema within 48 hours	Maintain dose
Persistent asymptomatic erythema over 48 hours	Decrease dose by 50 mJ/cm²
Persistent symptomatic erythema with pain or blister	Hold treatment until resolved, then reduce dose by 100 mJ/cm²
General treatment principle: • A dose that induces asymptomatic erythema for 24–48 hours after treatment is ideal • Treatment should be performed on two non-consecutive days per week • Sunscreens should be removed from the treatment area because they absorb ultraviolet B (UVB) light • For pediatric use, a dose reduction of 50 mJ/cm² from the initial dose is recommended	

- *Treatment protocol:* Sessions are usually performed twice a week. The exposure time is adjusted based on the minimal erythema dose (MED) and response of the treatment area **(Table 3)**.[15,16]
- *Advantages:* One of the key benefits of excimer laser therapy is its ability to target small, specific areas, making it particularly effective for facial vitiligo or localized small patches on the body.[17]
- Handheld excimer lamps are cheaper and cost-effective options and can be used for home-based phototherapy.

HOME PHOTOTHERAPY

Home phototherapy has become an increasingly popular option for patients seeking convenience and flexibility in their treatment regimen, hence saving patients' burden of making multiple visits to phototherapy centers and ensuring treatment adherence.[18]

- *Devices available:* There are various home phototherapy devices, such as handheld NB-UVB units and handheld excimer lamps. These devices allow patients to administer treatments in the comfort of their homes, which can enhance adherence and ease of use.[19]
- *Treatment protocol:* Similar to in-clinic treatments, home phototherapy typically involves sessions 2–3 times per week. Initial exposure times may begin at lower levels, gradually increasing as tolerated to achieve therapeutic doses.[20,21]
- *Patient education and monitoring:* Proper patient education is essential for the safe and effective use of home devices. Patients must understand how to

operate the equipment, adhere to recommended treatment schedules, and recognize signs of potential side effects, such as erythema or blistering.[22]
- *Benefits and challenges:* Home phototherapy can significantly improve treatment adherence and patient satisfaction. However, it may require more active participation from patients in their care, and there is a need for regular follow-up with healthcare providers to monitor progress and make necessary adjustments.[23,24]
- *Limitation:* The high initial cost of device, low-energy output of the device over time, lack of mechanical servicing, and unfamiliarity of patients with the modality are important limitations to the use of home-based units.

DOSE ESCALATION AND REDUCTION FOR HOME PHOTOTHERAPY

- *Dose escalation:* The concept of dose escalation is integral to optimizing treatment outcomes in NB-UVB therapy:
  - *Initial dosing strategy:* Treatment typically begins at a low-exposure time to gauge the patient's tolerance. For example, starting with 1–2 minutes of exposure allows clinicians to monitor skin reactions, such as erythema or discomfort.[25]
  - *Incremental increases:* After each session, the clinician may increase the exposure time by 10–20%, depending on the patient's skin reaction. The goal is to reach a therapeutic dose that induces mild erythema, which indicates effective stimulation of melanocytes without causing significant damage.[26,27]
- *Dose reduction:* Managing side effects is critical for maintaining patient adherence and achieving optimal outcomes:
  - *When to reduce doses:* If a patient experiences significant adverse reactions, such as severe erythema, blistering, or excessive pruritus, it may be necessary to reduce the dose for subsequent sessions. This can involve shortening exposure time or decreasing the frequency of treatments.[28,29]
  - *Long-term management:* Careful monitoring is essential, as inappropriate dosing can lead to inadequate repigmentation or increased side effects. Clinicians should educate patients about the importance of reporting any adverse reactions promptly.[30]

CONSEQUENCES OF MISSING SESSIONS ADHERENCE TO THE PRESCRIBED PHOTOTHERAPY SCHEDULE IS CRUCIAL FOR ACHIEVING THE DESIRED OUTCOMES

- *Impact of missed sessions:* Missing sessions can significantly hinder treatment progress. The skin may regress to its depigmented state, negating the benefits achieved prior to the missed appointments. Clinical studies indicate that treatment gaps of more than a week can lead to diminished repigmentation results.[31,32]

- *Guidance for rescheduling:* If patients miss multiple sessions, clinicians should evaluate whether to resume treatment at the previously established dose or start with a reduced dose to minimize the risk of skin irritation.[33]

SPECIAL CONSIDERATIONS FOR PHOTOTHERAPY

Certain populations, including pregnant individuals and children, may require tailored approaches to phototherapy:
- *Pregnancy:* NB-UVB and topical steroids in limited areas are reported to be safe during pregnancy and lactation. Monitoring for melasma and folate supplementation is recommended.[34,35]
- *Children:* Pediatric patients with vitiligo can benefit from phototherapy, but treatment protocols may need to be adjusted based on age, skin type, and emotional maturity. Specific eligibility considerations for NB-UVB use in children include the child's ability to comprehend basic instructions, ability to stand still for focal and whole body phototherapy and absence of known phobias for enclosed spaces. Involving caregivers in the treatment process and ensuring a supportive environment can enhance adherence and outcomes.[36,37]
- *Individuals prone to burns:* Conversely, some patients exhibit heightened sensitivity to NB-UVB light, resulting in burns at minimal doses. This phenomenon can be attributed to several factors:
  - *Skin type:* Individuals with fair skin (Fitzpatrick skin types I and II)[38,39]
  - *Prior skin damage:* Previous skin damage, such as sunburn or dermatologic procedures, can lead to increased sensitivity.[40,41]
  - *Photodermatoses:* Certain conditions, such as polymorphous light eruption or solar urticaria, can cause exaggerated reactions to UV exposure.[42,43]
  - *Immunosuppressive therapies:* Patients on immunosuppressive medications may exhibit altered skin responses to UV radiation, leading to increased sensitivity and a higher likelihood of burns.[44]

QUALITY OF LIFE IN PATIENTS WITH VITILIGO ON PHOTOTHERAPY

The psychological and social implications of vitiligo can be profound. Studies have shown that patients often experience social stigma, negative self-image, anxiety, depression, and social withdrawal, self-isolation due to the visible nature of their condition.[45,46] Effective treatment, including phototherapy, can lead to significant improvements in quality of life:
- *Psychosocial benefits:* Successful repigmentation through phototherapy can enhance self-esteem and social interactions, as patients feel more comfortable in their appearance. Health-related quality of life (HRQoL) assessments often show marked improvements following effective treatment. Patients report feeling more confident and less anxious about their appearance.[47,48]
- *Impact on daily life:* The visible nature of vitiligo can affect various aspects of daily life, including professional opportunities and interpersonal relationships. The requirement of regular treatment sessions may become a

double-edged sword and affect work and may be a monetary strain on the patient on one hand and may affect treatment results on the other. Positive treatment outcomes can lead to increased participation in social activities and improved mental well-being.[49]

- *Importance of comprehensive care:* Clinicians should incorporate psychosocial support into the management of vitiligo, providing resources, such as counseling or support groups to help patients navigate the emotional challenges associated with their condition.[50,51]

Quality of Life Assessments

Various tools, such as the Dermatology Life Quality Index (DLQI) and the Skindex-29, have been used to assess the quality of life in patients undergoing phototherapy for vitiligo. These instruments measure the extent to which skin conditions affect patients' daily lives, including emotional well-being, social interactions, and physical functioning.

Outcome measurements: Studies utilizing these tools have demonstrated statistically significant improvements in quality of life scores post-treatment, reflecting the effectiveness of phototherapy not only in achieving physical repigmentation but also in enhancing overall patient satisfaction and mental health.

NON-RESPONDERS TO PHOTOTHERAPY

- *Genetic factors:* Genetic predispositions may play a role in the variability of response to phototherapy. Some patients may have genetic polymorphisms affecting skin type, melanin production, or immune responses, which can hinder the effectiveness of NB-UVB treatment.[52,53]
- *Disease characteristics:* The extent and duration of vitiligo can influence treatment outcomes. Patients with long-standing or extensive vitiligo may have a diminished capacity for repigmentation compared to those with recent or localized lesions.[54] Certain clinical phenotypes, such as segmental vitiligo, may be less responsive to phototherapy.[55]
- *Underlying medical conditions:* Coexisting autoimmune diseases, such as thyroid disorders or psoriasis, can affect skin health and complicate treatment responses. Furthermore, patients undergoing immunosuppressive therapy may experience a reduced effectiveness of phototherapy.[56]
- *Adherence to treatment:* Patient adherence to prescribed treatment regimens is crucial for achieving optimal outcomes. Non-compliance, whether due to side effects, inconvenience, or lack of understanding, can lead to suboptimal results.[57,58]

ROLE OF IBUPROFEN IN NON-RESPONDERS

In vitiligo, inflammation may contribute to the persistence of depigmentation. Ibuprofen may help create a more favorable environment for repigmentation during phototherapy by reducing inflammation, and hence address the challenges faced by non-responders to phototherapy.[59,60]

Clinical Implications

- *Enhanced response to phototherapy:* The anti-inflammatory effects of ibuprofen could mitigate inflammatory responses triggered by UV exposure, potentially leading to better repigmentation results.[61,62]
- *Patient comfort:* Patients undergoing phototherapy often report discomfort, including erythema and pruritus. Ibuprofen can provide symptomatic relief, improving patient compliance with treatment regimens. Enhanced comfort may encourage patients to adhere to their phototherapy schedules, which is crucial for achieving optimal results.[63,64]

Adjunct therapy: For non-responders, ibuprofen can be considered as an adjunct to standard treatment protocols. Clinicians may recommend a short course of ibuprofen, particularly during the initial phases of phototherapy, to assess its impact on treatment efficacy.[65,66]

ROLE OF SUNSCREENS IN VITILIGO MANAGEMENT

Enhanced Sensitivity to Ultraviolet Exposure

Phototherapy, particularly NB-UVB and PUVA treatments, sensitizes the skin, making it more susceptible to sunburn and other forms of photodamage. As a result, patients with vitiligo undergoing these therapies must prioritize sun protection to avoid complications, such as increased pigmentation irregularities, erythema, and potential skin malignancies due to cumulative UV exposure.[67] Sunscreen use is crucial for patients undergoing phototherapy for several reasons.

Types of Sunscreens Recommended

- *Broad-spectrum formulations:* Patients should be encouraged to use broad-spectrum sunscreens with a sun protection factor (SPF) of 30 or higher. These formulations protect against both UVA and UVB rays, which is crucial for comprehensive sun protection.[68,69]
- *Physical versus chemical sunscreens:* While both types are effective, physical (mineral) sunscreens may be preferable due to their immediate protective effects and lower risk of skin irritation. Patients should be educated on selecting appropriate products based on their skin type and sensitivity.[70,71]

Application Guidelines

- *Routine application:* Sunscreen should be applied liberally to all exposed areas at least 15–30 minutes before sun exposure and reapplied every 2 hours, or immediately after swimming or sweating. This routine is particularly important during peak sun exposure hours.[72,73]
- *Integration with phototherapy sessions:* During phototherapy treatments, it is essential to apply sunscreen to areas not being treated with UV light, as these areas are still at risk for sunburn. This practice not only protects the skin but also enhances the overall comfort and safety of the patient during treatment sessions.[74-76]

CONCLUSION

Overall, phototherapy, as a modality, results in halting of depigmentation and initiation of repigmentation in vitiliginous skin. It is an excellent modality used for patients with extensive vitiligo or those who have not responded to topical treatments and to induce stability in active vitiligo. NB-UVB is more effective than PUVA in inducing stability and producing repigmentation in active vitiligo. Recent studies have indicated that early intervention with phototherapy can lead to better outcomes. Face and neck are showed best repigmentation, followed by trunk and limbs. A thorough understanding of practical aspects of treatment administration, dose management, and patient education is essential for optimizing outcomes. Additionally, addressing the psychosocial aspects of vitiligo and the importance of sun protection can enhance the overall quality of life for patients. As research continues to advance, the integration of novel therapies and personalized treatment approaches will likely improve the efficacy and safety of vitiligo management in the future.

REFERENCES

1. Esmat S, Hegazy RA, Shalaby S, Hu SC, Lan CC. Phototherapy and combination therapies for vitiligo. Dermatol Clin. 2017;35(2):171-92.
2. El-Mofty AM, Elsawalhy H, EL-Mofty ME. Clinical study of a new preparation of 8-methoxypsoralen in photochemotherapy. Int J Dermatol. 1994;33(8):588-92.
3. Hamzavi IH, Lim HW, Syed ZU. Ultraviolet-based therapy for vitiligo: what's new? Indian J Dermatol Venereol Leprol. 2012;78:42.
4. Shenoi SD, Prabhu S. Photochemotherapy (PUVA) in psoriasis and vitiligo. Indian J Dermatol Venereol Leprol. 2014;80:497.
5. Goren A, et al. Efficacy of a novel topical cream in the treatment of acrofacial vitiligo: A double-blind, placebo-controlled study. J Am Acad Dermatol. 2023;88(1):122-130.
6. Leite J, et al. PUVASOL therapy for vitiligo: A novel approach to treatment. J Dermatol. 2022;49(3):321-327.
7. Pai SB, Shetty S. Guidelines for bath PUVA, bathing suit PUVA and soak PUVA. Indian J Dermatol Venereol Leprol. 2015;81:559.
8. Balasaraswathy P, Kumar U, Srinivas CR, Nair S. UVA and UVB in sunlight, optimal utilization of UV rays in sunlight for phototherapy. Indian J Dermatol Venereol Leprol. 2002;68:198.
9. Mohammad TF, Al-Jamal M, Hamzavi IH, Harris JE, Leone G, Cabrera R, et al. The Vitiligo Working Group recommendations for narrowband ultraviolet B light phototherapy treatment of vitiligo. Journal of the American Academy of Dermatology. 2017;76(5):879-88.
10. Seneschal J, Speeckaert R, Taïeb A, Wolkerstorfer A, Passeron T, Pandya AG, et al. Worldwide expert recommendations for the diagnosis and management of vitiligo: Position statement from the international Vitiligo Task Force—Part 2: Specific treatment recommendations. J Eur Acad Dermato Venereol. 2023;37(11):2185-95.
11. Hearn RM, Kerr AC, Rahim KF, Ferguson J, Dawe RS. Incidence of skin cancers in 3867 patients treated with narrow-band ultraviolet B phototherapy. Brit J Dermatol. 2008;159(4):931-5.
12. Bae JM, Ju HJ, Lee RW, Oh SH, Shin JH, Kang HY, et al. Evaluation for skin cancer and precancer in patients with vitiligo treated with long-term narrowband UV-B phototherapy. JAMA Dermatol. 2020;156(5):529-37.
13. AlJasser M, Richer V, Ball N, Lui H, Zhou Y. Photolichenoid papules within vitiligo induced by narrowband UVB phototherapy. J Eur Acad Dermatol Venereol. 2016;30(8).
14. Tsoi LC, et al. Excimer laser for the treatment of vitiligo: A systematic review and meta-analysis. J Am Acad Dermatol. 2017;76(4):706-11.

15. Choi JH, et al. Efficacy of excimer laser treatment in patients with localized vitiligo: A systematic review and meta-analysis. J Dermatol. 2019;46(5):359-67.
16. Bae JM, Hann SK. Laser treatments for vitiligo. Medical Lasers. 2016;5(2):63-70.
17. Kim S, et al. Treatment of vitiligo with excimer laser: A 5-year experience. J Dermatol. 2020; 47(1):15-20.
18. Pariser DM, et al. Home phototherapy in patients with vitiligo: Efficacy and patient satisfaction. J Am Acad Dermatol. 2018;78(2):309-15.
19. Xu J, et al. Home phototherapy: A review of available devices for the treatment of vitiligo. J Dermatol. 2020;47(7):749-54.
20. Dainichi T, et al. Advances in home phototherapy for vitiligo: A review. J Dermatol. 2021; 48(1):1-7.
21. Matarazzo V, et al. The role of patient education in home phototherapy for vitiligo. J Dermatol Treat. 2019;30(1):68-73.
22. Nguyen J, et al. Home-based narrowband UVB phototherapy for vitiligo: A 10-year experience. J Dermatol Treat. 2021;32(2):179-85.
23. Sayal SK, et al. The importance of monitoring and adherence in phototherapy for vitiligo. J Dermatol Treat. 2022;33(3):222-8.
24. Bhawan J, et al. Patient adherence to home phototherapy for vitiligo: A study of factors influencing success. J Dermatol Treat. 2021;32(4):341-6.
25. Lim H, et al. Efficacy of combination therapy in vitiligo: A systematic review. J Dermatol Treat. 2021;32(5):474-80.
26. Ginsburg D, et al. Practical considerations in dose management during phototherapy for vitiligo. J Am Acad Dermatol. 2018;78(4):663-8.
27. Tolkachjov A, et al. Patient adherence and dose adjustments in narrowband UVB phototherapy for vitiligo. J Dermatol. 2021;48(3):392-6.
28. Xu X, et al. Adverse effects of narrowband ultraviolet B phototherapy: A systematic review. J Am Acad Dermatol. 2017;76(3):558-66.
29. Chen W, et al. Safety of phototherapy for vitiligo: A review of the literature. J Dermatol Treat. 2021;32(1):1-7.
30. Tohid H, et al. The effect of missed sessions on outcomes of phototherapy for vitiligo. J Dermatol. 2020;47(6):585-91.
31. Cline A, et al. Treatment interruptions and their impact on vitiligo management. J Am Acad Dermatol. 2021;84(4):931-3.
32. Pugliese S, et al. Long-term effects of missed treatments on the management of vitiligo. J Dermatol Treat. 2022;33(2):123-7.
33. Al-Mutairi N, et al. Factors influencing adherence to phototherapy in vitiligo patients. J Dermatol. 2021;48(5):623-8.
34. van Geel N, Speeckaert R, Taïeb A, Ezzedine K, Lim HW, Pandya AG, et al. Worldwide expert recommendations for the diagnosis and management of vitiligo: Position statement from the International Vitiligo Task Force Part 1: towards a new management algorithm. J Eur Acad Dermatol Venereol. 2023;37(11):2173-84.
35. Chi CC, Wang SH, Wojnarowska F, Kirtschig G, Davies E, Bennett C. Safety of topical corticosteroids in pregnancy. Cochrane Database Syst Rev. 2015(10):CD007346.
36. Pauls K, et al. Pediatric vitiligo: Considerations for phototherapy and patient management. J Am Acad Dermatol. 2021;84(2):389-95.
37. Alajlan A, et al. Phototherapy for vitiligo in children: An evidence-based review. J Dermatol Treat. 2022;33(1):13-9.
38. Dainichi T, et al. Skin types and responses to phototherapy in vitiligo: A clinical study. J Dermatol Treat. 2021;32(1):45-50.
39. Yoshida Y, et al. The impact of prior skin damage on phototherapy outcomes. J Dermatol. 2017;44(1):83-88.
40. Xu X, et al. Photodermatoses: Risk factors and their implications for phototherapy. J Am Acad Dermatol. 2016;75(6):1207-11.

41. Ghosh S, et al. Polymorphous light eruption and its implications for UV therapy. J Dermatol Treat. 2018;29(3):259-63.
42. Lim H, et al. Solar urticaria: A review of diagnosis and management. J Dermatol. 2020;47(2):122-28.
43. Gupta S, et al. Immunosuppressive therapy and its effect on skin sensitivity to UV radiation. J Am Acad Dermatol. 2020;83(4):974-9.
44. Koster T, et al. The interplay between immunosuppression and phototherapy in vitiligo. J Dermatol Treat. 2019;30(5):484-9.
45. Damsky W, et al. Psychosocial effects of vitiligo on patients: A systematic review. J Am Acad Dermatol. 2016;75(4):659-75.
46. Wu J, et al. Quality of life in patients with vitiligo: A review of the literature. J Dermatol Treat. 2021;32(4):396-403.
47. Lee YH, et al. The psychosocial impact of vitiligo: A study on quality of life and psychological distress. J Dermatol Treat. 2019;30(7):676-81.
48. Henningsen K, et al. Social and psychological effects of vitiligo: A study of patient perspectives. J Dermatol Treat. 2021;32(4):346-52.
49. Benmoussa M, et al. Impact of vitiligo treatment on quality of life: A systematic review. J Dermatol Treat. 2020;31(3):290-5.
50. Dufresne A, et al. Addressing the psychosocial needs of patients with vitiligo: A comprehensive approach. J Am Acad Dermatol. 2022;86(5):1063-70.
51. Patton S, et al. Counseling interventions for patients with vitiligo: Improving quality of life. J Dermatol Treat. 2021;32(4):404-9.
52. Alikhan A, et al. Genetic factors influencing the response to phototherapy in vitiligo. J Am Acad Dermatol. 2011;65(3):481-91.
53. Sinha S, et al. Genetic determinants of response to treatment in vitiligo: A review. J Dermatol Treat. 2020;31(5):480-7.
54. Ezzedine K, et al. Factors influencing repigmentation in vitiligo patients treated with narrowband ultraviolet B phototherapy. Br J Dermatol. 2015;172(6):1610-14.
55. Tsoi LC, et al. Segmental vitiligo: Clinical characteristics and treatment response. J Am Acad Dermatol. 2019;81(3):643-8.
56. Al-Mutairi N, et al. Autoimmune conditions in vitiligo: A review. J Dermatol. 2021;48(5):623-8.
57. Tolkachjov A, et al. Factors influencing patient adherence to phototherapy for vitiligo. J Dermatol Treat. 2020;31(4):401-6.
58. Manchanda R, et al. The role of patient education in adherence to vitiligo treatment. J Am Acad Dermatol. 2021;85(2):334-40.
59. Wu J, et al. The influence of NSAIDs on phototherapy outcomes in vitiligo: A preliminary study. J Dermatol. 2021;48(6):756-61.
60. Alikhan A, et al. The role of inflammation in the response to vitiligo treatment. J Dermatol Treat. 2015;26(3):252-7.
61. Choudhary R, et al. Efficacy of ibuprofen as an adjunct therapy in vitiligo patients undergoing phototherapy. J Dermatol Treat. 2021;32(6):563-9.
62. Lee YH, et al. Pain management in phototherapy: The role of NSAIDs. J Am Acad Dermatol. 2020;83(4):974-9.
63. Bhatia M, et al. Adjunct therapies in vitiligo: Clinical considerations and recommendations. J Dermatol Treat. 2020;31(3):290-5.
64. Ghosh S, et al. Managing side effects of phototherapy in vitiligo: NSAIDs as a therapeutic option. J Am Acad Dermatol. 2019;80(1):27-33.
65. Shukla P, et al. The role of adjunctive therapies in the management of vitiligo. Indian J Dermatol Venereol Leprol. 2022;88(3):364-73.
66. Gupta S, et al. The efficacy and safety of ibuprofen in the management of vitiligo. J Dermatol Treat. 2023;34(4):456-61.
67. Darsow U, et al. Patient education and sun protection for those undergoing phototherapy. J Eur Acad Dermatol Venereol. 2018;32(4):647-53.

68. Lim HW, et al. Sunscreen recommendations for patients undergoing phototherapy. J Dermatol. 2020;47(2):103-8.
69. Schmid K, et al. Sunscreens and their efficacy in preventing UV-induced damage in vitiligo patients. J Am Acad Dermatol. 2021;84(3):788-90.
70. Sinha S, et al. The role of sunscreens in the management of vitiligo: A review. Indian J Dermatol. 2016;61(1):18-23.
71. Gupta S, et al. Efficacy and safety of sunscreens in patients undergoing phototherapy for vitiligo. J Dermatol Treat. 2015;26(5):424-9.
72. Roy A, et al. Patient education on sun protection in vitiligo: A systematic review. J Dermatol. 2021;48(6):756-61.
73. Chaudhary R, et al. Impact of sunscreen use on the management of vitiligo: A clinical perspective. J Dermatol Treat. 2021;32(6):563-9
74. Bhorat S, et al. The importance of photoprotection in managing vitiligo: A review. J Dermatol Treat. 2022;33(4):456-62.
75. Wang G, et al. Sunscreen use in patients with vitiligo: An evidence-based review. J Dermatol. 2016;43(4):415-20.
76. Chiu HY, et al. Role of sunscreens in the management of vitiligo: A practical guide. Dermatol Ther. 2019;32(3).

CHAPTER 10

Vitiligo: Special Considerations

Ravina Surve, Mukesh D Shah

INTRODUCTION

Vitiligo affects 0.5–1% of population worldwide.[1] It is a complex disease with multifactorial nature. The pathogenesis is similar across different ethnic groups.[2] Destruction of melanocytes which are skin pigment producing cells causes depigmented patches. The contrast between the affected areas and normal skin is more pronounced in skin of color, making the depigmented patches more visible. The visibility of the condition can result in emotional distress, especially since vitiligo is sometimes misunderstood in certain communities. People may face stigmatization or social isolation. Effective management of vitiligo involves a holistic approach, combining medical treatment with psychosocial support, and awareness about the condition. Lot of advances have happened in terms of medical and surgical management of vitiligo, however special care needs to be taken while treating young children and pregnant women with vitiligo.

VITILIGO IN PREGNANCY

There are many hypotheses regarding vitiligo, however, autoimmune theory is the most accepted hypothesis. And various autoimmune conditions are believed to behave differently in pregnancy. There is improvement in few such as rheumatoid arthritis in pregnancy whereas there are associated maternal and fetal complications in some such as systemic lupus erythematosus.[3,4]

Considerations while Treating a Pregnant Female
Uncertain Course of Disease
- *Effect of pregnancy on vitiligo*: Autoimmune conditions are said to improve because of the relative state of immunosuppression in pregnancy. Vitiligo in pregnancy, however, has a variable and unpredictable outcome. During

pregnancy cortisol levels rise to three times also anti-inflammatory mediators such as interleukin-10 (IL-10) are raised.[5,6] Since low-dose steroid helps in stabilizing and repigmentation in vitiligo, these changes in pregnancy should lead to improvement in vitiligo. Yet, there are some patients who worsen during pregnancy, probably due to stress related to major bodily changes and changes in sleep patterns.[7] Percentage of patients worsening is lower since majority of patients stay stable or improve due to immunological alterations which occur in pregnancy.[8]

- *Effect of vitiligo on pregnancy*: According to Taiwanese and Korean cohort studies pregnant women with vitiligo have higher risk of spontaneous abortions.[1,9] Around 30% of vitiligo patients will be affected by at least one or more other autoimmune diseases. Systemic treatment before conception has shown to reduce the risk relatively. On other hand retrospective comparative study in Israel by Horev et al. from 1988–2006 had found that vitiligo is not associated with adverse pregnancy outcomes.[10]

Inheritability

Pathogenesis of vitiligo is complex. It is polygenic and multifactorial. It does not follow Mendelian law of inheritance. There are found to be variations in genes which are associated with increased risk of vitiligo. The participation of different loci of various genes has been described in families presenting with a high prevalence of vitiligo. Patients with a family history of vitiligo are at a higher risk of developing this disease at an early age compared with those without a family history of vitiligo.[11] However, most of the cases are sporadic and only 20% have an affected relative.[12-14] Patients should be counseled regarding avoiding consanguineous marriage to decrease risk of vitiligo in child.[15]

Psychosocial Impact

Vitiligo affects the person's psychological and social wellbeing. Patients with vitiligo often suffer from anxiety and depression.[16,17] It may have a negative impact on a person's quality of life. Stress, especially during pregnancy, may have a negative impact on growing fetus. It is important to create a supportive and encouraging environment to help women sail through pregnancy without exacerbation of vitiligo.

Treatment Options during Pregnancy

Treatment depends on factors like:
- *Type of vitiligo*: Generalized spreading vitiligo needs to be treated with systemic drugs or phototherapy. Localized vitiligo can be tackled with topical treatment modalities.
- *Trimester of pregnancy*: In the first trimester all forms of systemic treatment should be avoided. Once organogenesis is complete treatment options should be considered based on risk benefit ratio.
- *Oral medications*: Various systemic drugs are unsafe and not studied well in pregnancy. Patients treated with systemic drugs before conception have good

pregnancy outcome. Oral medications should be strictly avoided in the first trimester of pregnancy. Systemic and topical steroids are mainstay therapy for new onset or exacerbation of vitiligo lesions in pregnancy. However, they should be used sparingly since exposure to steroids in early pregnancy may lead to cleft palate deformities, preterm, or low birth weight babies etc.[18] Patient should be treated with minimal dosage and duration for treatment of active manifestation of the disease.

Topicals

- *Topical corticosteroids*: Although their bioavailability is low there were few studies showing fetal growth restriction in females using very potent topical steroids during pregnancy. Potent to very potent steroids should be avoided or used only for short period. The systemic effects of topical corticosteroids depend largely on the extent of skin absorption, which varies from 0.7 to 7% through intact skin.[19] Mid or low potency steroids may be used relatively safely for smaller patches. There is limited and inconclusive data on the safety of topical steroids in pregnancy. Misuse or prolonged use may even cause skin atrophy, striae, purpura, and milia.
- *Topical calcineurin inhibitors*: Although systemic tacrolimus is teratogenic, the absorption of the topical form is limited, and its use has not been associated with fetal anomalies.[20] It is safe to use topical tacrolimus in pregnancy as there is minimal systemic absorption and peak blood levels are undetectable.[21]
- *Phototherapy in pregnancy*: Psoralens—the theoretical mutagenic and teratogenic effect of PUVA treatment apparently does not carry any significant risk for abnormal delivery outcome.[22] Narrowband ultraviolet B (NB-UVB) therapy is generally considered by dermatologists as safe in pregnant women.[23] Some studies have suggested that NB-UVB phototherapy can diminish folate in humans, while other studies have shown that folate level is not affected by NB-UVB phototherapy.[24-28] Folate deficiency may cause neural tube defects in fetus. Pregnant females receiving phototherapy must receive folic acid supplements. Home-based units or excimer laser can be used for targeted therapy avoiding unnecessary exposure.

VITILIGO IN CHILDHOOD

Childhood vitiligo (CV) is defined as disease onset before the age of 12 years. Vitiligo may appear from shortly after birth to late adulthood. In about 50% of the cases the disease onset is before 20 years of age and, in 25% of the cases, it starts before the age of 10 years. Hence, CV should be focused on.[29] Most commonly CV shows a female preponderance and segmental variant is common. Children with nonsegmental vitiligo may develop other autoimmune disorders, especially thyroid disease.[30] Face and neck are the most common sites involved in CV **(Fig. 1)**. Children with vitiligo in the age group of 4–8 years are least affected socially. These being noticeable, young adults, teenagers often develop a negative self-image, they lack confidence. Hence, proper counseling and psychosocial support is important in this age group.

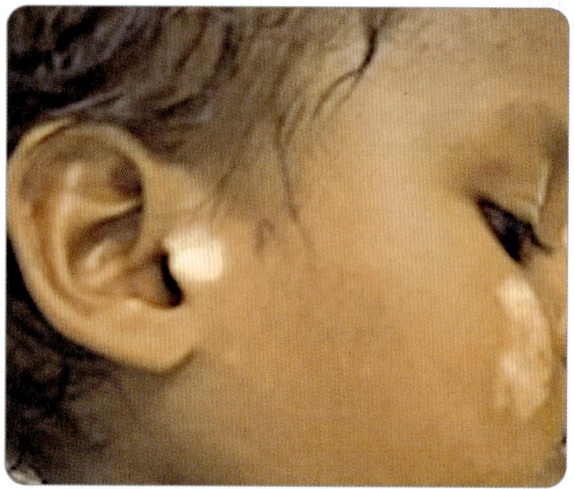

FIG. 1: Vitiligo in a child.

There are various treatment options for treating vitiligo, but not all can be used in children, and proper care needs to be taken.

Considerations while Treating Childhood Vitiligo

Differential Diagnosis
Very often parents come worried with their child to the doctor regarding light-colored patches the child develops on face. Firstly, proper examination should be done to rule out other possibilities such as pityriasis alba, pityriasis versicolor, polymorphic light eruptions or Hansen disease which may mimic previtiligo. Changed skin texture of the patches, scaling, itching, and mild redness all these prompt toward diagnosis other than vitiligo. Infants may have patches of nevus depigmentosus or nevus anemicus which should not be confused with vitiligo. In female child presenting with genital vitiligo, genital lichen sclerosus et atrophicus should be ruled out, later being more symptomatic.

Type and Duration of Vitiligo
Segmental type of vitiligo spreads only in dermatomal fashion, stabilizes early, and responds great to surgical management. Children with nonsegmental vitiligo may develop other autoimmune disorders. Nonsegmental vitiligo behaves in an unpredictable manner. It may regress spontaneously or exacerbate acutely. Acrofacial or lip tip vitiligo has slightly poor recovery rate and hence should be treated at earliest to stabilize and prevent new lesions.

Safety of Treatment Options
Topical corticosteroids, calcineurin inhibitors, and phototherapy are most commonly used drugs in CV.
- *Topical corticosteroids*: High-potency topical steroids should be used for increasing or new lesions. However, they should not be used for longer

periods or on larger surface area due to the risk of hypothalamic pituitary axis suppression in children. Most guidelines suggest mid- or low-potency topical corticosteroids to be used in children due to increased risk of side effects and higher body surface area in pediatric patients. Topical steroids used in periorbital region may very rarely cause glaucoma.[31] There are also studies which suggest there is no risk of glaucoma with topical steroids used in periorbital region.[32] However, potent steroids should be rarely used in this region. Due to thinner skin of children as compared to adults, they are at increased risk of developing atrophy, striae, and milia. To avoid these side effects, use them in tapering fashion, use them for not >2–4 months continuously.

- *Topical calcineurin inhibitors*: There are studies showing comparable efficacy of topical calcineurin inhibitors with topical steroids. Topical calcineurin inhibitors are a good steroid sparing alternative.[33] They might cause slight burning sensation, but other side effects such as skin atrophy, purpura are avoided. Pimecrolimus and tacrolimus 0.03% can be used in younger children. Black box warning on topical calcineurin inhibitors cautions against prolonged use due to risk of skin cancer or lymphoma. There is a lack of extensive experience with the use of topical calcineurin inhibitors over longer periods. Regular use of these agents, particularly in children <2 years of age due to their developing immune systems and the potential increased absorption of the medication through their skin, should be undertaken only after careful consideration.
- *Topical Janus kinase (JAK) inhibitors*: Topical tofacitinib has been used for various conditions such as atopic dermatitis, psoriasis, and alopecia areata. It has been used in vitiligo in children as well, and good repigmentation is seen specially in lesions on face.
- *Phototherapy*: Phototherapy alone as well as an adjunct with topical therapies gives great results. Ultraviolet radiations (UVR), both in the range of UVB and UVA, are considered as a first-line therapy especially for extensive vitiligo, because of their good efficacy and tolerance. Oral psoralens are avoided in children due to gastric and ocular toxicity. Topical psoralen ultraviolet A (PUVA) or topical psoralen and UVA obtained by solar light (PUVASOL) are commonly used options. NB-UVB is safer and gives persistent repigmentation similar to color of unaffected skin.[34]
- Children who have extensive vitiligo NB-UVB is treatment of choice with minimal side effects. Children >5 years who are capable of standing on their own and can comprehend to wear goggles inside light chamber can be safely given NB-UVB therapy. Targeted phototherapy such as excimer light therapy has added advantage of the treatment of smaller patches, difficult sites without unnecessary exposure to normal skin. Phototherapy when combined with other topical medications can give better response **(Figs. 2A and B)**.
- *Oral therapy*: In children with unstable vitiligo, or rapidly progressing lesions, oral steroid therapy can help in stabilizing the condition as well as help in repigmentation. It can be given in mini pulse dose form to minimize side effects of steroids. Oral steroids for prolonged period may cause growth suppression, adrenal insufficiency, osteoporosis, etc. Other systemic therapies such as methotrexate, azathioprine, etc., should be used considering risk benefit

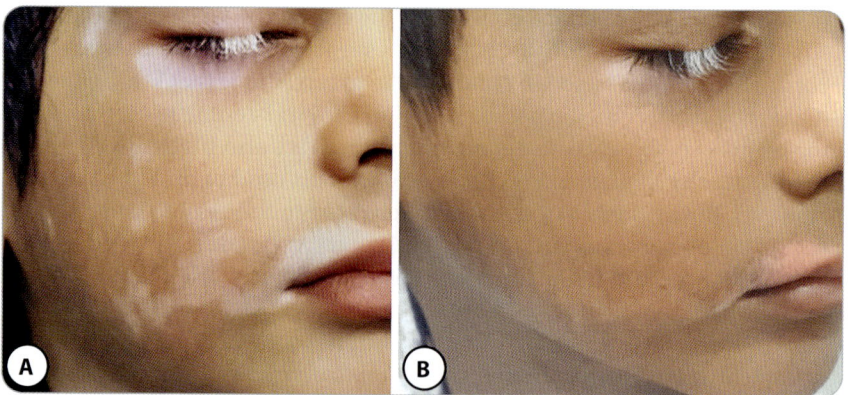

FIGS. 2A AND B: (A) Vitiliginous patches on face of a child; (B) Repigmentation after 4 months of narrowband ultraviolet B (NB-UVB) and topical calcineurin inhibitors.

ratio. Cyclosporine apart from immunomodulation, i.e., halting progression of disease also helps in the activation of melanogenesis. Oral JAK inhibitors such as tofacitinib have also been tried in vitiligo in adults, studies on CV are sparce.[35] Oral JAK inhibitors when used with phototherapy have superior results. Oral solutions are available for children >2 years of age. Long-term studies are not available, hence, can be used only to tide over crisis in young children.[36]

- *Surgical modalities*: Surgeries can be done in CV where lesions are localized and unresponsive to conventional treatment. They should be avoided in very young children because lesions might extend along with their natural body growth. Also, they are difficult to immobilize in the postoperative time.[12,37] Among all the surgical options, suction blister grafting and mini punch grafting are most commonly done procedures since they are convenient and effective procedures **(Figs. 3A and B)**. Noncultured melanocyte transfer is also preferred for larger lesions.

Difficult to Treat Sites

Certain areas such as the acral sites, lips, eyelids, nipples, and areolas are difficult to treat areas. They are challenging due to their anatomical and physiological characteristics. These sites being non hairy have lesser melanocyte reservoir, hence repigmentation is slower. Also, these sites are difficult to immobilize and there is constant friction which may hamper the results of surgical therapy. Palms and soles are thicker and penetration of topicals is not easy. Skin grafting procedures are also difficult in these areas.

TIPS AND TRICKS

Lips

Lip vitiligo is challenging to treat due to lack of hair follicle and lesser concentration of melanocytes. Surgical management is the mainstay for treatment of

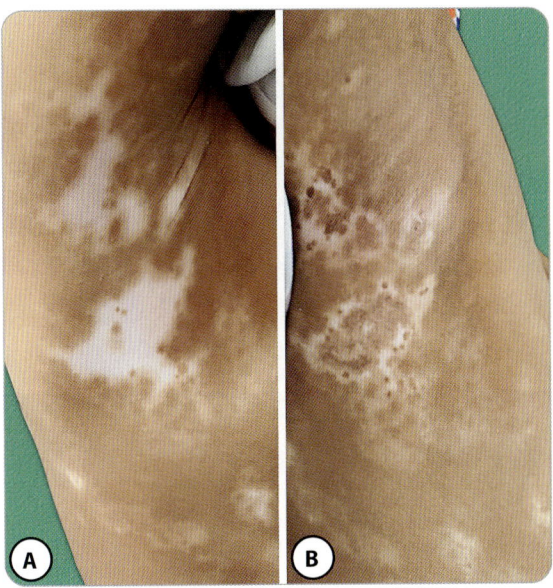

FIGS. 3A AND B: (A) Segmental vitiligo in a child; (B) Repigmentation after 3 months of suction blister grafting and topical psoralen and UVA obtained by solar light (PUVASOL) therapy.

lip vitiligo. Suction blister grafting is recommended procedure here with good repigmentation rate and good color match. Keeping the graft in place is difficult in angle of mouth region, since lips are constantly used for talking and eating. Mini punch grafting also gives good color match on lips, but there is risk of cobblestoning if grafts are not placed properly. Cyanoacrylate gels are liquids that polymerize in the presence of moisture to form adhesives. They can be used to keep grafts of suction blister grafting and punch grafting in place **(Figs. 4A and B)**. They have antimicrobial properties so glued wounds are less likely to develop infections.[38] When only upper one-third portion of lower lip is involved, excision of vitiliginous lesion is an instant and cosmetically acceptable treatment option.

Eyelids

The skin of eyelids is delicate and thin and hence topical therapies such as calcineurin inhibitors and topical steroids should be used carefully since they may cause skin irritation. Surgical treatment options give good results but proper bandaging over a closed eye is required for optimal results.[39] Dermabrasion is difficult in this region, as there is no underlying bony support. Hence, mini punch grafting is better option **(Figs. 5A and B)**. Mini punch grafting with cyanoacrylate gel can be done for better graft uptake. Noncultured melanocyte transfer can also be done, recipient area is prepared by CO_2 laser dermabrasion with corneal shield or the skin is pulled on bony ridge and manual or motor dermabrader is used.

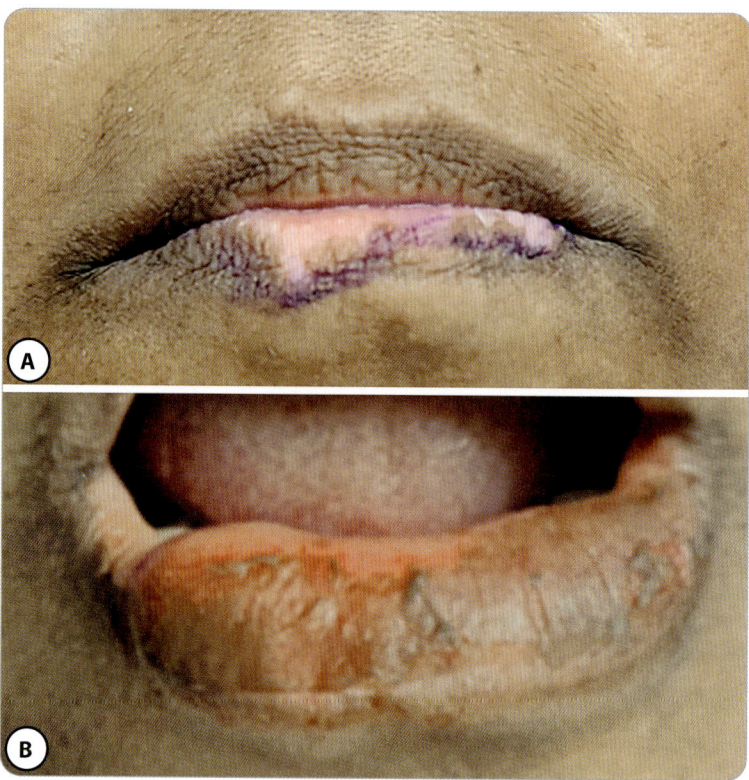

FIGS. 4A AND B: (A) Lip vitiligo; (B) Suction blister grafting with cyanoacrylate gel (for stabilization of graft).

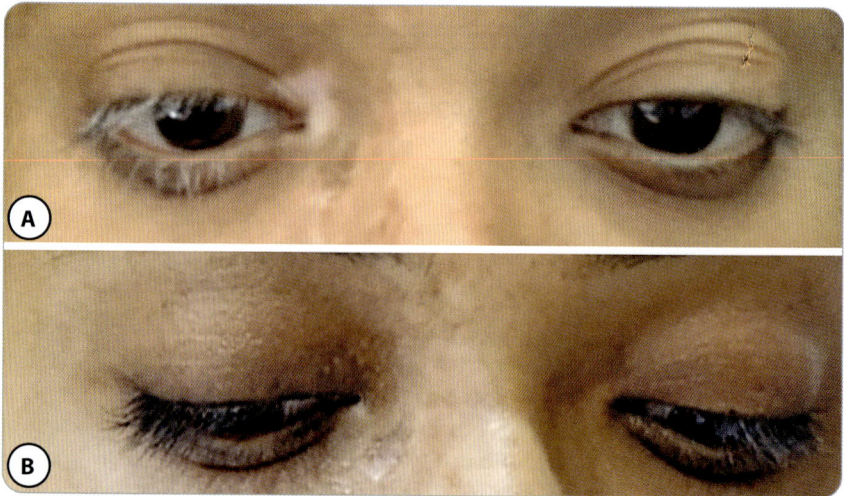

FIGS. 5A AND B: (A) Vitiligo patch on medial canthus region; (B) Repigmentation after 3 months of mini punch grafting procedure.

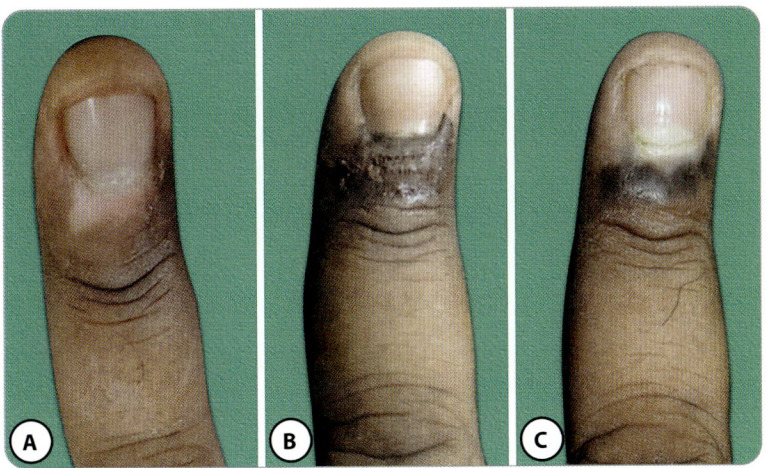

FIGS. 6A TO C: Micropigmentation over vitiligo patch on fingertip (A) before procedure (B) immediately after (C) post 6 months of treatment.[41]

Eyebrow

Leucotrichia is resistant and difficult to treat. Even after surgical procedures, surrounding skin gets repigmented but hair remain white. Follicular unit transplantation will help in repigmentation of skin as well as transplanted hair unit gives pigmented hair.[40]

Acral Area

Acral region is recalcitrant to treatment because of constant mobility and relatively lower density or absence of pilosebaceous follicles, the reservoirs from which the melanocytes migrate. Surgical therapies including noncultured melanocyte transfer, suction blister grafting, and mini punch grafting may give good results. Splinting of the region treated for at least 5–7 days postsurgery will help in better outcome. Micropigmentation also is helpful for instant cosmetic results **(Figs. 6A to C)**.[41] However, results with it are not long lasting, color starts fading after 6 months. 5-Fluorouracil with CO_2 laser has been tried in acral regions, where fractional CO_2 laser treatment is followed by 5-fluorouracil topical application for 5 days and same cycle is repeated monthly. It is novel, safe, and effective method.[42]

Palms and soles being thicker than the rest of the body parts topical medical management is often ineffective. Punch grafting may be done, however, the donor site should be taken from palms or soles, since grafts from other body region may not show a good color match and often will lead to cobblestoning **(Fig. 7)**.[43]

Vitiligo management involves thorough clinical evaluation, followed by personalized treatment based on the extent of the disease, site, its activity, and the patient's condition and preferences.

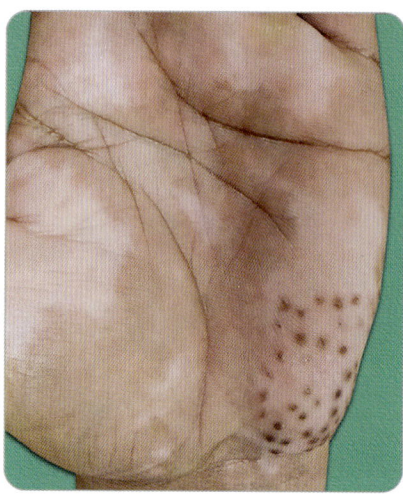

FIG. 7: Cobblestoning appearance and poor color match after mini punch grafting from thigh as donor area.

CONCLUSION

Vitiligo is a complex and multifactorial disease that requires a comprehensive approach for effective management. While its pathogenesis remains the same across different ethnicities, its impact varies, particularly in skin of color where the depigmented patches are more noticeable. Special considerations are needed in specific populations, such as pregnant women and children, where treatment options must be carefully tailored to ensure safety and efficacy. Vitiligo management demands a patient-centered approach that not only focuses on medical and surgical interventions but also addresses the psychological and social impact of the disease.

REFERENCES

1. Park KY, Kwon HJ, Wie JH. Pregnancy outcomes in patients with vitiligo: a nationwide population-based cohort study from Korea. J Am Acad Dermatol. 2018;79(5):836-42.
2. Krüger C, Schallreuter KU. A review of the worldwide prevalence of vitiligo in children/adolescents and adults. Int J Dermatol. 2012;51:1206-12.
3. Merz WM, Fischer-Betz R, Hellwig K, Lamprecht G, Gembruch U. Pregnancy and autoimmune disease. Dtsch Arztebl Int. 2022;119(9):145-56.
4. Jeon C, Agbai O, Butler D, Murase J. Dermatologic conditions in patients of color who are pregnant. Int J Womens Dermatol. 2017;3(1):30-6.
5. Soldin OP, Guo T, Weiderpass E, Tractenberg RE, Hilakivi-Clarke L, Soldin SJ. Steroid hormone levels in pregnancy and 1 year postpartum using isotope dilution tandem mass spectrometry. Fertil Steril. 2005;84(3):701-10.
6. Lin H, Mosmann TR, Guilbert L, Tuntipopipat S, Wegmann TG. Synthesis of T helper 2-type cytokines at the maternal-fetal interface. J Immunol. 1993;151(9):4562-73.
7. Manolache L, Benea V. Stress in patients with alopecia areata and vitiligo. J Eur Acad Dermatol Venereol. 2007;21(7):921-8.
8. Webb KC, Lyon S, Nardone B, West DP, Kundu RV. Influence of Pregnancy on Vitiligo Activity. J Clin Aesthet Dermatol. 2016;9(12):21-5.

9. Hung CT, Huang HH, Wang CK, Chung CH, Tsao CH, Chien WC, et al. Pregnancy outcomes in women with vitiligo: A Taiwanese nationwide cohort study. PLoS One. 2021;16(3):e0248651.
10. Horev A, Weintraub AY, Sergienko R, Wiznitzer A, Halevy S, Sheiner E. Pregnancy outcome in women with vitiligo. Int J Dermatol. 2011;50(9):1083-5.
11. Spritz RA. The genetics of generalized vitiligo and associated autoimmune diseases. J Dermatol Sci. 2006;41:3-10.
12. Gianfaldoni S, Tchernev G, Wollina U, Lotti J, Satolli F, França K, et al. Vitiligo in Children: A Better Understanding of the Disease. Open Access Maced J Med Sci. 2018;6(1):181-4.
13. Bhatia PS, Mohan L, Pandey ON, Singh KK, Arora SK, Mukhija RD. Genetic nature of vitiligo. J Dermatol Sci. 1992;4:180-4.
14. Nath SK, Majumder PP, Nordlund JJ. Genetic epidemiology of vitiligo: multilocus recessivity cross-validated. Am J Hum Genet. 1994;55:981-90.
15. Alenizi DA. Consanguinity pattern and heritability of vitiligo in Arar, Saudi Arabia. J Family Community Med. 2014;21:13-6.
16. Kussainova A, Kassym L, Akhmetova A, Glushkova N, Sabirov U, Adilgozhina S, et al. Vitiligo and anxiety: a systematic review and meta-analysis. PLoS One. 2020;15(11):e0241445.
17. Lai YC, Yew YW, Kennedy C, Schwartz RA. Vitiligo and depression: a systematic review and meta-analysis of observational studies. Br J Dermatol. 2017;177(3):708-18.
18. Park-Wyllie L, Mazzotta P, Pastuszak A, Moretti ME, Beique L, Hunnisett L, et al. Birth defects after maternal exposure to corticosteroids: prospective cohort study and meta-analysis of epidemiological studies. Teratology. 2000;62:385-92.
19. Chi CC, Wang SH, Wojnarowska F, Kirtschig G, Davies E, Bennett C. Safety of topical corticosteroids in pregnancy. Cochrane Database Syst Rev. 2015;(10):CD007346.
20. Christopher V, Al-Chalabi T, Richardson PD, Muiesan P, Rela M, Heaton ND, et al. Pregnancy outcome after liver transplantation: a single-center experience of 71 pregnancies in 45 recipients. Liver Transpl. 2006;12:1138-43.
21. McMullan P, Yaghi M, Truong TM, Rothe M, Murase J, Grant-Kels JM. Safety of dermatologic medications in pregnancy and lactation: An update—Part I: Pregnancy. J Am Acad Dermatol. 2024;91(4):619-648.
22. Gunnarskog JG, Källén AJB, Lindelöf BG, Sigurgeirsson B. Psoralen Photochemotherapy (PUVA) and Pregnancy. Arch Dermatol. 1993;129(3):320-3.
23. Ibbotson SH, Bilsland D, Cox NH, Dawe RS, Diffey B, Edwards C, et al. An update and guidance on narrowband ultraviolet B phototherapy: a British Photodermatology Group Workshop Report. Br J Dermatol. 2004;151:283-97.
24. Shaheen MA, Abdel Fattah NS, El-Berhamy MI. Analysis of serum folate levels after narrowband UVB exposure. Egypt Dermatol Online J. 2006;2:13.
25. El-Saie LT, Rabie AR, Kamel MI, Seddeik AK, Elsaie ML. Effect of narrowband ultraviolet B phototherapy on serum folic acid levels in patients with psoriasis. Lasers Med Sci. 2011;26:481-5.
26. Rose RF, Batchelor RJ, Turned D, Goulden V. Narrowband ultraviolet B phototherapy does not influence serum and red cell folate levels in patients with psoriasis. J Am Acad Dermatol. 2009;61:259-62.
27. Cicarma E, Mork C, Porojnicu AC, Juzeniene A, Tam TT, Dahlback A, et al. Influence of narrowband UVB phototherapy on vitamin D and folate status. Exp Dermatol. 2010;19: e67-72.
28. Lajevardi V, Ghiasi M, Hejazi P, Ansar M, Akbar Z, Shakiba H, et al. The effect of narrow band UVB on levels of folate: trial on patients with dermatologic disorders. Iran J Dermatol. 2015;18:36-37.
29. Lacovelli P, Sinagra JL, Vidolin AP, Marenda S, Capitanio B, Leone G, et al. Relevance of thyroiditis and other autoimmune diseases in children with vitiligo. Dermatology. 2005;210:26-30.
30. Pajvani U, Ahmad N, Wiley A, Levy RM, Kundu R, Mancini AJ, et al. The relationship between family medical history and childhood vitiligo. J Am Acad Dermatol. 2006;55:238-44.

31. Sahni D, Darley CR, Hawk JLM. Glaucoma induced by periorbital topical steroid use—a rare complication. Clin Experiment Dermatol. 2004;29(6):617-19.
32. Haeck IM, Rouwen TJ, Timmer-de Mik L, de Bruin-Weller MS, Bruijnzeel-Koomen CA. Topical corticosteroids in atopic dermatitis and the risk of glaucoma and cataracts. J Am Acad Dermatol. 2011;64(2):275-81.
33. Lee JH, Kwon HS, Jung HM, Lee H, Kim GM, Yim HW, et al. Treatment outcomes of topical calcineurin inhibitor therapy for patients with vitiligo: a systematic review and meta-analysis. JAMA Dermatol. 2019;155(8):929-38.
34. Scherschun L, Kim JJ, Lim HW. Narrow-band ultraviolet B is a useful and well-tolerated treatment for vitiligo. J Am Acad Dermatol. 2001;44(6):999-1003.
35. Qi F, Liu F, Gao L. Janus Kinase Inhibitors in the Treatment of Vitiligo: A Review. Front Immunol. 2021;12:790125.
36. Biswal A, Agrawal I, Panda M. Use of Oral Tofacitinib in the Treatment of Pediatric Vitiligo: A Case Series. J Dermatol. 2024;69(4):366.
37. Tamesis ME, Morelli JG. Vitiligo treatment in childhood: A state-of-the-art review. Paediatr Dermatol. 2010;27:437-45.
38. Bhingradia YM, Chaudhary NR, Patel NK. Mini Punch Grafting Involving Angle of Lip Using Cyanoacrylate Glue. J Cutan Aesthet Surg. 2023;16(1):69-70.
39. Nanda S, Relhan V, Grover C, Reddy BS. Suction blister epidermal grafting for management of eyelid vitiligo: special considerations. Dermatol Surg. 2006;32(3):387-91; discussion 391-2.
40. Pangti R, Gupta V, Gupta S. Follicular unit extraction of leukotrichia and replacement with follicular units from the scalp in combination with epidermal cell suspension in a case of vitiligo. Dermatol Ther. 2020;33(6):e13916.
41. Sharma A, Agrawal S, Dhurat R, Mhatre M, Surve R, Kerure A. Micropigmentation—a revived therapeutic tool for recalcitrant, difficult-to-treat periungual vitiligo. Dermatol Ther. 2020;33(4):e13568.
42. Weshahy R, Abdelhamid MF, Sayed KS, El Desouky ED, Ramez SA. Efficacy and safety of combined fractional ablative CO_2 laser and 5 fluorouracil in the treatment of acral vitiligo: An open, uncontrolled study. J Cosmet Dermatol. 2022;21(11):5636-41.
43. Kumar P. Autologous punch grafting for vitiligo of the palm. Dermatol Surg. 2005;31(3):368-70.

CHAPTER 11

Psychosocial Aspects of Vitiligo

Pradnya Prakash Manwatkar

INTRODUCTION

Vitiligo is an autoimmune condition that leads to the progressive loss of melanocytes which leads to depigmented patches on the skin. There are ample studies and data on the pathophysiological aspects of the disease. However, the psychosocial implications of this condition have been understudied, albeit being equally significant. Vitiligo influences the quality of life and mental health of affected individuals, and this chapter explores the relationship between vitiligo, stress, and psychosocial factors. This chapter is an attempt on shedding light on the intricate interplay between skin health and psychological well-being.

MELANOCYTE DEVELOPMENT AND FUNCTION

Ectodermal Origin of Melanocytes

The epidermis and neuronal cells come from the same of cells called the ectodermal cells. Melanocytes originate from neural crest cells which are multipotent cells that migrate from the neural tube. These neural crest cells arise from the ectoderm during embryonic development. It gives rise to various structures, including the skin, hair follicles, and the nervous system.[1]

Upon migration, as these cells reach the dermal-epidermal junction, they differentiate into melanoblasts, which are the precursors to melanocytes. Several signaling pathways such as the bone morphogenic protein (BMP) and Wnt help to regulate the proliferation and differentiation of these cells.

Transcription factors also play a role in the development of melanocytes. The microphthalmia-associated transcription factor (MITF) is a master regulator that propentiates melanocyte development and function. The MITF also regulates genes involved in melanin synthesis, such as tyrosinase.[2] Furthermore, melanoblasts interact with keratinocytes in the epidermis, which is vital for their maturation and survival.[3]

Role of Stress Hormones on the Melanocytes

Research indicates that stress hormones, particularly cortisol, can significantly influence the function and survival of melanocytes. Elevated cortisol levels result from chronic stress and they can inhibit melanocyte proliferation and function. Thereby, leading to increased susceptibility to their death that leads to depigmentation of the skin.[4] Cortisol exerts its effects, such as modulation of key signaling pathways that include the mitogen-activated protein kinase (MAPK) pathway, which is critical for melanocyte survival. Cortisol is also secreted at the level of epidermis through the keratinocyte corticotropin-releasing hormone (CRH), every time there is stressful trigger perceived by the individual. Thus, stress and the cortisol released in these conditions have a direct role to play in the triggering of the depigmentation that occurs in cases of vitiligo.

STRESS, VITILIGO, AND MELANOCYTE DEATH

Cycle of Stress and Vitiligo

The relationship between stress and vitiligo is cyclical; stress can exacerbate the condition, while the condition itself can induce stress. Chronic stress elevates cortisol levels, which can lead to the apoptosis (programmed cell death) of melanocytes through various receptor-mediated processes.[5] Elevated levels of proinflammatory cytokines, such as tumor necrosis factor-α (TNF-α) and interleukin-6 (IL-6), can further contribute to melanocyte loss.

Stress-induced catecholamines can produce reactive oxygen species (ROS). Abnormally increased catecholamine can produce vasoconstriction that leads to epidermal-dermal hypoxia. Further leading to possibly formation of quinones, semiquinone radicals, and oxyradicals. Catecholamines can produce H_2O_2 that alters calcium homeostasis leading to faulty uptake of L-phenylalanine, the amino acid precursor of tyrosine in melanocytes. It is reasonable to suggest that the increased levels of these oxidative radicals might contribute to melanocyte damage in the early phase of vitiligo.

Epidermal cells have fully functional serotonin and melatoninergic systems. They themselves also express steroidogenic activity. It is proven that melatonin modulates melanogenesis and shows involvement in stress response system of the skin. There is a complex relationship between pigment-producing mechanism and 5-hydroxytryptamine (5-HT, serotonin).

Study showed that the plasma levels of 5-HT (serotonin), 5-hydroxyindoleacetic acid (5-HIAA), and melatonin significantly increased either in vitiligo groups than the control group.[6] The levels of both serotonin and melatonin in females were significantly higher than males within all groups. There was no effect of the sex on 5-HIAA levels within all studied groups.

Receptor-mediated Processes

Melanocyte apoptosis in vitiligo can occur via several receptor-mediated pathways. For instance, the activation of the Fas/Fas ligand system has been implicated in the autoimmune component of vitiligo. The activated immune cells trigger the death of melanocytes.[7] Additionally, stress-induced activation of the hypothalamic-pituitary-adrenal (HPA) axis results in an increase in adrenal corticotropic hormone (ACTH) and cortisol, which can negatively impact melanocyte survival.[8]

Chemical Mediators of Melanocyte Death

In addition to stress hormones, other chemical mediators, such as ROS, play a crucial role in melanocyte death. Increased oxidative stress in the skin has been observed in vitiligo patients, leading to damage of melanocytes and furthering the cycle of depigmentation.[9] Furthermore, nitric oxide (NO), a signaling molecule involved in various physiological processes, has been implicated in melanocyte apoptosis, highlighting the complex biochemical environment surrounding this condition.

PSYCHOSOCIAL IMPACT OF VITILIGO

Stigma and Social Perception

There have been a lot of social stigmas associated with vitiligo. This can lead to feelings of embarrassment, anxiety, and depression. Because of the visible nature of the condition, it can provoke negative reactions from peers. Thereby leading to social withdrawal and a decline in self-esteem. A study highlighted that individuals with vitiligo reported higher levels of psychosocial distress compared to those with other dermatological conditions. Add to it the societal standards of beauty and you see the distress in individuals with vitiligo exponentially rising.

Psychological Distress and Quality of Life

Vitiligo has also been known to significantly impact quality of life. Conditions, such as body dysmorphic disorder (BDD) can occur in patients. Patients often experience emotional turmoil due to changes in their appearance, leading to conditions, such as social anxiety disorder and BDD. Research has shown that the severity of vitiligo correlates with increased levels of depression and anxiety, indicating that the extent of skin involvement can exacerbate psychosocial issues.[10]

That stress or stressful event can also vitiligo has also been proven time and again. Death of a family member was stated to be the cause of vitiligo 22% of patients in a study.[11] These stressors preceded the incidence of vitiligo for even as long as 2 years. There was no correlation of the stressor and the area of involvement in the vitiliginous patches.[12]

MANAGEMENT STRATEGIES

Psychological Interventions

Addressing the psychosocial aspects of vitiligo is essential in managing the overall well-being of affected individuals. Psychological interventions, including cognitive-behavioral therapy (CBT), have shown promise in alleviating the emotional distress associated with vitiligo. A randomized controlled trial demonstrated that participants receiving CBT experienced significant reductions in anxiety and depressive symptoms compared to control groups.

REBT or rational emotive behavior therapy can also help to address not only the stress that is a result of the vitiligo but can also help to deal with the stressful event that leads to the occurrence of it.[13] It is important to address these vital preceding events, as they can lead to the aggravation of the disease or can lead to treatment failures. REBT helps identify the dysfunctional thoughts that lead to emotions of shame, anxiety, and depression which can lead to the changes in the 5-HT, cortisol, etc., levels that lead to the activation of the peripheral HPA axis or the triggering of CRH production by the keratinocytes that can start the cascading event of melanocytic death as is seen in vitiligo.

Rational emotive behavior therapy basically uses a simple model called the ABC model to be able to address these dysfunctional thoughts. A is the activating event (not restricted to a timeline), B is the dysfunctional belief system about that event, and C is the consequence (vitiligo as is being discussed in this textbook). REBT states that A does not cause C. It is the B/dysfunctional belief about the A that leads to the C. ABC model looks like: A + B = C.

Here is an example:
If we identified in our patients of vitiligo their A as unemployment, it is not the state of unemployment that led to the changes in the 5-HT levels or in the peripheral HPA. It was their belief about being unemployed that led to these changes in their cortisol levels that subsequently led to the occurrence of the melanocytic death. Here, if we are to identify the dysfunctional B about unemployment that our patient carries, these could look like the following:
- I must be worthless to have lost my Job.
- If I do not have a job, I will never be able to gain respect from my family ever.
- A jobless man/woman never has any respect in society. What will the society think of me? That I am a big failure forever.

And many more such automatic negative thoughts (ANTs) can arise due to the single activating event of unemployment. REBT helps us in identifying these thoughts and further changing them to helpful functional ones which can look like the following:
- I may not have a job now but that does not mean I have no worth and will never have a job again.
- My job does not define my worth. It is a part of who I am and not the whole of me. I can stand it.
- My family loves me for who I am and not for the job that I do.

Rational emotive behavior therapy is a process-oriented therapy with the goal of creating what is called a "therapeutic insight" in the patient. Therapeutic insights help the patient realize that the disease did not happen out of nowhere. It helps one to gain some sense of control, thereby leading to a state of mind where the notion is that the power of the disease reversing may well be within reach.

CASE EXAMPLE

A 32-year-old female presented with a loss of color under left breast in the first 1-month postpartum. She noticed the patch after which she decided to take

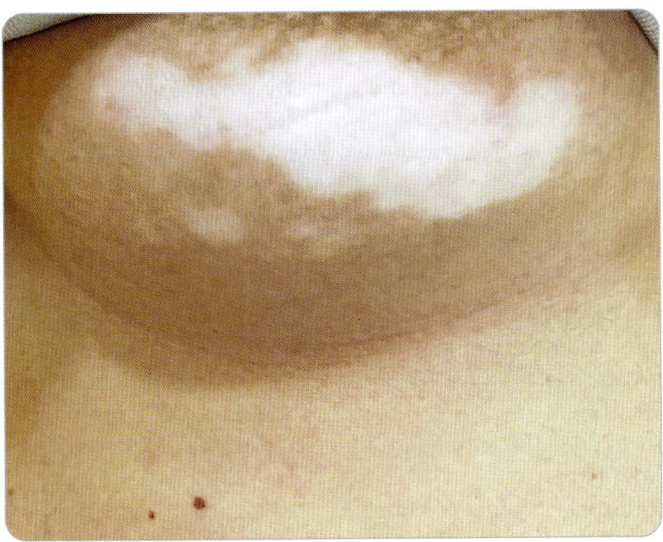

FIG. 1: Development of melanocyte.

treatment. She was medically and surgically fit. She had delivered twins through cesarean section and the babies were on bottle feeding as she was not able to lactate efficiently **(Fig. 1)**.

Upon detail history, we were able to find out her As:
- Turns out that she had a history of two miscarriages over the 1 year that she was planning to conceive.
- These twins were precious and that added to her anxiety during pregnancy.
- To add to this, she was on a sabbatical from her job due to the restrictions that were imposed on her by her gynecologist owing to the miscarriages. She felt that she was not doing enough income-wise and she missed her work and the value it created in her life.
- Her husband was supportive but mostly absent due to his busy work schedule.
- Her body had changed drastically, and she had added extra kilos and was not used to seeing herself like this.

Her Cs were:
- The appearance of the depigmented patch under her left breast
- Anxiety that led to insomnia
- Sadness that was leading to her spontaneous bouts of crying.
- Anger that she was bound down and was not able to return to her routine life where she was thriving and achieving her goals.
- Fear that her body would never go back to what it was prepregnancy.

The routine line of medical treatment was started. Topical application of steroid cream, tacrolimus, and decapeptide lotion, as she was not breastfeeding. And we started on working on identifying her dysfunctional Bs:
- She must have done something wrong, and she must be responsible for the miscarriages that happened.
- It was must that these two babies turn out to be healthy no matter what or she would not be able to forgive herself.

- Her husband must take the responsibility always and be around her no matter what. After all she too had given up her routine for these babies.
- She would falter and lag behind all her colleagues at work and she would never be able to catch up for lost work and lost time at work, ever. She would be then sidelined and colleagues would not remember the value she added to their team.
- She would never ever be able to get back to previous body weight and shape. It would be impossible, and it was unachievable no matter what she would do eventually to get back to her original shape.

Over a period of 2 months, we were now able to change these dysfunctional Bs into functional and healthy Bs:

- Although she would have liked for an uneventful pregnancy, because she had miscarriages does not mean that she had done something wrong. A miscarriage does not signify fault in the mother. It is okay and she would be able to stand it.
- She would make a sincere effort on taking care of herself during and post pregnancy. The effort mattered more. Because the only factor that was within her control to ensure healthy babies was she took care of herself?
- She would ask for help from her husband and not assume he understood.
- Her sabbatical did not erase all the success that she had achieved in the past at her work. That this was just a pause in her job and not a decline in her worth as an employee or person.
- She would again make a sincere effort to return back to her weight. And her weight again or appearance had no bearing on her qualities as a mother, employee, or person.

If you look at all the Bs, in almost all cases, they are related to self-worth of the person. Helping the patient in realizing that human worth is inherent, no value can be attached to it, and to devoid of validation is the key to helping change dysfunctional Bs to functional ones.

Patient ended up coming for follow-up three times over 2 months from December 2023 till January 2024. She was lost to follow-up for 8 months post which she consulted in September 2024 to check if the lesion had subsided despite not applying medicines. There was remission seen.

To conclude, the future dermatologist should incorporate a thorough psychoanalytical evaluation of the patient along with the comprehensive medical history.

Dermatological Treatments

Dermatological management of vitiligo has been discussed time and again. They include topical treatments, phototherapy, and surgical options, such as melanocyte transplantation. However, A holistic approach that incorporates REBT with these treatments is crucial for optimal outcomes **(Fig. 2)**.

Support Groups and Community Resources

Engaging in support groups has always been helpful. It reduces the feeling of isolation and loneliness that the disease can result in. The feeling of

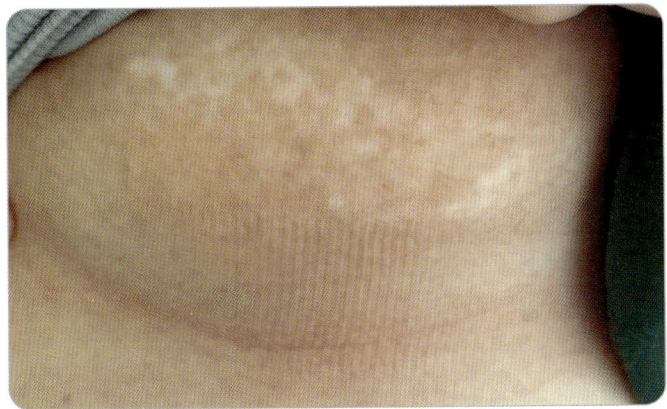

FIG. 2: There are other psychological interventions that can be used. Neurolinguistic programming (NLP), transactional analysis (TA), and also hypnotherapy[14] are known to help to create a thought-based change and change in the emotional dysregulation that can lead to sustainable treatment outcomes postmedical line of management.

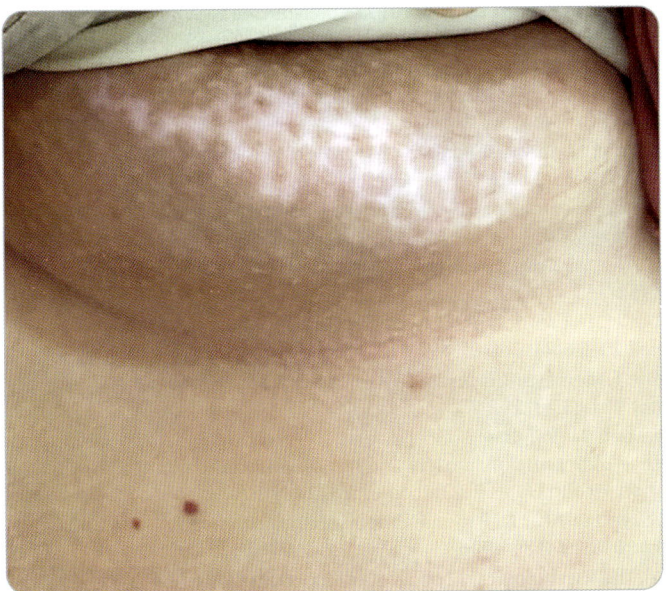

FIG. 3: Improvement of melanocyte.

marginalization reduces when a group comes together and tries to face the challenges of the disease together **(Fig. 3)**. Basically, it can provide individuals with vitiligo a platform to share experiences, learn coping strategies, and gain emotional support. Community resources, including educational materials and workshops, can empower patients.

According to a study, patients who engage in support networks report better psychological outcomes, proving the importance of social support in such conditions.[15]

CONCLUSION

Vitiligo is not merely a cosmetic condition; it encompasses complex psychosocial dimensions. The interplay between stress and melanocyte death, and psychological well-being underscores the need for comprehensive management strategies. These strategies need to address both the physical and emotional aspects of vitiligo. By fostering a deeper understanding of these psychosocial factors, healthcare providers can better support individuals living with vitiligo, ultimately improving their quality of life.

REFERENCES

1. Gilbert SF. Developmental Biology, 6th edition. Sunderland (MA): Sinauer Associates; 2000.
2. Hemesath TJ, et al. Transcription factor MITF links stem cell maintenance and melanocyte differentiation. Nature. 1998;391(6662):707-11.
3. Levy C, et al. The role of keratinocytes in the development and function of the epidermal melanocyte. J Investig Dermatol. 2005;125(6):1071-9.
4. Klein L, et al. Impact of stress on melanocyte biology. J Investig Dermatol. 2015;135(6):1485-93.
5. Bai Y, et al. Cortisol-induced apoptosis of melanocytes in vitiligo. J Dermatol Sc. 2020;98(2):93-100.
6. Kotb El-Sayed MI, Abd El-Ghany AA, Mohamed RR. Neural and Endocrinal Pathobiochemistry of Vitiligo: Comparative Study for a Hypothesized Mechanism. Front Endocrinol (Lausanne). 2018;9:197.
7. Harris S, et al. Immune-mediated destruction of melanocytes in vitiligo. Clin Rev Allergy Immunol. 2017;53(2):263-72.
8. Lee J, et al. The role of HPA axis in the pathogenesis of vitiligo. Arch Dermatol Res. 2018;310(5):407-14.
9. Mandal A, et al. Oxidative stress in vitiligo: A comprehensive review. J Dermatol Treat. 2022;33(5).
10. Garg T, et al. Depression and anxiety in vitiligo patients: A cross-sectional study. Indian J Dermatol. 2019;64(4):340-5.
11. Cupertino F, Niemeyer-Corbellini JP, Ramos-E-Silva M. Psychosomatic aspects of vitiligo. Clin Dermatol. 2017;35(3):292-7.
12. Hamidizadeh N, Ranjbar S, Ghanizadeh A, Parvizi MM, Jafari P, Handjani F. Evaluating prevalence of depression, anxiety and hopelessness in patients with vitiligo on an Iranian population. Health Qual Life Outcomes. 2020;18(1):20.
13. Şahin ES, Voltan Acar N. Rational emotive behavior therapy from a new perspective. Int J Hum Sci. 2019;16(4):894-906.
14. Silvan M. The Psychological Aspects of Vitiligo. Cutis. 2004;73:163-7.
15. Benani O, et al. The role of social support in managing vitiligo: A qualitative study. Int J Dermatol. 2021;60(6):727-33.

CHAPTER 12

Camouflaging Techniques for Vitiligo

Kanika Sahni, Shivangi Garg

INTRODUCTION

Vitiligo impacts approximately 0.5–2% of the global population and 8.8% in India.[1,2] The stark contrast between depigmented patches and normal skin, particularly in individuals with darker skin phototypes, can cause severe psychological distress, leading to significant emotional challenges, especially among women and those with darker skin making them seek treatment more often.[3] Such vitiligo patients often experience higher levels of social anxiety, depression, low self-esteem, and poor body image compared to healthy individuals. They may also face discrimination and stigmatization.[4-6]

A key goal in patient-centered care is to alleviate the psychosocial burden and improve the quality of life impacted by vitiligo. Enhancing quality of life is linked to patient satisfaction which can positively influence treatment adherence and outcomes.[7-9]

Camouflage therapy is the temporary or permanent concealment of disfiguring lesions of skin, hair, and nails. The goal of the therapy is to provide cosmetically acceptable outcome. Skin camouflage is the term used for specially formulated product to conceal color or contour defects of the skin. It is a viable option for patients who are awaiting treatment response or when treatment does not yield the desired results. It has been seen that camouflage can enhance the quality of life for individuals with vitiligo, promoting social and psychological well-being by minimizing the visibility of depigmentation. **Flowchart 1** depicts the classification of skin camouflage techniques.

Cosmetic camouflage using specialized products designed to reproduce and blend in with the natural colors of skin is the most frequently used camouflaging technique.

COSMETIC CAMOUFLAGE

Camouflage makeup is designed to be waterproof and effective at concealment. It needs to be carefully selected to match the patient's skin tone. The uniform

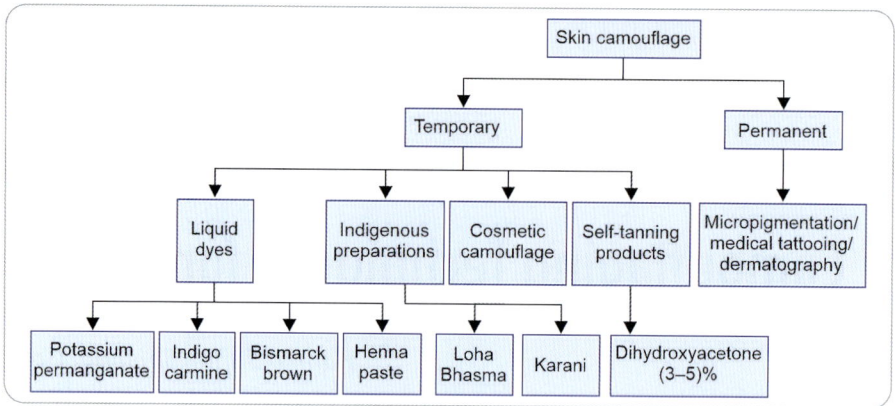

FLOWCHART 1: Classification of skin camouflage techniques.

application of thin layers of selected opaque cosmetics with light-reflecting ingredients is highly effective in covering or minimizing the visual impact of depigmentation.

The ideal camouflage material should have the following characteristics:[10,11]

- *Color matching:* The makeup should blend seamlessly with the patient's skin tone, ensuring it matches the surrounding skin on the face.
- *Opacity:* The makeup must effectively conceal all types of skin discolorations, providing a natural and normal appearance.
- *Waterproof:* Ideally, camouflage makeup should be waterproof.
- *Sweat resistance:* The makeup should be resistant to smudging or washing away due to sweating.
- *Adhesion:* The makeup should adhere well to the skin, staying in place without sliding off.
- *Long wear:* The makeup should offer long-lasting coverage with the ability to reapply easily if needed.
- *Ease of application:* The makeup should be simple to apply. Complicated color combinations or steps may discourage daily use by patients.
- *Non-allergenic/non-comedogenic/non-photosensitizing:* Ideally, the makeup should be inert, not causing allergic reactions, photodermatitis, or acne.
- *Sun protection:* As an opaque substance, the makeup will naturally offer some sun protection. A good camouflage should provide uniform sun protection.
- *Ease of removal:* The makeup should be easy to remove at the end of the day using non-alcoholic and non-acetone-based makeup removers.
- *Cost-effectiveness:* All desirable properties of the product should be considered in the context of affordability.

There are various types of camouflage cosmetics, including:[12]

- *Full concealment:* High-coverage foundation creams or cover creams designed for complete coverage of affected area, extending beyond the affected area (e.g., Dermablend Cover Crème Foundation, Covermark Classic Cover).
- *Pigment blending:* Cover creams that match the patient's foundation color (e.g., Dermablend Smooth Liquid Camo Hydrating Foundation).

TABLE 1: Ingredients of a camouflage preparation.

Ingredient type	Examples	Purpose
Pigments	Iron oxides and titanium dioxide	Imparting color to the product and skin
Fillers	Talc, mica, kaolin, polymeric, or silicone fillers	Esthetics on skin; ease of application; oil control; optical effects; lastingness; thickening/texture
Emulsifiers	PEG-10 dimethicone, cetyl/PEG/PPG-10/1 dimethicone, and polyglyceryl-4 isostearate	Allow oils (silicone or hydrocarbons) and water phases to mix and form an emulsion
Emollients	Dimethicone and isonoyl isononanoate	Ease of application and for dispersion of actives and solid particles
Thickeners	Gums, waxes, carbomer, and disteardimonium hectorite	Texturizing for oil, water, or both within the formula and provide structure
Other polymers	Various	Thickening; lastingness; esthetics; oil control; optical effects; ease of application

- *Subtle coverage:* Light application of foundation cream or fluid for moderate concealment (e.g., Dermablend Intense Powder Camo® Mattifying Foundation, a buildable coverage mattifying powder foundation).

TYPICAL INGREDIENTS

The various important constituents of a camouflage preparation responsible for its various properties are listed in **Table 1**.[12]

The incorporation of volatile oils, either siliconated or carbonated, has led to the development of long-lasting foundations. As the volatile component evaporates, the tinted film becomes more concentrated on the skin. This film adheres to the skin during drying, resisting friction and avoiding transfer onto clothing.

BASIC FOUNDATION FORMULATIONS[13]

- *Oil-based foundations:* These foundations are primarily designed for dry skin. They are water-in-oil emulsions where pigments are suspended in oil, such as mineral oil, lanolin alcohol, vegetable oils (e.g., coconut, sesame, and safflower), or synthetic esters (e.g., isopropyl myristate and octyl palmitate). These foundations mix with sebum, creating a moist feeling after water evaporates, making them easy to apply and ideal for patients with dry skin. Microskin's simulated second skin lotion is an oil-based foundation that also contains alcohol with ethanol as a solvent.
- *Water-based foundations:* Designed for dry to normal skin, these are oil-in-water emulsions with a higher water content and less oil, where pigments are suspended in the emulsion. They include primary emulsifiers such as

triethanolamine or nonionic surfactants and secondary emulsifiers such as glyceryl stearate or propylene glycol stearate. Though less stable than oil-based foundations, they are more popular.

- *Oil-free foundations:* These are formulated for oily skin and do not contain animal, vegetable, or mineral oils. Instead, they use silicone derivatives such as dimethicone or cyclomethicone, which are non-comedogenic. They typically come in liquid form, packaged in bottles. For example, Glo Skin Beauty oil-free camouflage.
- *Water-free or anhydrous foundations:* These foundations mix different oils (vegetable, mineral, lanolin alcohol, and synthetic esters) with waxes to create a cream, into which high concentrations of pigment are incorporated. Titanium dioxide, along with iron oxide and sometimes ultramarine blue, serve as the coloring agents. These foundations, which can be applied from a compact or stick, are waterproof and opaque, making them well-suited for cosmetic camouflage purposes.

Foundations are manufactured with various finishes, such as matte, semi-matte, moist semi-matte, and shiny. For cosmetic camouflage, matte-finish foundations are generally preferred. Foundations are also available in diverse forms such as liquid, mousse, water-containing cream, soufflé, anhydrous cream, stick, cake, and shake lotion. Most camouflage products are formulated as creams, as this allows for a higher concentration of iron oxide, enhancing coverage.

REVIEW OF CAMOUFLAGE TECHNIQUES

Among various camouflage techniques used over 19 years, liquidized simulated second skin technology (Microskin) has shown significant promise. This technology involves color matching and a spray/stippling application that binds to the skin's epidermis, addressing concerns about color, coverage, and application in camouflage bases. Two studies demonstrated that this innovative method boosted confidence, happiness, and social experiences in children and adolescents with burn scarring.

For example, an 8-week Microskin[TM] skin camouflaging program significantly improved quality of life, particularly in socialization and school appearance, for children with burn scars. Another study found that a 5-week Microskin[TM] program enhanced psychosocial functioning and family dynamics for children with mature burn scars. Microskin[TM] was applied approximately every 4 days, with 95% of participants expressing a desire to continue using it. Despite minor side effects such as skin itching, this method appears to be a promising treatment, helping children feel happier, more self-assured, and more comfortable in social situations. Overall, simulated second skin technology seems to be an important and effective therapy for individuals with skin disorders.

Microskin[TM] skin camouflage kit: The kit includes a camouflage solution (Microskin simulated second skin, 30 mL), fixing powder (Microseal powder, 30 g), removing serum, and a Microskin red rubber sponge. The solution typically lasts about 3 days, though it wears off more quickly on the hands or with rubbing, contact, washing, or use of alcohol-based products such as hand sanitizers.

Melanin extraction from hair for camouflage cream: Research is ongoing to develop camouflage creams using melanin extracted from a patient's hair. The process involves an acid-base method known as Bolt's procedure. Hair is cleaned with detergent, water, and acetone, then digested in 1M NaOH overnight. Concentrated HCl is added to precipitate a brown gum called crude melanoprotein, which is further purified through repeated cycles of base solubilization and acid precipitation. This yields a dark brown powder, representing approximately 4.8% of the original hair mass. The powder is then incorporated into colloidal carrier systems for better skin penetration. A portion of the hair is bleached with hydrogen peroxide to produce melanin in various shades of brown, which can be mixed to match the patient's skin tone. These melanin-loaded solid lipid nanoparticles (SLN) and nanostructural lipid carriers (NLC) are then used as camouflage creams or pigments for tattooing vitiliginous skin.[14]

INDICATIONS

Cosmetic camouflage has been used and studied for a number of pigmentary and disfiguring dermatoses as described in **Table 2**.[15-17]

TECHNIQUES OF CAMOUFLAGE APPLICATION

- *Selection of appropriate camouflage*:
  - *Color matching:* Always match the camouflage color directly on the patient's skin. Consider underlying tones that influence skin color—hemoglobin contributes red, keratin contributes yellow, and melanin contributes brown. Thinner skin has more red tones, while thicker skin appears more yellow, making it nearly impossible to mimic natural skin color with only one shade.
  - *Three color coordinates:*
    - *Hue:* It refers to the pure spectrum colors, commonly identified by names such as red, orange, yellow, blue, green, and violet. Each hue represents a different wavelength of reflected light, as seen in the color circle or rainbow.
    - *Value:* It defines the relative lightness or darkness of a color. Adding white to a hue results in a high-value color (tint), while adding black results in a low-value color (shade).
    - *Intensity (chroma or saturation)*: It refers to the brightness of a color. A color is at full intensity when not mixed with black or white—a pure hue. Intensity can be altered by adding gray, making the color duller or more neutral.
  - *Color matching challenges:* Matching colors from different manufacturers is difficult due to the variety of shades that can be created by combining

TABLE 2: Indications of cosmetic camouflage in dermatology.

Vascular lesions (LOE: 2B)	Pigmentary disorders (LOE: 2B)	Scars (LOE: 2B)	Chronic skin diseases	Transient postsurgical
• Vascular malformations (port-wine stains and hemangiomas) • Telangiectasias • Rosacea • Varicose veins	• Vitiligo (LE: 1B) • Post-inflammatory hyper/hypopigmentation • Melasma • Lentigines • Solar lentigo • Nevi • Café-au lait-spots • Periorbital hyperpigmentation • Tattoos	• Atrophic • Hypertrophic • Stretch marks • Burn scars (LOE: 1B)	• Acne • Acne (LOE: 2B) • Scleroderma • Lupus erythematosus (LOE: 1B)	• Laser • Dermabrasion • Chemical peels • Surgical procedures (rhytidectomy, rhinoplasty, etc.)

(LOE: level of evidence)

different colors and varying the amount of white. Always judge color on the skin, not in the container, as the appearance may differ.
- *Tools for application:*
  - *Application methods:* Camouflage products can be applied with a sponge, brush, or fingertips using a patting motion, which ensures that the product stays on the skin's surface without clogging pores, allowing the skin to retain its natural characteristics. Edges should be blended to eliminate distinct borders.
  - *Airbrush technique:* A specialized tool where a compressor sprays an ultrafine mist onto the skin, providing even coverage, especially useful for textured skin areas.
- *Pre-camouflage counseling:*
  - *Patient consultation:* Inquire about the patient's prior experience with camouflage creams and counsel them about the limitations of the product. Understand their expectations, hobbies, and outdoor activities. Check if any topical medication is being used that might affect skin color. Assess the skin texture and area involved thoroughly.
- *Stepwise application*:
  - *Preparation:* The area is cleaned with a gentle cleanser and patted dry.
  - *Color selection:* The camouflage shade is chosen based on the patient's skin tone. The product is warmed on the back of the hand to make it more malleable for easier application. If an exact match is not obtained with one shade, two or three shades can be mixed for a better match.
  - *Application:* The selected shade is applied onto the vitiligo lesion from the center outward using a sponge or fingertip in a patting motion to ensure that the product does not clog pores, allowing the skin to retain its natural characteristics. The edges are blended into the surrounding skin for a seamless cosmetic match.
  - *Setting the camouflage:* A fixing powder is applied with a sponge to set the makeup, prevent smudging, and make it waterproof. These powders typically contain talc (hydrated magnesium silicate) and pigments such as iron oxide, ultramarine, chrome oxide, and chrome hydrate. The powder should be translucent to avoid altering the color of the camouflage product. For patients with very dry skin, powder may be unnecessary as the oils are quickly absorbed. Alternatively, a fixing spray can be used. Excess powder is brushed off after 10 minutes.
- *Camouflage application considerations:*
  - *Selective application:* Camouflage is not usually applied over the entire face such as regular foundation; instead, it should closely match the surrounding skin. Different areas of the body may require different camouflage shades due to variations in skin tone.
- *Removal of the camouflage:*
  - *Cleansing:* Standard facial cleansing methods, such as using water and soap, are insufficient for removing oil-based camouflage makeup. A water-in-oil-based cleansing solution is recommended to break down

and dislodge the oil and wax coating. Afterward, a regular water and soap cleanse is recommended to fully clean the skin.

IMPACT OF COSMETIC CAMOUFLAGE ON QUALITY OF LIFE IN VITILIGO PATIENTS

- *Improvement in quality of life:*
  - Cosmetic camouflage has been shown to significantly enhance the quality of life in vitiligo patients, improving their appearance, and reducing the focus on skin discoloration, which in turn boosts confidence and self-esteem.
- *Qualitative improvement*:
  - A qualitative study by Pasterfield and colleagues[18] examined the experiences of individuals with visible skin conditions who used skin camouflage. The study found that camouflage helped participants feel more presentable and was closely linked to gender identity. For many, the use of camouflage became part of their routine, helping to reduce the avoidance of social situations and providing a sense of control.
  - The frequency of usage of cosmetic camouflage has been associated with increased confidence and decreased avoidance as assessed by Kent.[19]
- *Quantitative improvement*:
  - A cohort study involving 78 vitiligo patients conducted by Ongenae et al.[15] revealed that the Dermatology Life Quality Index (DLQI) scores improved after the use of camouflage. The study particularly noted improvements in feelings of embarrassment, self-consciousness, and clothing choices. The study recommended the use of camouflage for patients with higher DLQI scores, especially those with minor facial involvement.
  - Rao et al.[20] studied a cohort of 14 Indian patients with acrofacial vitiligo and reported similar significant improvement in quality-of-life scores as assessed with DLQI scores.
- *Author's experience:*
  - In a randomized controlled trial on patients with predominantly acrofacial vitiligo using cosmetic camouflage in addition to their ongoing medical treatment, the patients in the intervention arm reported significant improvement in DLQI and vitiligo impact scale (VIS-22) scores with high patient satisfaction scores as well. The use of cosmetic camouflage also led to significant reduction in participation restriction and stigmatization experienced by patients along with improvement in quality of life scores of family members as well. The camouflage product was effective and safe as an adjuvant treatment method.
- *Effectiveness in resistant areas:*
  - Vitiligo in certain body areas, such as acral regions (hands and feet), **(Figs. 1 and 2)** lips, elbows, and knees, often proves resistant to therapy. These areas can be effectively concealed using cosmetic camouflage.

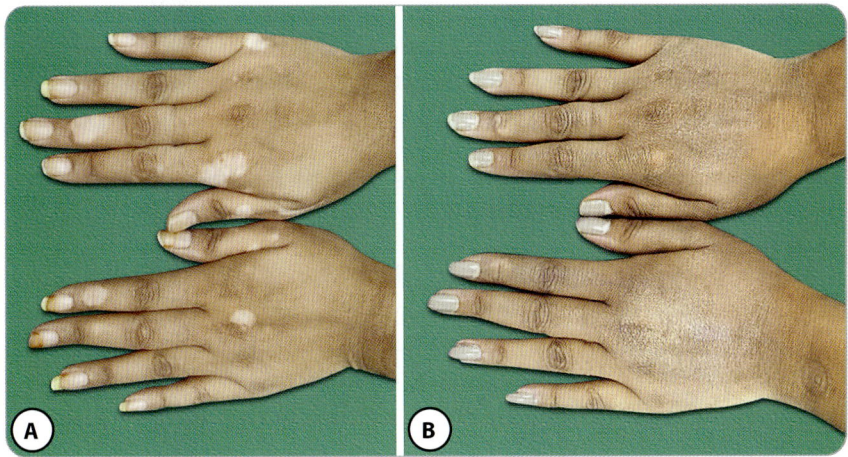

FIGS. 1A AND B: Vitiligo over hands (A) before and (B) after application of cosmetic camouflage.

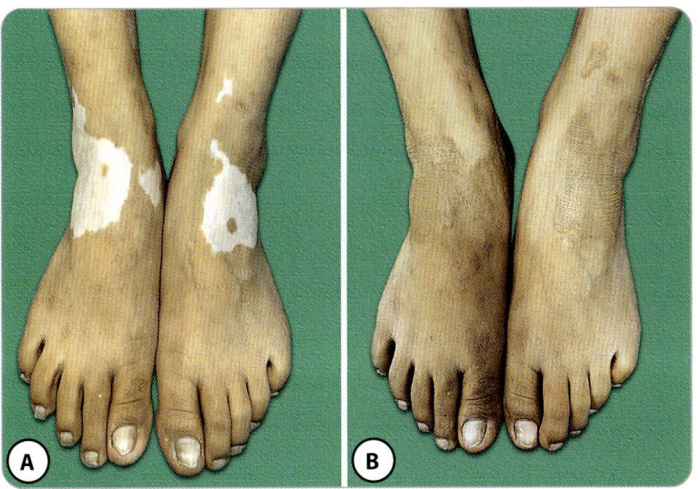

FIGS. 2A AND B: Vitiligo over feet (A) before and (B) after application of cosmetic camouflage.

PRACTICAL PEARLS FOR THE APPLICATION OF CAMOUFLAGE

When applying cosmetic camouflage, especially for conditions such as vitiligo, consider the following practical tips to ensure optimal results:
- *Skin tone variations*:
  - The face and other body areas often have different color tones, necessitating the use of various shades of camouflage. For extensive facial vitiligo, it may be necessary to replicate common skin imperfections to create a natural appearance and avoid a mask-like effect.

- *Application technique*:
  - Camouflage cream should be dabbed onto the skin, not rubbed. This method helps to maintain the product's integrity and ensures even coverage.
- *Feathering borders*:
  - After covering the lesion, the edges must be blended smoothly into the surrounding skin for a more natural look.
- *Mirror and lighting*:
  - The color matching as well as final application are best performed in a room with good lighting, and ideally, the cosmetic appearance must also be evaluated in natural daylight before finalizing the shade or product. It is ideal to use a mirror during the application process to assess patient satisfaction with the camouflage.
- *Blurring borders for large lesions*:
  - For larger vitiligo lesions, instead of covering the entire area, blurring the borders with the camouflage product to subtly reduce the contrast between the depigmented lesion and normal skin may be considered.
- *Sunscreen application*:
  - If the patient requires sunscreen, it should be applied before the camouflage cream, especially if the camouflage does not contain sunscreen.
- *Cleaning camouflage cream*:
  - An oily cleanser is ideal to remove the product and may be followed by soap and water cleansing. It is best to avoid using alcohol or acetone containing products due to their potential to irritate the skin.
- *Phototherapy considerations*:
  - Patients undergoing phototherapy must remove all camouflage cream before ultraviolet light treatment to ensure the effectiveness of the therapy. They can reapply the camouflage immediately after the phototherapy session and in our experience, patients have not found this to be a hindrance to camouflage use.
- *Enhancing facial features:*
  - Eye shadow, mascara, and eyeliner can be used to hide vitiligo on the eyelids and leukotrichia of the eyelashes. Lipstick can be applied to cover vitiligo on the lips.
- *Handling sweat and friction*:
  - Sweat or friction may cause camouflage creams to smudge or wear off, leading to anxiety or stress. To mitigate this, patients can apply henna or DHA (dihydroxyacetone) as a base to mask depigmentation, followed by a green and then brown camouflage cream for a natural look.

LIMITATIONS OF COSMETIC CAMOUFLAGE

- *Application challenges:*
  - It can be difficult to apply camouflage products over large surface areas, which may require significant time and effort.

CHAPTER 13

Vitiligo Future Trends and Diet

Samkit Shah, Mansi M Bhatt

INTRODUCTION

Vitiligo is one of the acquired disorders of pigmentation presented as well-defined depigmented macules or patches on our skin. Biopsies of the lesional skin show an absence of epidermal melanocytes.

Multiple theories have been proffered for melanocyte destruction, including genetic, viral, biochemical, autoimmune, and melanocyte detachment mechanisms.[1-3]

Current research data suggest that autoimmune conditions and oxidative stress are the main factors contributing to the destruction of melanocytes in vitiligo.[4,5] Oxidative stress may initiate the cycle of destruction of melanocytes.[4] An altered intracellular redox status and depletion of enzymatic and nonenzymatic antioxidants have been documented in the epidermis of patients with vitiligo.[6-8] Hence, the generation of reactive oxygen species (ROS) may begin the cycle of destruction of melanocytes in genetically susceptible individuals by activation of the innate and adaptive immune response.[1,2,6]

A variety of humoral and CMI (cell-mediated immunity) defects are reported in patients with vitiligo.[2,5,9] Multiple studies document the role of activated cytotoxic CD81 T lymphocytes and the interferon gamma (IFN-γ)-induced chemokine CXCL10 as key immune mediators of destruction of the melanocyte.[10-12] Thus, the interplay between immune system and oxidative stress may represent important pathways in vitiligo. It is a novel strategy to address the role of diet, lifestyle modifications, and oral vitamins, minerals, botanicals, etc., as adjunctive approaches in this therapeutically challenging condition.

ROLE OF DIET

A review of literature revealed no studies assessing the role of diet in the prevention and management of patients with vitiligo. There are multiple books, web sites, and nonmedical publications recommending unsubstantiated diets and supplements for all the autoimmune diseases, including vitiligo. In India, patients having vitiligo are advised to avoid citrus fruits, sour yogurt, vitamin C products, milk, and fish; however, this is not substantiated in controlled studies.[13,14]

Although, per se food may not appear to play an important role in vitiligo management, there are certain dietary recommendations based on the antioxidant, micronutrient, and vitamin composition of foods. For example, vegetable oils that are high in omega-6 may increase the production of ROS and proinflammatory cytokines that may play a role in vitiligo.[15,16]

Because many diets do not provide vitamins and minerals in enough quantities or types to take over the oxidative stress or modulate the immune system, there is increasing demand and need in supplementation.

Diet

- Gluten—many patients showed improvement after stopping gluten.
- Fatty acids—stopping a diet rich in fatty acids showed improvement in vitiligo lesions.
- *Alpha-lipoic acid*: It plays a role in biological mitochondrial reactions; it is also an antioxidant. In its reduced form, dihydrolipoate, it reacts with ROS, and protects the cell membranes with its involvement with vitamin C and E pathways. It has been shown to have some beneficial effects in oxidative stress models and several other clinical conditions characterized by inflammation.
- *Phenylalanine*: It is an amino acid which is shown to work as a potential treatment for vitiligo by playing a central regulatory role in melanin, catecholamine, and antibody synthesis, thus contributing to the hypotheses of autoimmune and neural theories of vitiligo pathogenesis.

ORAL SUPPLEMENTS[15-20]

- *Vitamin B12/folic acid*—DNA repair, synthesis, methylation of DNA
- *Vitamin C*:
    - Antioxidant
    - Immunomodulatory
- *Vitamin D*:
    - Melanocyte/keratinocyte growth and differentiation[21]
    - Inhibits T-cell activation
    - Increases melanogenesis
    - Immunomodulatory
- *Vitamin E*:
    - Free radical scavenger
    - Inhibits platelet coagulation
    - Antioxidant/anti-inflammatory
- *Zinc*:
    - Antioxidant
    - Regulates gene expression
    - Cofactor for superoxide dismutase

- *Cost:*
  - High-quality camouflage products are often expensive, making them less accessible for some patients.
- *Smudging and wear-off:*
  - Camouflage creams are prone to smudging or wearing off, especially on the hands and feet due to friction.
- *Suitability issues:*
  - Application can be challenging in patients with open lesions, severe acne, or infectious skin conditions, as these issues can interfere with the smooth application of the product.

CONCLUSION

Camouflage is an underutilized modality in the management of vitiligo. However, there is sufficient data to show that it has the potential to significantly improve quality of life and self-esteem in vitiligo patients. Enhancing physician and patient awareness regarding this modality can offer a ray of hope for patients with vitiligo lesions on visible sites, especially those that are particularly resistant to medical and surgical treatments.

REFERENCES

1. Krüger C, Schallreuter KU. A review of the worldwide prevalence of vitiligo in children/adolescents and adults. Int J Dermatol. 2012;5:1206-12.
2. Shajil EM, Agrawal D, Vagadia K, Marfatia YS, Begum R. Vitiligo: clinical profiles in Vadodara, Gujarat. Indian J Dermatol. 2006;51:100.
3. Obioha O, Heath C, Grimes PE. Vitiligo and Skin of Color. In: Picardo M, Taïeb A (Eds). Vitiligo, 2nd edition. Cham.: Springer; 2019. pp. 153-61.
4. Kent G, al-Abadie M. Factors affecting responses on Dermatology Life Quality Index items among vitiligo sufferers. Clin Exp Dermatol. 1996;21:330-3.
5. Porter J, Beuf AH, Lerner A, Nordlund J. Response to cosmetic disfigurement: patients with vitiligo. Cutis. 1987;39:493-4.
6. Porter JR, Beuf AH, Lerner A, Nordlund J. Psychosocial effect of vitiligo: a comparison of vitiligo patients with "normal" control subjects, with psoriasis patients, and with patients with other pigmentary disorders. J Am Acad Dermatol. 1986;15:220-4.
7. Renzi C, Picardi A, Abeni D, Agostini E, Baliva G, Pasquini P, et al. Association of dissatisfaction with care and psychiatric morbidity with poor treatment compliance. Arch Dermatol. 2002;138:337-42.
8. Boehncke WH, Ochsendorf F, Paeslack I, Kaufmann R, Zollner TM. Decorative cosmetics improve the quality of life in patients with disfiguring skin diseases. Eur J Dermatol. 2002;12:577-80.
9. Parsad D, Pandhi R, Dogra S, Kanwar AJ, Kumar B. Dermatology Life Quality Index score in vitiligo and its impact on the treatment outcome. Br J Dermatol. 2003;148:373-4.
10. Bouloc A. Camouflage Techniques. In: Draelos ZD (Ed). Cosmetic Dermatology: Products and Procedures, 2nd edition. Oxford, UK: John Wiley & Sons; 2015. pp. 186-92.
11. Westmore MG. Camouflage and makeup preparations. Clin Dermatol. 2001;19:406-12.
12. Guichard S, Roulier V. Facial foundation. In: Draelos ZD (Ed). Cosmetic dermatology: products and procedures. Hoboken, NJ, USA: John Wiley & Sons; 2022. pp. 177-85.
13. Draelos ZD. Colored facial cosmetics. Dermatol Clin. 2000;18:621-31.

14. Gupta S, Olsson MJ, Parsad D, Lim HW, van Geel N, Pandya AG (Eds). Vitiligo: medical and surgical management. John Wiley & Sons; 2018.
15. Ongenae K, Dierckxsens L, Brochez L, van Geel N, Naeyaert JM. Quality of life and stigmatization profile in a cohort of vitiligo patients and effect of the use of camouflage. Dermatology. 2005;210:279-85.
16. Araviiskaia E, Le Pillouer Prost A, Kosmadaki M, Kerob D, Roo E. Recommendations for the use of corrective makeup after dermatological procedures. J Cosmet Dermatol. 2022;21:1554-8.
17. Antoniou C, Stefanaki C. Cosmetic camouflage. J Cosmet Dermatol. 2006;5:297-301.
18. Pasterfield M, Clarke SA, Thompson AR. A qualitative examination of the experience of skin camouflage by people living with visible skin conditions. Br J Dermatol. 2019;180:1531-2.
19. Kent G. Testing a model of disfigurement: effects of a skin camouflage service on well-being and appearance anxiety. Psychol Health. 2002;17:377-86.
20. Rao PN, Vellala M, Potharaju AR, Kiran U. Cosmetic camouflage of visible skin lesions enhances life quality indices in leprosy as in vitiligo patients: An effective stigma reduction strategy. Lepr Rev. 2020;91:343-52.

HERBAL SUPPLEMENTS

- *Phyllanthus emblica*:
    - Antioxidant
    - Anti-inflammatory
    - Antimicrobial
    - Antiviral
- *Ginkgo biloba*:
    - Antioxidant
    - Anti-inflammatory
    - Platelet-activating factor antagonist
- *Polypodium leucotomos*:
    - Protection
    - Antioxidant
    - Inhibition of apoptosis
    - Immune modulation
    - Decreases proinflammatory cytokines
- *Piperine (animal studies)*:
    - Melanocyte replication
    - Induces formation of melanocytic dendrites
    - *Green tea (epigallocatechin-3-gallate)*:
        - Antioxidant
        - Anti-inflammatory
        - Antiatherogenesis
        - Anticancer
- *Capsaicin*: It is an ingredient found in hot chili pepper and commonly used in spices, food additives, and drugs.
    - Antioxidant
    - Inhibits apoptosis by inhibiting caspase activation and increased total antioxidant capacity.
- *Nigella sativa seed oil*: It is an annual flowering plant that produces black seeds (black cumin) whose oil extracts have been used for a variety of skin disorders. Its major component is the thymoquinone, which has been studied as the major component providing many medicinal properties.
    - Anti-inflammatory
    - Anticancer
    - Immunomodulating agent
- *Picrorhiza kurroa*: It is a well-known Ayurvedic herb, traditionally known as Kutki.
    - Hepatoprotective properties
    - Immunomodulating effects on cell-mediated and humoral immunity
    - Active ingredient apocynin—an effective antioxidant by inhibiting NADPH oxidase in neutrophils and microglia.
- *Khellin*: Khellin is a crystalline extract of herb *Ammi visnaga*. When it is combined with ultraviolet (UV) therapy,
    - Stimulate melanogenesis and melanocyte proliferation

PLANT-DERIVED COMPOUNDS

- *Flavonoids*:
  - Baicalein:
    - It is a flavonoid extracted from the roots of *Scutellaria baicalensis*, Georgi.
    - Strong antioxidant properties—scavenges ROS by oxidative consumption of the three 5, 6, 7-position OH–groups—form stable semiquinone radicals—powerful antioxidant activity.
  - Quercetin:
    - It is a type of polyhydroxy flavonoid, which is chemically named 3,3,4,5,7-pentahydroxyflavone.
    - It has high content in apple, onion, and green tea, *Asparagus racemosus*.
    - One of the most consumed flavonoids in people's daily diet.
      » Antioxidant and scavenging free radicals
      » Anticancer
      » Antiaging
      » Anti-inflammatory
      » Antiviral and antibacterial
      » Immune regulation
      » Reducing lipid levels
  - Kaempferol: It is a type of flavonoid, which mainly comes from the rhizome of *Kaempferia galanga L*. It widely exists in all kinds of fruits, vegetables and beverages, hazelnut, tea, propolis, broccoli, and grapefruit.
- Apigenin
- Galangin
- Naringenin and hesperetin
- Afzelin
- Fisetin
- Puerarin
- Butin
- Liquiritin and liquiritigenin
- Vitexin
- Hyperoside
- Baicalin
- Polyphenol
- Epigallocatechin-3-gallate
- Cannabidiol
- 1,5-dicaffeoylquinic acid
- 3,5-diCQA

The **Figure 1** shows nanodrug delivery system in the treatment of vitiligo.

One of the biggest challenges of transdermal delivery to treat conditions, such as vitiligo is that only a few therapeutic compounds possess an ideal penetration behavior and characteristics. The best technology also only allows drugs with a molecular mass of 100 Da and good lipophilicity to permeate through the skin. Also, another obstacle to achieve the desired therapeutic effects is incompetence

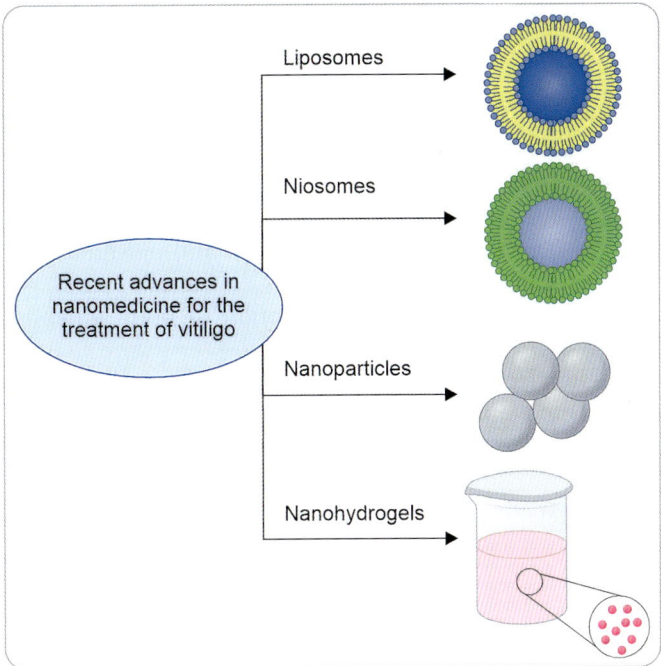

FIG. 1: Nanodrug delivery system in the treatment of vitiligo.

of current dosage forms, such as creams, ointments, lotions, gels, and other vectors. Generally, all the issues associated with conventional topical preparations suggest the reform and innovation of transdermal drug delivery for the treatment of vitiligo.

Recent advancements in cutting-edge nanotechnology provide a great opportunity to overcome short-comings related to conventional methods **(Fig. 1)**.

By taking advantage of the properties of the stratum corneum, there is a potential for use of a nanodrug delivery system that can enhance the transdermal penetration of drugs and increase their therapeutic effects. A large number of nanodrug delivery systems carrying therapeutic agents are being developed, such as liposomes, polymeric nanoparticles, microspheres, solid lipid nanoparticles, and nanofibrous structures.

- Liposomes—8-methoxypsoralen
- Deformable liposomes—baicalin and berberine
- Deformable liposomes—resveratrol and psoralen
- Cationic niosomes—human tyrosinase plasmid in mouse melanoma cells by Tat peptide
- Cationic niosomes—tyrosinase plasmid pMEL
- Microemulsion-based gel—clobetasol propionate
- Nanosized ethosomes-based hydrogel—8-methoxypsoralen
- Nanoparticles—palladium and platinum
- Nanoparticles—polydopamine

Principles of Nanodrug Delivery Systems Designed for Vitiligo Therapy

Enhancing the Penetrate Capacity of Therapeutic Agents

Similarities between lipid particles and the stratum corneum make liposomes excellent vectors for delivery of therapeutics. Conventional liposomes are thought to be inadequate for transdermal delivery, but more advanced liposomes, such as invasomes, transferosomes, ethosomes, and niosomes can overcome disadvantages seen with original methods.
- Invasomes enhance transdermal absorption of both aqueous and lipid-soluble drugs.
- Ethosomes—smaller particle size; fusion with skin lipids and increase the penetration of ethosomes
- Niosomes—a greater bioavailability; more stable than liposomes in oxidizing environment
- Transfersomes greatly improve the deformability and elasticity of the carriers; migrate into deeper skin layers.

JAK Inhibitors

Surgical interventions:
- Thin skin grafting
- Punch grafting
- Suction blister grafting
- Follicular unit transplantation
- Noncultured epidermal cell suspension transplantation
- Noncultured hair follicle cell suspension transplantation
- Cultured epidermal suspension transplantation
- Jodhpur technique

Transcutaneous Drug Delivery and Repigmentation by Fractional CO_2 Laser

Fractional CO_2 laser has been introduced as an add-on treatment for vitiligo.

Mechanism of action—various cytokines and growth factors are released during wound repair. Thus, fractional CO_2 may help induce melanocyte migration during the inflammation and the healing phases. It also increases IL-4, IL-10, IL-17, and IL-23 levels, which demonstrates the restoration of the Th balance of the immune system.

Combination Drugs of Fractional CO_2 Laser Therapy

This is effective in recalcitrant, acral, and vitiligo on bony prominences.
- 5-fluorouracil (5-FU) is used for skin tumors, which may improve melanocyte migration through activation of the CXCL12/CXCR4 axis. Patient was asked to apply 5% 5-FU cream for five days consecutively following every laser treatment session.

- Bimatoprost is a prostaglandin F2α analog, which is seen to improve cutaneous pigmentation by activating the prostaglandin F receptor and melanosome uptake by the keratinocytes. The bimatoprost 0.01% solution is prepared by dissolving bimatoprost powder in an ethanol/water base. Apply one drop over the treatment area of 4 cm², twice a day for 12 weeks. Conducting three sessions of fractional CO_2 laser at monthly intervals was seen to be effective in repigmentation.
- Platelet-rich plasma (PRP) is effective in healing and regeneration since it contains a variety of mitogenic/chemotactic growth factors and stimulates the process of melanogenesis.

Promotion of Melanocytes and Melanocyte Stem Cell Activation

- *Afamelanotide*: Alpha melanocyte-stimulating hormone (α-MSH) is a critical regulatory protein that promotes melanogenesis and melanocyte proliferation. Afamelanotide is a potent α-MSH analog, which is reported to be an effective treatment option for vitiligo. Subcutaneous implants have shown to increase the repigmentation rate and total area for vitiligo patients treated with NB-UVB.
- *Mesenchymal stem cells*: They maintain the immune homeostasis of the local environment. They have been found to promote melanocyte proliferation and show antiapoptosis property by targeting the phosphatase and tensin homolog/phosphatidylinositol 3 kinase/protein kinase B pathway.
- *Adipose tissue extracellular fraction*: It is detected to ameliorate the capability to counteract oxidative stress and activate the Wnt/β-catenin pathway. Microinjury caused by fractional laser has been identified to improve the pigmentation in vitiligo via the Wnt/β-catenin pathway.

Promising advanced therapy medicinal products (ATMPs) for the treatment of vitiligo, new comings:
- Mesenchymal stromal cells (MSCs)
- Induced pluripotent stem cells
- Multilineage differentiating stress enduring cells

FUTURE DEVELOPMENTS IN VITILIGO

Ritlecitinib

Vitiligo is an autoimmune condition characterized by depigmentation of skin, hair, or both together.

In patients having vitiligo, the CD8+ T cells attack the melanocytes, which result in nonscaly chalky-white depigmented lesions.

This leads to an abnormal adaptive immune response from the cytotoxic CD8+ T cells and produces cytokines typical of T helper Types 1, 2, and 17 (Th1, Th2, and Th17) immune responses, including IFN-γ The Th1 and Th2 immune responses thus activate the Janus kinase/signal transducers and activators of transcription (JAK/STAT) pathway, in turn leading to increased levels of IFN-γ, that drives decreased melanocyte adhesion.

Additionally, chemokines, such as C-X-C motif chemokine ligand (CXCL) 9, CXCL10, and CXCL11 are released, leading to a positive feedback loop.[22]

In multiple studies over the past few years, patients with active lesions (compared to patients with stable lesions) showed decreased blood regulatory T cells (Tregs) and CD4+/CD8+ T-cell ratio, increased serum CXCL9 and CXCL10, increased serum CCL20, CD8+ T cells and expression of E-cadherin in the epidermis and dermis, increased CXCL10 in perilesional skin and raised CXCL9 and CXCL10 in suction blister fluid. These findings indicate that active and stable lesions display different profiles of immune cells and activation of the JAK/STAT pathway.

The new and interesting observation of the JAK/STAT pathway inhibition downstream the disease-associated cytokines, such as IFN-γ can be used as a potential treatment for vitiligo and resulted in several clinical trials, thus having an of ruxolitinib cream, a topical JAK1/2 inhibitor for the treatment of nonsegmental vitiligo (NSV).

Ritlecitinib is an oral selective inhibitor of JAK3 and the tyrosine kinase expressed in hepatocellular carcinoma (TEC) family kinases, which is approved for treatment of alopecia areata. It is currently under investigation for the treatment of nonsegmental vitiligo. In a phase 2b trial (NCT03715829), ritlecitinib demonstrated significant improvement in the Facial Vitiligo Area Scoring Index and immune and melanocyte biomarkers at week 24 in patients with active NSV.

Dose: Daily 50 mg (with or without 4-week 100-mg or 200-mg loading dose), 30 mg, or 10 mg for 24 weeks.

At week 24, 50 mg significantly stabilized the mean percent change from baseline in depigmentation extent in both active lesions and stable lesions.

After 24 weeks of treatment, 50 mg increased the expression of melanocyte markers in stable lesions, while Th1/Th2-related and costimulatory molecules decreased significantly in both stable and active lesions.

Vitilinex

Vitilinex® consists of two products—(1) skin prep lotion (containing—*Centipeda cunninghamii*, aloe vera, terpinen-4-ol, and dihydroavenanthramide D) and (2) emollient (containing black cumin seed oil, black pepper *Coleus forskohlii*, *Psoralea corylifolia*, thyme oil, myrrh and neroli extracts. These oil extracts have shown to have very strong antioxidant properties.[23]

The skin prep lotion was applied to the affected areas and allowed to dry, followed by the application of the emollient. The area was then irradiated weekly week over 12 weeks at 311 nm, with a starting dose of 20% less than the minimal erythema dose (MED) for each patient, evaluated on a vitiliginous lesion seven days before the start of treatment. The irradiation dose was progressively increased by 20%. In cases where erythema was noted, we reduced the dose by 20% in the following treatment.

Centipeda cunninghamii in the prep lotion, contains caffeic acid and sesquiterpene lactones, having strong anti-inflammatory and antioxidant activity.

Terpinol-4-on, a potent constituent of tea tree oil, possesses antioxidant and anti-inflammatory properties by suppressing superoxide production and proinflammatory cytokines—tumor necrosis factor alpha (TNF-α), interleukin 1β (IL-1β), IL-8, IL-10, and prostaglandin E2 (PGE2).

The antioxidant benefit of aloe vera is well documented and believed to impart its benefit in vitiligo treatment by inhibiting cyclooxygenase 2 (COX2) and PGE2 whilst dihydroavenanthramide D has been shown to prevent UV-irradiated generation of ROS and expression of matrix metalloproteinase-1 and -3 in human dermal fibroblasts at 5 ppm.

Black cumin seed oil (*Nigella sativa*), used in the embodiment, contains thymoquinone which has been shown to induce melanin production and dispersion. Piperine, from Piper nigrum, and its synthetic analogs, have been shown to stimulate mouse and human melanocyte proliferation. Thyme oil, myrrh, and neroli extracts have shown to have very strong antioxidant properties in cell culture studies.

The repigmentation in vitiligo is believed to be linked to a synergistic effect of all the antioxidant action of these herbal bioactives. The availability of any new treatment that can reduce the use of UVB from high to low, and still be efficacious, is of immense benefit to both patients and treating physicians

ReCell

It is a patented kit for transferring cells from the donor site to the recipient site. The major difference between the ReCell technique and conventional cellular transplantation techniques is the use of a sodium lactate which is patented as a cell delivery system and for dilution of the cell suspension, which gives a donor/recipient ratio of about 1:80. It is thought that this medium plays an important role in both survival and multiplication of the pigment cells.

JACE

It is an epidermal-derived cell sheet which was used in Japan Pharmaceuticals and Medical Devices Agency (PMDA) in 2007 for vitiligo. This product has also been used for treating giant congenital melanocytic nevus (GCMN). It is reported that most of the grafts survived, and the dark brown color of the nevus lightened significantly. Also, its application was seen to contribute to the patients survival up to seven weeks after burns.

Renewcell

Administrating cell-based products, such as autologous melanocytes for the treatment of vitiligo has been associated with great results in the recent decades. In addition, given the immunomodulatory properties of MSCs, cell-based therapies are a potential targeted therapy for patients having vitiligo. It is shown that MSCs can ameliorate the underlying pathology of vitiligo through regulating phosphatase, tensin homolog (PTEN) expression, and improving melanocyte proliferation in experimental models. Transplantation of cultured melanocytes or noncultured melanocytes–keratinocytes has been used for cell-based therapies in clinical settings. Autologous cell-based products were firstly used by Guerra et al. in a clinical trial in 2003 and associated with significant repigmentation rate in stable lesions. In Iran, cell-based therapy for vitiligo was firstly conducted at Royan institute through intraepidermal transplantation of autologous epidermal cells in suspension for 10 vitiligo patients in 2010. This study associated with no side effects and significant repigmentation in 40% of patients with mild-to-moderate repigmentation in the other patients. The second study in Royan institute that assessed the long-term efficacy of autologous epidermal cells transplantation in 300 patients with stable vitiligo published in 2018, associated with effective repigmentation (>50%) in almost 30% of the patients in the majority of treated patches over the 36 months follow-up. These two clinical trials suggested the safety and efficacy of this innovative cell-based approach and this product called ReColorCell®.

In February 6th, 2018, Cell Tech Pharmed™ Co. applied ReColorCell® as a novel cellular/gene-based therapeutic product to be registered in the Iranian drug list (IDL). Production line and process of this live cell-based product was already GMP-certified by IR-FDA at Cell Tech Pharmed™ Co.

REFERENCES

1. Alikhan A, Felsten LM, Daly M, Petronic-Rosic V. Vitiligo: A comprehensive overview Part I. Introduction, epidemiology, quality of life, diagnosis, differential diagnosis, associations, histopathology, etiology, and work-up. J Am Acad Dermatol. 2011;65:473-91.
2. Rodrigues M, Ezzedine K, Hamzavi I, Pandya AG, Harris JE; Vitiligo Working Group. New discoveries in the pathogenesis and classification of vitiligo. J Am Acad Dermatol. 2017;77:1-13.
3. Speeckaert R, van Geel N. Vitiligo: An update on pathophysiology and treatment options. Am J Clin Dermatol. 2017;18:733-44.
4. Lerner AB. Vitiligo. J Invest Dermatol. 1959;32(Part 2):285-310.
5. Al'Abadie MS, Senior HJ, Bleehen SS, Gawkrodger DJ. Neuropeptide and neuronal marker studies in vitiligo. Br J Dermatol. 1994;131:160-5.
6. Morrone A, Picardo M, de Luca C, Terminali O, Passi S, Ippolito F. Catecholamines and vitiligo. Pigment Cell Res. 1992;5:65-9.
7. Wu CS, Yu HS, Chang HR, Yu CL, Yu CL, Wu BN. Cutaneous blood flow and adrenoceptor response increase in segmental-type vitiligo lesions. J Dermatol Sci. 2000;23:53-62.
8. Malhotra N, Dytoc M. The pathogenesis of vitiligo. J Cutan Med Surg. 2013;17:153-72.
9. Khan R, Satyam A, Gupta S, Sharma VK, Sharma A. Circulatory levels of antioxidants and lipid peroxidation in Indian patients with generalized and localized vitiligo. Arch Dermatol Res. 2009;301:731-7.
10. Gauthier Y, Cario Andre M, Taieb A. A critical appraisal of vitiligo etiologic theories. Is melanocyte loss a mela- nocytorrhagy? Pigment Cell Res. 2003;16:322-32.
11. Adotama P, Zapata L, Jr, Currimbhoy S, Hynan LS, Pandya AG. Patient satisfaction with different treatment modalities for vitiligo. J Am Acad Dermatol. 2015;72:732–3.
12. Jadad AR, Moore RA, Carroll D, Jenkinson C, Reynolds DJ, Gavaghan DJ, et al. Assessing the quality of reports of randomized clinical trials: Is blinding necessary? Control Clin Trials. 1996;17:1-12.
13. Dutta RR, Kumar T, Ingole N. Diet and Vitiligo: The Story So Far. Cureus. 2022;14(8):e28516.
14. Di Nardo V, Barygina V, França K, Tirant M, Valle Y, Lotti T. Functional nutrition as integrated approach in vitiligo management. Dermatol Ther. 2019;32:e12625.

15. Shipton MJ, Thachil J. Vitamin B12 deficiency—a 21st century perspective Clin Med (Lond). 2015;15:145-50.
16. Carmel R. How I treat cobalamin (vitamin B12) deficiency. Blood. 2008;112:2214-21.
17. Antony AC. Vegetarianism and vitamin B-12 (cobalamin) deficiency. J Clin Nutr. 2003;78:3-6.
18. Carr AC, Maggini S. Vitamin C and immune function. Nutrients. 2017;9(11):1211.
19. Pullar JM, Carr AC, Vissers MC. The roles of vitamin C in skin health. Nutrients. 2017;9(8):866.
20. AlGhamdi K, Kumar A, Moussa N. The role of vitamin D in melanogenesis with an emphasis on vitiligo. Indian J Dermatol Venereol Leprol. 2013;79:750-8.
21. Prietl B, Treiber G, Pieber TR, Amrein K. Vitamin D and immune function. Nutrients. 2013;5:2502-21.
22. Ezzedine K, Peeva E, Yamaguchi Y, Cox LA, Banerjee A, Han G, et al. Efficacy and safety of oral ritlecitinib for the treatment of active nonsegmental vitiligo: A randomized phase 2b clinical trial. J Am Acad Dermatol. 2023;88(2):395-403.
23. Van TN, Minh TT, Huu DL, Huu SN, Thanh TV, Huu ND, et al. Successful Treatment of Vitiligo Vietnamese Patients with Vitilinex® Herbal Bio-Actives in Combination with Phototherapy. Open Access Maced J Med Sci. 2019;7(2):283-6.

14A CHAPTER

Resources: Guidelines for Practitioners—Algorithmic Approach

Neha Akhoon

INTRODUCTION

Vitiligo is classified into various types, depending upon its clinical characteristics and distribution patterns, which also determines its management. A correct assessment of disease activity, vitiligo extent and involved sites is crucial to frame patient expectations concerning the natural evolution and treatment results. This chapter is presented as a review of the guidelines with highlighted recommendations on how to approach a patient of vitiligo.

- *Undertake a comprehensive history*:[1]
    - Age of onset
    - Stability/progression of disease
    - Speed of onset
    - Triggering factors
    - Psychological/psychosocial impact
    - Personal/family history: Thyroid dysfunction/autoimmune diseases
- *Examination*:
    - Classification of lesions (site and type)
    - Disease extent [body surface area (BSA) affected]
    - Skin phototype
    - Wood's lamp examination
- *Assess and monitor quality of life (QoL) and level of psychological distress*:
    - *General measures*: Patient Health Questionnaires (PHQ-4 and PHQ-9) and Dermatological Life Quality Index (DLQI)
    - *Targeted approach*: Vitiligo Impact Patient Scale (VIPS) and Vitiligo-specific QoL scale (VitiQoL)
- Take *clinical photographs* on first visit and on follow-up visits for monitoring
- *Investigations*:
    - Measure vitamin D levels for those avoiding sun-exposure
    - Evaluate for thyroid disorder (antithyroid antibodies), pernicious anemia, and Addison's disease
- *Management of vitiligo: Define the goal of treatment* which can be—
    - Stabilization
    - Repigmentation
    - Depigmentation

- *Counseling of the patient:*
  - Discuss the expectations of the patient and prognosis (shared decision)
  - Discuss the disease impact and regarding treatment (onset of action, duration of treatment, and adverse effects)

CLASSIFICATION OF THE LESIONS (FLOWCHART 1)

- *Nonsegmental vitiligo (NSV):*
  - Acrofacial
  - Mucosal (>1 mucosal site)
  - Generalized
  - Universal
  - Mixed [associated with segmental vitiligo (SV)]
  - Rare variants
- *Segmental vitiligo:*
  - Unisegmental
  - Bisegmental
  - Plurisegmental
- *Undetermined/unclassified:*
  - Focal
  - Mucosal (one site)

In the recent clinical guidelines, there has been emphasis on shared decisions between the patient and the treating physician regarding the treatment of vitiligo, keeping in consideration the skin type of the patient, disease duration, presence of comorbidities, and extent of disease including visible/sensitive areas and geographical region **(Flowcharts 2 and 3)**.

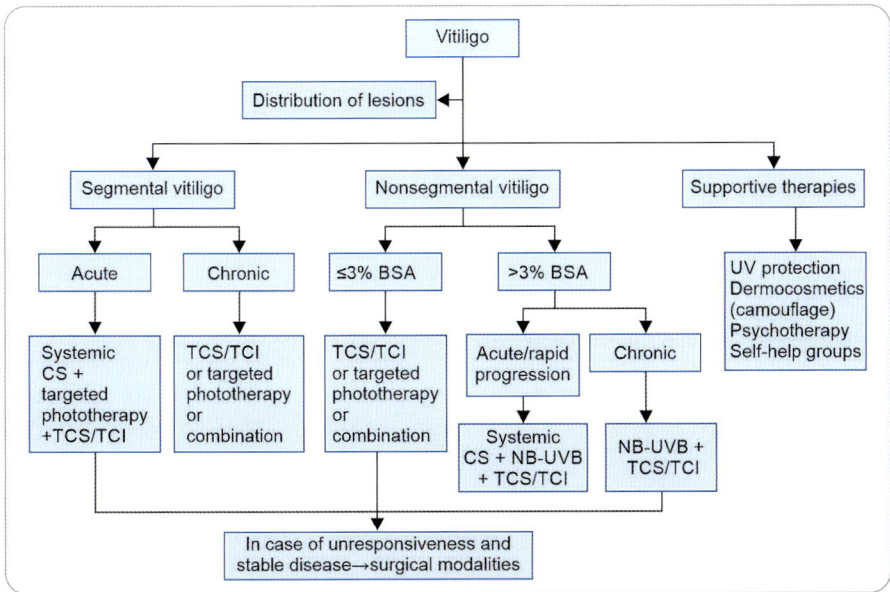

FLOWCHART 1: Simplified overview of therapeutic algorithm for vitiligo.[2,3]

(BSA: body surface area; CS: corticosteroid; TCS: topical corticosteroid; TCI: topical calcineurin inhibitor; NB-UVB: narrowband ultraviolet B)

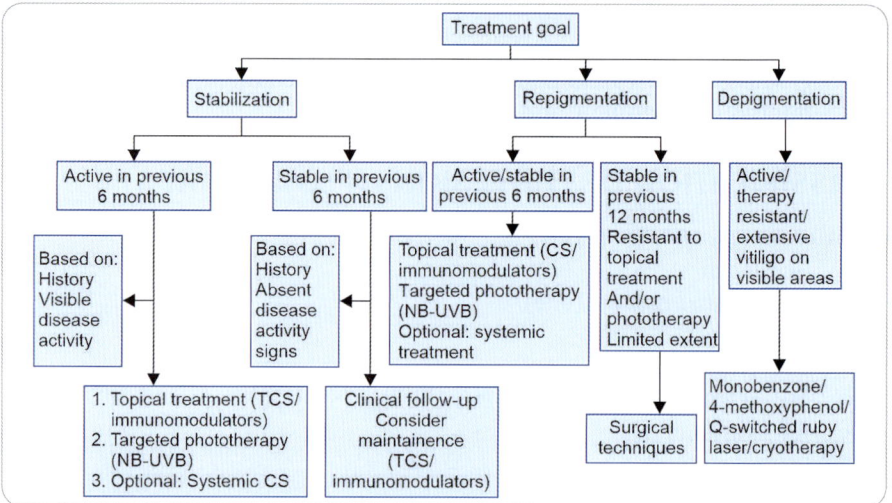

FLOWCHART 2: Treatment guideline for nonsegmental vitiligo.
(CS: corticosteroid; NB-UVB: narrowband ultraviolet B)

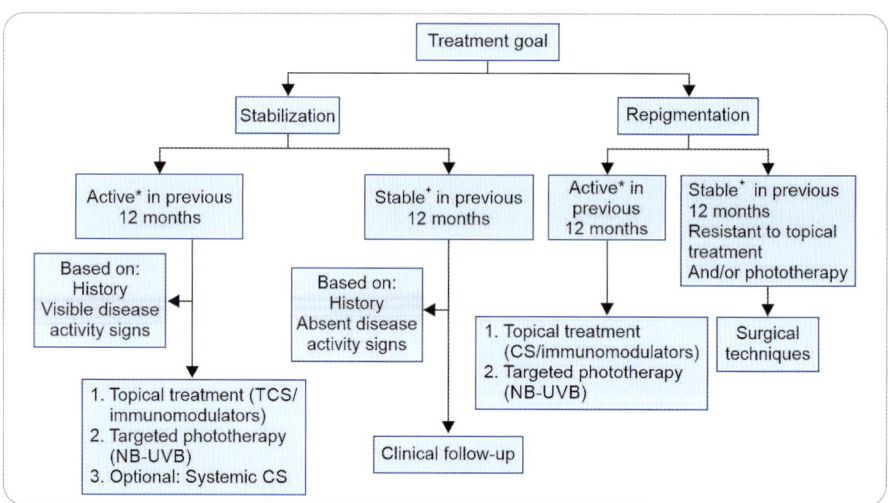

*Active lesions: New lesions or increase in number and extent of existing lesions.
+Stable lesions: No new lesions or no increase in number and extent of existing lesions.

FLOWCHART 3: Treatment guideline for segmental vitiligo.

Note:
Disease activity signs: Clear presence of confetti-like depigmentation, hypochromic borders, and areas of Koebner's phenomenon.

(CS: corticosteroid; TCS: topical corticosteroid; NB-UVB: narrowband ultraviolet B)

It is pertinent to explain to the patients regarding the relation between location and expected results: best to worse results are expected on the face > other body sites > hands/feet. Also, explain the expectations and limitations of therapy.

Other immunosuppressants, such as methotrexate, cyclosporine, azathioprine, and minocycline, are discussed. The lack of studies with robust methodology for most of these drugs/combinations is mentioned **(Table 1)**.

TABLE 1: Various treatment modalities for vitiligo.[4,5]

Type of vitiligo	Subtype	First line	Second line	Third line	Fourth line	Other modalities
NSV	Localized	• Once daily TCS for up to 3 months (continuous/intermittent) • *Head and neck:* Twice daily TCI initially for up to 6 months	• Localized phototherapy (NB-UVB) • Excimer lamp/laser	Surgical techniques (if Koebner phenomenon is negative)		• UV protection • Dermatocosmetics (camouflage-self-tanning agents, dermal pigmentation, cosmetic tattoos) • Psychotherapy
	Generalized	NB-UVB therapy for maximum of 1–2 years (if no response after 3 months → stop)	• Oral psoralen + UVA (PUVA) • Phototherapy + potent TCS/TCI	*Surgical treatment if:* • Nonresponsive to other treatment modalities (no repigmentation) • Stable • Negative Koebner phenomenon *Combination therapy:* Phototherapy 3–4 weeks after surgical procedure (to enhance repigmentation)	*Depigmentation therapy, if:* • Nonresponding to other treatment modalities • Widespread BSA (>70%) • Highly visible recalcitrant areas like face/hands • Positive Koebner phenomenon *With:* • Monobenzone • 4-methoxy phenol • Q-switched ruby laser • Cryotherapy	
	Rapidly progressive disease	*Oral minipulse (OMP) therapy:* • Betamethasone 0.1 mg/kg weekly 2 consecutive days × 3 months → decrease dose by 1 mg/month × 3 months • Equivalent dose of alternative oral CS: Dexamethasone/prednisolone/methylprednisolone				
	NSV stable for 6 months	• Clinical follow-up • Maintenance treatment: TCS/TCI at least twice a week for 6 months				

Continued

Continued

Type of vitiligo	Subtype	First line	Second line	Third line	Fourth line	Other modalities
SV		• Once daily TCS for up to 3 months (continuous/ intermittent) • Head and neck: Twice daily TCI initially for up to 6 months OMP (not mentioned in the guidelines for SV) can be given	• Localized NB-UVB • Excimer lamp/ laser	*Surgical techniques if:* • Stabilization without repigmentation • Negative Koebner		• Avoid triggering factors • Camouflage
	SV stable for 12 months	• *For goal of stabilization:* Only follow-up • *For goal of repigmentation and resistance to topical treatment and/or phototherapy:* Surgical techniques				

(NB-UVB: narrowband ultraviolet B; NSV: nonsegmental vitiligo; SV: segmental vitiligo; TCI: topical calcineurin inhibitor; TCS: topical corticosteroid)

CONCLUSION

These algorithms are intended to guide decision-making in clinical practice. The treatment goal should be clearly discussed with the patients, given the different approaches for disease stabilization and repigmentation. The evaluation of disease activity remains a cornerstone in the tailor-made approach to treat vitiligo patients.

REFERENCES

1. Eleftheriadou V, Atkar R, Batchelor J, McDonald B, Novakovic L, Patel JV, et al. British Association of Dermatologists guidelines for the management of people with vitiligo 2021. Br J Dermatol. 2022;186(1):18-29.
2. van Geel N, Speeckaert R, Taïeb A, Ezzedine K, Lim HW, Pandya AG, et al. Worldwide expert recommendations for the diagnosis and management of vitiligo: Position statement from the International Vitiligo Task Force Part 1: towards a new management algorithm. J Eur Acad Dermatol Venereol. 2023;37(11):2173-84.
3. Seneschal J, Speeckaert R, Taïeb A, Wolkerstorfer A, Passeron T, Pandya AG, et al. Worldwide expert recommendations for the diagnosis and management of vitiligo: Position statement from the international Vitiligo Task Force—Part 2: Specific treatment recommendations. J Eur Acad Dermatol Venereol. 2023;37(11):2185-95.
4. Marzano AV, Alberti-Violetti S, Maronese CA, Avallone G, Jommi C. Vitiligo: Unmet Need, Management and Treatment Guidelines. Dermatol Pract Concept. 2023;13(4S2):e2023316S.
5. Böhm M, Schunter JA, Fritz K, Salavastru C, Dargatz S, Augustin M, et al. S1 Guideline: Diagnosis and therapy of vitiligo. J Dtsch Dermatol Ges. 2022;20(3):365-78.

CHAPTER 14B

Resources: Role of Patient Education and Support Groups in Vitiligo

Maya Shriram Tulpule, Mukta Tulpule

INTRODUCTION

Vitiligo is a chronic skin condition with a protracted treatment course.

Usually, the first contact of a vitiligo patient is a general practitioner, physician, or pediatrician instead of a dermatologist or specialist **(Fig. 1)**. Patients reach out to unqualified sources and social media for information about their condition and often get the wrong advice. The delay in seeking treatment from a qualified dermatologist affects or worsens their condition making it more difficult to treat.[1]

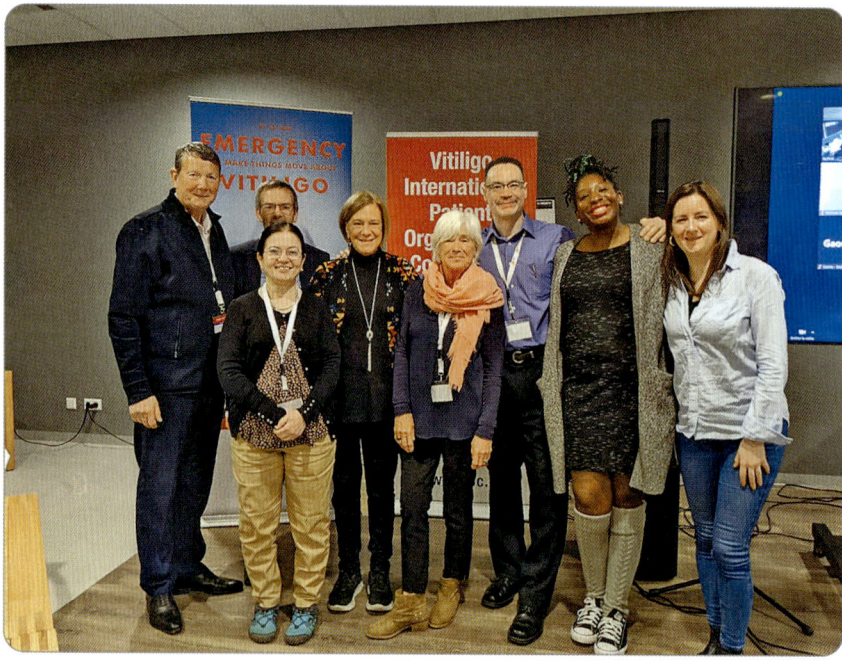

FIG. 1: Vitiligo patient support group board members.

The role of patient education begins with creating awareness at the grassroot level. Screening for vitiligo should begin in schools. Many times, children with vitiligo face bias or even bullying. Creating more awareness about the noncontagious and harmless nature of the condition will go a long way in easing social integration. Though vitiligo is categorized as a cosmetic condition, it creates a large psychological burden in patients. The stress is due to looking different from peers, having a condition that may be visible to others and a stigma attached to the same, especially in the Indian subcontinent.

Parents and teachers of children having vitiligo should have accessible information about how to counsel the children and how to deal with societal interpretations regarding the same. Trained counselors can help to build a positive outlook, prevent depression or social regression, and improve treatment compliance in children. Often, parents are more stressed than children about the diagnosis and counseling family members will reduce anxiety for the child.

Educating general practitioners about the latest technologies and treatment options available with dermatologists creates awareness to refer patients early to specialists.

Building a local community of support in the form of patient self-help support groups has many advantages:
- Patients have access to authentic information and research.
- Patients get more time to discuss their condition, treatment outcomes, and communicate with others going through the same issues. This network builds resilience, provides coping strategies, and also builds hope.[2]
- Improved compliance to treatments through each other's encouragement, feeling of belonging, and providing a safe environment to voice their concerns.
- Finding specialists treating vitiligo
- Locating centers which provide phototherapy machines in areas accessible to them
- Vitiligo patients require support beyond a prescription. This can be in the form of cosmetic camouflage or demonstration of using the same, correct and regular use of sunscreens, dietary counseling, etc.
- Difficulty in finding a marriage partner is a major concern in the vitiligo community in India. Patient support groups have created marriage bureau platforms online and offline (specifically for vitiligo patients or children of patients having vitiligo) to help with this issue.
- Raising awareness about vitiligo in the society by conducting awareness drives regularly

Patient support groups are a new concept in India. Vitiligo patient support groups from across the world such as USA, France, Germany, India, South Africa, Ghana, Egypt, and many more have joined hands to form an International organization called Vitiligo International Patient Organizations Committee (VIPOC). They hold an annual conference and discuss various ways to raise more awareness for vitiligo. They educate their patient leaders about the latest research conducted internationally about vitiligo so that information can be passed on to patients and members. Patient leaders are trained about advanced counseling techniques, communication skills, fund raising, etc. In some countries such as

France and Germany, patient leaders have successfully lobbied with governments to make the latest medication to treat vitiligo like ruxolitinib available in their countries. Patient leaders work toward making vitiligo treatment more affordable, more accessible, and bring it under the scope of insurance cover.

Recently, articles have been published by dermatologists with patient leaders.[3]

What can dermatologists with high footfall of vitiligo patients do?[4]

- Dermatologists should provide information about vitiligo self-help support groups to patients to help them tide over. Screening for depression and anxiety in patients should be done when assessing vulvar quality of life index (VQLI), and at risk, individuals should be guided toward appropriate treatment and support.
- Clinics can make their own patient support system, by making a WhatsApp group of their regular patients. Organizing a quarterly meeting with patients if possible. This motivates patients to bond with each other and motivate each other to continue treatment.
- Patient information leaflets about vitiligo treatment can be made available along with information about support groups.
- Online support groups are also popular among patients for sharing information with each other.
- Patients who are a part of a support group report significantly higher quality of life indices **(Fig. 2)**.[5]

Vitiligo patients need more hand-holding, hope, and emotional or financial support along with medicines and treatment. This gap can be filled successfully by patient support groups.[6]

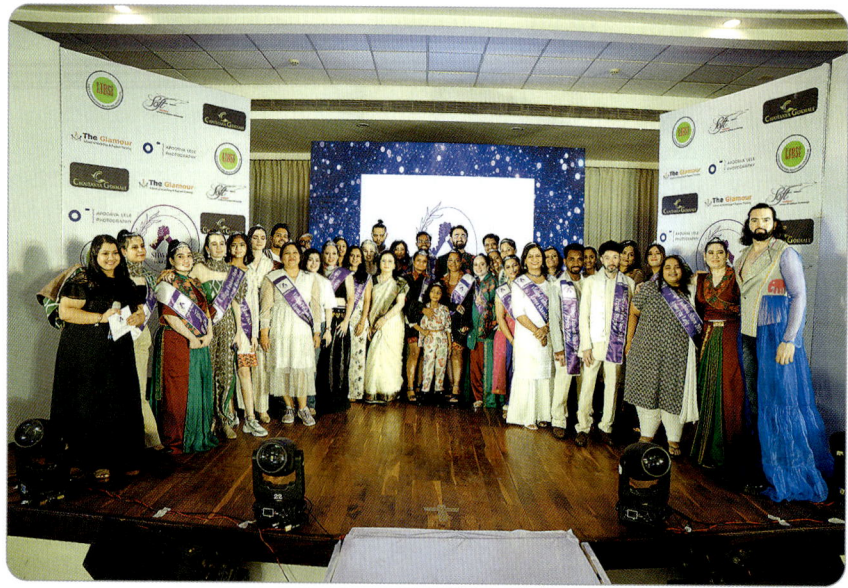

FIG. 2: NBUVB and excimer is available at my clinic at Sahawas hospital.

CONCLUSION

A patient support group is integral to creating awareness and to cope with the multiple aspects of vitiligo other than skin treatments.

REFERENCES

1. Chen T, Grau C, Suprun M, Silverberg NB. Vitiligo patients experience barriers in accessing care. Cutis. 2016;98(6):385-88.
2. Rzepecki AK, McLellan BN, Elbuluk N. Beyond traditional treatment: The importance of psychosocial therapy in vitiligo. J Drugs Dermatol. 2018;17(6):688-91.
3. Hamzavi IH, Bibeau K, Grimes P, Harris JE, van Geel N, Parsad D, et al. Exploring the natural and treatment history of vitiligo: perceptions of patients and healthcare professionals from the global VALIANT study. Br J Dermatol. 2023;189(5):569-77.
4. Geisler A, O'Connell KA, Pandya R, Milburn A, Robinson C, Parks-Miller A, et al. Importance of and instruction for starting a vitiligo patient support group. Dermatol Online J. 2022;28(6).
5. Zabetian S, Jacobson G, Lim HW, Eide MJ, Huggins RH. Quality of life in a vitiligo support group. J Drugs Dermatol. 2017;16(4):344-50.
6. Smith ZI, Wang JF, Elbuluk N, Huggins RH, Birnbaum MR, Rzepecki A, et al. A multi-centered case-control study of vitiligo support groups and quality of life. J Drugs Dermatol. 2021;20(6):672-5.

14C CHAPTER

Resources: List of Phototherapy Chambers and Excimer Lamps in India

Deepti Ghia

INTRODUCTION

Phototherapy remains a cornerstone in the management of vitiligo, with narrowband ultraviolet B (NBUVB) light and 308 nm excimer light being among the most effective modalities. Access to these treatments is crucial for optimizing patient outcomes, yet finding specialized centers offering these services can be challenging.

This chapter provides a comprehensive directory of clinics and dermatologists across India who offer NBUVB and excimer laser therapy for vitiligo. The compilation aims to assist both patients and referring physicians in locating reliable treatment centers, thereby improving access to quality care. The listed details include clinic addresses, contact information, and available treatment modalities, serving as a valuable resource for individuals seeking phototherapy options.

CHAPTER 14C: Resources: List of Phototherapy Chambers and Excimer Lamps in India

State	Name	Complete clinic address	Narrow-band full body UVB chamber	Excimer laser	Comments, if any
Andhra Pradesh	Dr Mallina Krishna Rao	Srinivasa Skin Hospital Rastrapathi Road, Opposite Paparao Petrol Bunk, Tanuku, West Godavari, Andhra Pradesh, Pin: 534211, India Ph: 9502844445	Yes	Yes	NBUVB Hand and Foot Unit available
	Dr Neelakanta Rasineni	Dr Neelakanta Skin, Hair and Laser centre, Vijayawada, Andhra Pradesh, India Ph: 9963234094, 8686225085	Yes	No	NBUVB Hand and Foot Unit
	Dr Chandana	Dr Chandana's La Skin 360 Hospital, Rajahmundry, Andhra Pradesh, India Ph: 8970360360	No	Yes	Excimer and vitiligo surgery services available
	Dr Prathyusha Yakkala	Prakrithi Skin Hair and Laser Clinic, Besides Mk Gold Coast, Yendada, Visakhapatnam Andhra Pradesh, India Ph: 8712782191/ 9391592593	No	Yes	
	Dr Pellakuru Preethi	Siddartha Endocrine and Dermatology Hospital, 16-14-286/3, Srihari Nagar, Revenue Ward 16-III, Nellore: 524003, India Ph: 7981554994	No	Yes	–
	Dr Vijay Kumar Raju	Vijaya Skin Hospital. 60 Feet Road, Ongole, AP: 523002, India Ph: 9849343391	Yes	No	
	Dr Manjari Malladi	Sri Satya Skin Centre, College Road, Amalapuram, Andhra Pradesh: 533201, India Ph: 9160817100	Yes	No	NBUVB excimer and vitiligo surgery
Assam	Dr Saloni Katoch	Dr KN Barua Institute of Dermatological Sciences, 5th floor, Roodraksh Mall, Bhangagarh, Guwahati, Assam, India Ph: 7035356043, 9531189752	Yes	No	Phototherapy, Excimer laser and Vitiligo surgery, https://knbaruabids.com/?fbclid=IwAR32Z0KW8jL4lx7wwGWCdFJd23mLBU_8H4a7aFndJoh8S7nJGUYdqb3X6GE

Continued

Continued

State	Name	Complete clinic address	Narrow-band full body UVB chamber	Excimer laser	Comments, if any
Tamil Nadu	Dr N Anand	M 53/2, New 6, Indira Nagar 1st Main Road, Besant Nagar, Chennai, Tamil Nadu: 600090, India Ph: 9962565628	Yes	No	
Chhattisgarh	Dr Ajit Kumar	Sparsh Skin and Dental Clinic, Near Hotel Guru, Opposite Pandri, Raipur, Chhattisgarh, India Ph: 0771-4014382, 9795224877	Yes	No	
	Dr Piyush Agrawal	Skin Zone, 1st floor, Landmark: Gauri Shankar Mandir Road, Above Union Bank, Itwari Bazar, Raigarh, Chhattisgarh: 496001, India Ph: 9770098384	Yes	Yes	NBUVB whole body chamber, Excimer laser and vitiligo surgery available
	Dr Piyush Agrawal	1st floor, Above Union Bank, Itwari Bazar, Raigarh, Chhattisgarh, India Ph: 8462033550	Yes	Yes	
Haryana	Dr Vinay Singh	B-70, Sector 57, Sushant Lok III, Gurugram, Haryana, India Ph: 9811066509	Yes	Yes	
New Delhi	Dr Sujay Khandpur	Department of Dermatology and Venereology, AIIMS, New Delhi: 110029, India Ph: 011-26593217	Yes	Yes	Hand and foot PUVA also available
	Dr Ashok Gupta	Leelawanti Skin and Laser Institute, E-5/21, near ICICI bank, Krishna Nagar, New Delhi: 110051, India Ph: 9718478829	Yes	Yes	
	Dr Sumit Gupta	Excel Hospital, BN-56, East Shalimar Bagh, New Delhi: 110088, India Ph: 9811341350	Yes	Yes	Whole Body NBUVB, Hand and Foot NBUVB, Excimer lamp, UVA Panel (Total Four Devices)
	Dr Priyanka Jaju	Leelawanti Skin and Laser Institute, E-8A/1, Krishna Nagar, New Delhi: 100051, India Ph: 011-22096324, 9718478829	Yes	Yes	
	Dr Rahul Arora	SkinMedics Skin Hair and Laser Clinic, BE-1, Shalimar Bagh, New Delhi, India Ph: 9253025302	No	Yes	

Continued

Continued

State	Name	Complete clinic address	Narrowband full body UVB chamber	Excimer laser	Comments, if any
New Delhi	Dr Sandeep Gupta	Balaji Skin Clinic, New Delhi, India Ph: 9780881808	No	Yes	
	Dr Jyoti Gupta	B-43, Soami Nagar, Near Panchsheel Enclave, South Delhi, India Ph: 9999739066	No	Yes	
Uttar Pradesh	Dr Mohna Chauhan	Clairederma, Center for Skin, Hair and Laser in Prakash Hospital, Sector-33, Noida, Uttar Pradesh, India Ph: 9319603344	Yes	Yes	Phototherapy chamber and excimer
Gujarat	Dr Janak Thakkar	OrnaSkin, Nakshatra IV, Near Kathiawar Gymkhana, Rajkot, Gujarat, India Ph: 9998127171	Yes	Yes	
	Dr Bhavesh Devani	Drashti Skin and Eye Hospital, Mangla Main Road, Rajkot, Gujarat, India Ph: 9408094081	Yes	Yes	NBUVB Panel
	Dr Jagdish Sakhiya	5th floor, 507, Autograph The Commercial Hub, Bhatar Rd, opp. Rajhans Olympia, Sanskar Nagar, Athwa, Surat, Gujarat: 395017, India Ph: 1800 1200 70000	Yes	Yes	Whole body phototherapy
	Dr Jagdish Sakhiya	Shital Varsha Complex, 5, Shivranjani Char Rasta, 201-202, Satellite Rd, Suryapooja Block B, Satellite, Ahmedabad, Gujarat: 380015, India Ph: 1800 1200 70000	Yes	Yes	Whole body phototherapy
	GMERS Medical College, Sola, Ahmedabad c/o Dr Krina Patel (Professor)	A block 202, Department of Dermatology, GMERS Medical College and Sola Civil Hospital, SG Highway, Ahmedabad: 380060, India Ph: 7927661187	Yes	No	
	Dr Pooja Modi	Dermatouch Clinic, Shlok Infinity, 1st floor, A block, Gota Road, opp. Vishwakarma Mandir, Chandlodiya, Ahmedabad, India Ph: 7777992003, 7996228744	No	Yes	Excimer laser

Continued

Continued

State	Name	Complete clinic address	Narrow-band full body UVB chamber	Excimer laser	Comments, if any
Gujarat	Dr Archana Oswal	Dr Archana's Skin Care Clinic, 201, 2nd floor, Labh Icon, Near Bansal Mall, Gotri Vasna Connecting Road, Gotri, Vadodara: 390021, India Ph: 9426270479	No	Yes	Both Excimer laser and PUVA available
	Dr Nirali Modi	Sparsh Skin Clinic, Opposite Lokhandwala Complex, LIC Road, Godhra 389001, Gujarat, India Ph: 9265899668	No	No	
	Dr Seema Jain	2nd floor, Body Care Complex, Opp. Bus Stop, Ashram Road, Gujarat, India Ph: 9376106275	Yes	No	NBUVB whole body chamber
	Dr Samkit Shah	Urmil Skin Clinic, Raymond Circle, Madhu Apartment, Charwada Road Gunjan, Vapi, Gujarat, India Ph: 800054083, 7971290000	Yes	Yes	
	Dr Chetan Lalseta	Shraddha Hospital, 1 Jagannath Park, Ckowk, Near Shree Giriraj Hospital,150 Ft Ring Road, Rajkot: 360005, Gujarat, India Ph: 9825199585	No	Yes	NVUVB Hand and Foot Therapy, Excimer light
	Dr Jagdish Sakhiya	1101, Infinity Tower, Lal Darwaja Station Rd, near Ayurvedic College, Suryapur Gate, Varachha, Surat, Gujarat: 395003, India Ph: 8155900010	Yes	Yes	Whole body phototherapy
	Dr Saurabh Kapadia	Perfect Skin Sare, 2nd floor, Shubh Complex, Opp. Petrol Pump, Sector 21, Gandhinagar, Gujarat, India Ph: 7923260097, 9265489235	No	Yes	Excimer and Surgery both services available
	Dr Pooja Chowdhary Jagati	Twachaa Skin and Hair Clinic, 15/16, Axiom Amrapali Complex, Near Bhopal Ambli Circle, Above Dominos Pizza, SP Ring Road, Bhopal, Ahmedabad, India Ph: 8511023793, 9099044639	Yes	No	www.twachaaskinclinic.com Whole body chamber, Surgery available

Continued

CHAPTER 14C: Resources: List of Phototherapy Chambers and Excimer Lamps in India

Continued

State	Name	Complete clinic address	Narrow-band full body UVB chamber	Excimer laser	Comments, if any
Haryana	Dr Kartikay Aggarwal	Aggarwal Hospital, Main Road, Near Sapphire Hotel, Jagadhri, Haryana, India Ph: 9603250000	Yes	Yes	Hand and Feet NBUVB and Excimer Laser
	Dr Radhika Khurana	Prolife Hospital, Sector 21, Panchkula. Dr Radhika Khurana MNs mind and Skincare Clinic, House No. 1513, Opp. Grain Market, Sector 21, Panchkula: 134112, Haryana, India Ph: 7300873102	No	Yes	
	Dr Rajat Mehta	Mehta Skin and Laser Clinic, SCO 130, 1st floor, Sector 25, Panchkula, Haryana, India Ph: 8264565650	Yes	No	
	Dr Vivek Aggarwal	Vivek Skin Clinic, Near Grand Taj Hotel, Sector 10, Kurukshetra, Haryana 136119, India Ph: 9416782008	Yes	No	
Himachal Pradesh	Neelkanth Hospital	Neelkanth Hospital, 93/1, Zonal Hospital Road, Mandi, Himachal Pradesh, India Ph: 8278726347	Yes	No	
Jammu and Kashmir	Dr Cheena Langer	Aastha Skin and Dermatocosmetic Centre, Lane 2, Karan Nagar, Amphalla, Opposite Vridhashram, Jammu (J&K), India Ph: 9796676541	Yes	No	
	Dr Ummer Yaseen	Dr Ummer Yaseen Medical Centre, near Masjid Usman Budshah Nagar, Natipora, Jammu and Kashmir, India Ph: 7006717110	Yes	Yes	Hand and Phototherapy also available
Jharkhand	Dr Nikita Gupta	Carderm Clinic, Golmuri Market, Jamshedpur, Jharkhand, India Ph: 9008449377	No	Yes	Excimer
	Dr Ravishankar Dwivedi	Shanti Skin and Laser Centre, 1st floor, Shri Laxmi Tower, Hinoo, Ranchi, Jharkhand, India Ph: 9835331002	Yes	Yes	We are also having hand and foot panels. We are conducting entire range of vitiligo surgeries—PG/SBG/STG/MKT

Continued

Continued

State	Name	Complete clinic address	Narrow-band full body UVB chamber	Excimer laser	Comments, if any
Karnataka	Dr Venkataram Mysore	Venkat Center for Skin and Plastic Surgery, 3437, 1G Cross, 7th Main Road, Subbanna Garden, Vijayanagar, Bengaluru: 560040, India Ph: 9611842627	Yes	No	Vitiligo surgeries, phototherapy
	Dr KN Shivaswamy	Department of Dermatology MS Ramaiah Medical College and Hospitals, Bengaluru, Karnataka, India Ph: 8062153400	Yes	No	Daavlin UVB, UVA Chamber
	Dr Harsha Siddappa	Ziva Skin and Hair cCenter, #2, 1st floor, hHesaraghatta mMain rRoad, T Dasarahalli, Benagluru: 560073, Karnataka, India Ph: 9611256888	No	Yes	
	Dr Harish Prasad BR	Vitals klinic, BTM 2nd stage, Bengaluru, Karnataka, India Ph: 9206869610	Yes	Yes	Melanocyte transplant surgeries
	Dr Venkataram Mysore	Venkat Center for Skin and Plastic Surgery, Banashankari Bengaluru, Karnataka, India Ph: 7022101689	Yes	Yes	
	Dr Swetha K Hegde	Skin Care Clinic, #209, 50th Cross, 3rd Block, Rajajinagar, Opposite BWSSB Office, Bengaluru: 560010, Karnataka, India Ph: 7795054791	Yes	Yes	Hand and foot PUVA, full body UVA also available
	Dr Sujala Sacchidanand Aradhya	Sujala Polyclinic and Laboratory, #64 Supraja Towers, Siddaiah Puranik Road, Near Shankarmutt signal, Basaveshwaranagar, Bengaluru: 560079, India Ph: 9035415007, 9845306221	No	Yes	Vitiligo surgeries and an Excimer
	Dr Vathsala Gowda	Shridevi Institute of Medical Sciences and Research Hospital, Sira Road, NH4, Tumkur, Karnataka, India Ph: 7942686456	Yes	No	Whole body NBUVB available

Continued

Continued

State	Name	Complete clinic address	Narrow-band full body UVB chamber	Excimer laser	Comments, if any
Karnataka	Dr Chethana SG	JSS Hospital, Mysuru, Karnataka, India Ph: 8312473777	Yes	No	Full body NBUVB, targeted phototherapy, hand and foot phototherapy and all vitiligo surgeries
	Dr Santosh Shinde	Vijayalaxmi Arcade, Narvekar Galli, Near Khade Bazar Police Station, Belagavi: 590001, Karnataka, India Ph: 6366207070	Yes	Yes	Phototherapy UVA and NBUVB (Daavlin)
	Dr Shashikiran	Jayashree Multispeciality Hospital, Begur Road, Vishwapriya Layout, Bengaluru: 560076, Karnataka, India Ph: 9845466161	No	No	Hand and feet unit. Vitiligo surgeries
	Dr Vathsala S	SkinMed Advanced Skin Clinic, MG Road, 1st Cross, Tumkur, Karnataka, India Ph: 8073959949	Yes	Yes	NBUVB and Excimer available
	Dr Bhavana Dalvi	KLE Hospital, Belagavi	Yes	Yes	Full body NBUVB, targeted phototherapy (excimer light), and vitiligo surgeries
	Dr Smitha Warrier	Fortis Hospital, Bannerghatta Road, Bengaluru, Karnataka, India Ph: 9205010100	Yes	No	UVA chamber
	Dr Vijay Aithal	Department of Dermatology, St John's Medical College Hospital, Bengaluru, Karnataka, India Ph: 22065027, 22065028, 22065029	Yes	Yes	UVA chamber, hand foot unit
	Dr Hari Kishan Kumar	Dr Kishan's Skin Care and Aesthetic Research Centre, Bengaluru, Karnataka, India Ph: 8277414467	Yes	No	
	KMC, Manipal	Tiger Circle Road, Madhav Nagar, Eshwar Nagar, Manipal, Udupi, Karnataka: 576104, India Ph: 8202922276	Yes	No	Targeted UVB, hand and foot unit, PUVA, bath PUVA

Continued

Continued

State	Name	Complete clinic address	Narrow-band full body UVB chamber	Excimer laser	Comments, if any
Karnataka	Dr K Srinivasa Murthy	Skin and Cosmetology Centre, 32/4, 1-B, 1st floor, Alsa Glenridge Apts, Langford Road, Shantinagar, Bengaluru: 560025, India Ph: 9148765923	Yes	No	Daavlin whole body NBUVB and UVA and targeted phototherapy unit
	Dr Venkatram Mysore	Venkat Centre for Skin and Plastic Surgery, 3437, 1G Cross, 7th Main Road, Subbanna Garden, Vijayanagar, Bengaluru: 560025, India Ph: 8023392788	Yes	Yes	
Kerala	Dr CP Thajudheen	Dr THAJ LASER SKIN AND HAIR CLINIC, Thaj Land, Jubilee Road, Tellicherry, Kerala, India Ph: 9744441100	Yes	Yes	
	Dr Ashique KT	Amanza Skin Clinic, Queens Complex, 4/220, Ooty Road, Above Axis Bank, Valiyangadi, Perinthalmanna, Malappuram, Kerala, India Ph: 9048800010	No	Yes	Hand and Foot unit and panel light
	Dr Jazeem Mahamood, Dr Thansiha Nargis	Prime Skin Clinic, Chenoli Junction, South Bazaar, Kannur, Kerala, India Ph: 9539333359	No	Yes	Excimer laser and Vitiligo surgery
	Dr Eby Chacko	Skinpase Skin Care, Near Maharani Theatre, Pala, Kottayam, Kerala, India Ph: 9846011133	No	Yes	Excimer laser
	Dr Boby Krishna	Near SAP camp, Peroorkada, Thiruvananthapuram, Kerala, India Ph: 9539744330	Yes	Yes	Phototherapy
	Dr Mohammed Naseef K	Premier Skin Care Center, 1st floor, Above Federal Bank, Shola Complex, Ramanattukara, Calicut, Kerala, India Ph: 9633154254	Yes	No	NBUVB phototherapy unit
Madhya Pradesh	Dr Sidharth Oswal	Oswal Skin Clinic, Dr Barat Road, Near Russel Square, Napier Town, Jabalpur, MP: 482001, India Ph: 9425387714	Yes	Yes	Hand and Foot panel. NBUVB also available

Continued

Continued

State	Name	Complete clinic address	Narrow-band full body UVB chamber	Excimer laser	Comments, if any
Madhya Pradesh	Dr Deepak Mohana, MD	Dr Mohana's Skin Laser and Hair Transplant Center, 201, Juhi Plaza, Kanchanbagh, Geeta Bhawan Square, Indore, Madhya Pradesh, India Ph: 9009858803	Yes	Yes	
	Dr Hitesh Bhalavi	Sukoon Skin and Mind Clinic, Infront of Raja Ki Bagia, Nagpur Road, Chhindwara, Madhya Pradesh, India Ph: 7389082853	No	No	Facility of vitiligo surgery available
	Dr Kanhaiya Patidar	Mayra Skin and Aesthetics Clinic, 102, Sanrachna Avenue, (Above Sampoorna Sodani Diagnostics), Satya Sai Square, Vijay Nagar, Indore: 452010, Madhya Pradesh, India Ph: 8982337464	Yes	Yes	Whole body NBUVB chamber and Excimer lamp available
	Dr Anna Alex	Skin OPD, 2nd floor, old OPD block, Hamidia Hospital , Sultania Road, Bhopal, Madhya Pradesh, India Ph: 7225971112	Yes	No	
Maharashtra	Dr Deepti Ghia	G-38-39, South Mumbai Dermatology, Hughes Road, Next to Dharam Palace, Mumbai: 400007, Maharashtra, India Ph: 7977281031	Yes	Yes	Targeted therapy also available
	Dr Madhulika Mhatre	Skin Saga, 104, Sai Iconic, Opp. Kokilaben Hospital, Four Bungalows, Andheri West, Mumbai, Maharashtra: 400053, India Ph: 9819166344	Yes	Yes	Excimer available
	Dr Manish Shah	Comprehensive Skin Clinic, 26/27, Labh Nivas, Khetwadi 4th Lane, Off S.V.P. Rd, Near Alankar Cinema, Close to Wilson School, Opposite Shiv Sena Shakha, Mumbai: 400004, Maharashtra, India Ph: 8793768131	Yes	Yes	

Continued

Continued

State	Name	Complete clinic address	Narrow-band full body UVB chamber	Excimer laser	Comments, if any
Maharashtra	Dr Anil Bhokare	Apex Skin Clinic, Trimbak Naka, Nashik, Malegaon, Maharashtra, India Ph: 9422246188	Yes	Yes	Having both UVA and UVB chamber
	Dr Swapnil Shah	441, Shukrawar Peth, Solapur, Maharashtra, India Ph: 9923456780	Yes	Yes	Hand and foot unit are also available
	Dr Bhavna Chandwani	Dermashine Skin Clinic, Pimple Saudagar, PCMC, Pune, Maharashtra, India Ph: 7218989553, 7080809075	No	Yes	
	Dr Harsh Shah	Sharda's Skin and Hair Clinic, 101, Maithili Chs, Opp. Subway, Near Talwalkars Gym, Panch Pakhadi, Thane (West), Maharashtra, India Ph: 8591245979	Yes	No	
	Dr Prashant Palwade	Satej Skin Hair Laser Center, Above UCO Bank, Samarth Nagar, Aurangabad: 431001, Maharashtra, India Ph: 9067238171	Yes	Yes	Hand and foot NBUVB unit also available
	Dr Jay D Gupte	Dr Gupte's Skin Clinic, Ram Nivas, A-Wing, 1st floor, Above Wellness Medical Stores, Gokhale Road, Naupada, Thane (West), Maharashtra: 400602, India Ph: 9769644401	No	No	NBUVB hand and foot unit available
	Dr Jyotsna Vinayak Deo	Cutis Skin and Laser Centre, Row House 1, Plot 182C, Punit Park, Cosmopolitan II CHS, Savitribai Phule Marg, Sector 17, Nerul (East), Navi Mumbai: 400706, Maharashtra, India Ph: 9987536454	Yes	Yes	Clinic timings are 10.30 AM to 6.30 PM. Monday to Saturday
	Dr Sushil Satish Savant	The Humanitarian Clinic: Skin Hair and Laser Centere, 1st floor, Ratnagar CHS, Four Bunglows Signal, Above Airtel Gallery, Andheri West, Mumbai: 400053, Maharashtra, India Ph: 9321652496, 9702891624	Yes	Yes	Composite whole body UVA and NBUVB chamber

Continued

CHAPTER 14C: Resources: List of Phototherapy Chambers and Excimer Lamps in India

Continued

State	Name	Complete clinic address	Narrow-band full body UVB chamber	Excimer laser	Comments, if any
Maharashtra	Dr Navin Modi	Modi Skin Clinic, A/108, Everest Tower, Karnik Road, Kalyan West, Thane, Maharashtra, India Ph: 9769349707	No	Yes	Hand foot portable available
	Dr Meghana Phiske	MGM Medical College, Kamothe, Navi Mumbai, Maharashtra, India Ph: 9819030429	Yes	No	Full body NBUVB available at the hospital where I am attached as Associate Professor
	Dr Raghunandan Torsekar	Disha Skin and Laser Institute, 101, Srushti Prime, Gokhale Road, Naupada, Thane West, Thane, Maharashtra: 400602, India Ph: 9321632000	Yes	Yes	We have two whole body units with UVA and NBUVB lights. We have Excimer lamp and Hand and foot phototherapy unit also
	Dr Nilesh Goyal	Juvenis Clinic, 4 Adarsh, Behind Archies Gallery, SV Road, Santacruz (W), Mumbai: 54, Maharashtra, India Ph: 9769966696	Yes	No	Targeted UVB phototherapy available
	Dr Supriya Deshmukh	301, Ashar Millennia, Above MI Mobiles, Kapurbawdi Junction, Thane west, Maharashtra, India Ph: 8691922225	No	Yes	Facility of Excimer available
	Dr Mithila Gadekar	Skinn Remedy, Laxmi Karanja Chowk, Ahmednagar, Maharashtra, India Ph: 8329442664	No	Yes	Excimer and Surgery both services available
	Dr Shveta Sharma	Dr Shveta's Skin and Hair Clinic, 2nd floor, Manipal Hospital, Kharadi, Pune: 411014, India Ph: 9967174444	No	Yes	Excimer available
	Dr Amit Shah	Shobhana Skin Cosmetic and Laser Clinic, Ram Mandir to Civil Hospital Road, South Shivajinagar, Sangli, Maharashtra: 416416, India Ph: 9370414849	Yes	No	NBUVB and PUVA, Exciplex laser, vitiligo surgery

Continued

Continued

State	Name	Complete clinic address	Narrow-band full body UVB chamber	Excimer laser	Comments, if any
Maharashtra	Dr Poonam Kabra	Kabra Skin, 1st Floor, RK Towers, Behind Harsh Sankul, Civil Line Road, Opposite to SA College, Akola, Maharashtra 444001, India Ph: 9146341241	No	Yes	
	Dr Parikshit Satpute	AVDHOOT SKIN CARE AND LASER CLINIC, Nageshwarwadi, Aurangabad: 431001, Maharashtra, India Ph: 9028036113	No	Yes	
	Dr Anil Bhokare	Apex Skin Clinic, Opp. MSG college, Near MG Petrol Pump, Malegaon, Nashik: 423203, Maharashtra, India Ph: 9422246188	No	Yes	
	Dr Anjali Dalal	The Skin Galaxy, 4B, Tank Road, Mini Land, Opposite Mahavir Banquet Hall, Off LBS Road, Bhandup West, Mumbai: 400078, Maharashtra, India Ph: 9833010901	No	No	Handheld NBUVB light
	Dr Pallavi Rathi	My Skin My Health Clinic, A 407 Pranik Chambers, Saki Vihar Road, Sakinaka Junction, Andheri East, Mumbai, Maharashtra: 400072, India Ph: 9513731569	Yes	Yes	UVB phototherapy, Excimer laser
	Dr Esha Agarwal	Cutis ENT and Laser Centre, 1st floor, Vijay Bhavan, Lokmat Square, Dhantoli, Nagpur, Maharashtra: 440012, India Ph: 0712-2996614, 8390657666	No	Yes	Excimer laser and vitiligo surgeries including melanocyte culture
	Dr Deesha Sonarkhan	Marvel Skin Hair and Laser Clinic, IFO Bus Stand, Above Raj Medical, Chandranagar, Latur, Maharashtra: 413512, India	Yes	No	Full body NBUVB phototherapy, vitiligo surgeries
	Dr Bhushan Madke	Jawaharlal Nehru Medical College, Wardha, Maharashtra, India Ph: 7066887353	Yes	Yes	

Continued

Continued

State	Name	Complete clinic address	Narrow-band full body UVB chamber	Excimer laser	Comments, if any
Maharashtra	Dr Sunita Patel	Skin Care Clinic, 175, Rd Number 11, Jawahar Nagar, Goregaon West, Mumbai, Maharashtra 400104, India Ph: 7710969483, 8291056114	No	No	NBUVB hand and foot unit available
	Dr Deepam Shah	Viva Aesthetic Clinic, Mumbai, Maharashtra, India Ph: 9324589084	No	Yes	
	Deenanath Mangeshkar Hospital	Erandwane, Pune: 411004, Maharashtra, India Ph: 2040151375	Yes	Yes	Also UVA
	Symbiosis University Hospital and Research Centre	Symbiosis University Hospital and Research Centre, Symbiosis International (Deemed University) Campus, Hill Base, Lavale, Pune, Maharashtra, India	Yes	Yes	
	Dr Anil Kolhe	Asian Institute of Dermatology, Savewadi, Dinanath Nagar, Latur: 413512, Maharashtra, India Ph: 2382248934	Yes	Yes	
	Dr Vijay Zawar	Shreeram Sankul, Opp. Hotel Panchavati, Vakilwadi, Nashik, Maharashtra, India Ph: 8780335029	Yes	No	Quite useful in well-selected patients
Odisha	Kalinga Institute of Medical Sciences (KIMS)	Kusabhadra Campus, KIMS Rd, Chandaka Industrial Estate, KIIT University, Patia, Bhubaneswar, Odisha: 751024, India Ph: 9937055325	Yes	No	Hand foot Unit also available
	Dr Chinmoy Raj	Department of Dermatology, Venereology and Leprosy, Kalinga Institute of Medical Sciences, Bhubaneswar: 751024, Odisha, India Ph: 9692261294	Yes	No	
	Dr Monali Pattnaik	Tattva Skin Clinic, Kalinga Hospital Square, Bhubaneswar, Odisha, India Ph: 7008624033	No	Yes	
	Dr Manoj Ram	Dr Manoj Ram Skin Care, Kathgola Phandi Road, Mangalabag, Cuttack, Odisha: 753007, India Ph: 8117048936	Yes	No	NBUVB phototherapy

Continued

Continued

State	Name	Complete clinic address	Narrow-band full body UVB chamber	Excimer laser	Comments, if any
Punjab	Dr Rakesh Bharti	Bharti Derma Care and Research Centre, Amritsar, Punjab, India Ph: 9814044213	No	Yes	
	Dr Aastha Sharma	Department of Dermatology, Sohana Hospital, Sector-77, SAS Nagar, Mohali, Punjab: 140308, India Ph: 9115551432, 0172-2295000	Yes	No	
	Dr Jasleen Kaur	Jagmohan Hospital, Near Khalsa College, Amritsar 143002, Punjab, India Ph: 7947151251	Yes	No	UVB phototherapy
	Dr Isha V Mittal	The Skin Zeal, Sco 29, 1st floor, B Block, VIP Road, Zirakpur, Punjab, India Ph: 7293939326	No	Yes	Facility of vitiligo surgeries and excimer laser available
	Dr Manmit Kaur	Ludhiana: 141001, Punjab, India Ph: 7407798278	No	Yes	Excimer available
Rajasthan	Dr Saurabh Singh	Department of Dermatology, Venereology and Leprology, AIIMS Jodhpur, Rajasthan: 342005, India Ph: 0291-2740742	Yes	No	Composite whole body NBUVB and UVA chamber. Make: Daavlin
	Dr Rohit Kataria	K-6, Govind Nagar Housing Board Colony, Near RK Govt. Hospital, Kankroli, Rajsamand, Rajasthan, India Ph: 9116536161	Yes	Yes	All types of facilities for vitiligo available
	Dr Shail Agarwal	House Number 11, Durga Vihar Colony, Jhalawar, Rajasthan, India Ph: 8619335044	No	Yes	Hand and foot NBUVB unit are also available
	Dr Shail Agarwal	House Number 11, Durga Vihar Colony, in front of Jhalawar Medical College, Jhalawar, Rajasthan, India Ph: 8619335044	No	Yes	Hand and foot unit NBUVB available
Tamil Nadu	Dr Maya Vedamurthy	9/5 Mahalingam, 2nd Cross Street, Mahalingapuram, Chennai: 600034, Tamil Nadu, India Ph: 9840062115	Yes	Yes	

Continued

CHAPTER 14C: Resources: List of Phototherapy Chambers and Excimer Lamps in India

Continued

State	Name	Complete clinic address	Narrow-band full body UVB chamber	Excimer laser	Comments, if any
Tamil Nadu	Dr Pallavi Dhanyan	CODE Skin Clinic, Anna Nagar, Madurai, Tamil Nadu, India Ph: 9444043210	Yes	Yes	Full body photo-therapy unit, Hand foot unit and Excimer
	Dr T Pari	Dr. Pari's Skin and Hair Clinic 4, Sarathy Nagar, Opp. Vijaya Nagar Bus Stand, Velachery, Chennai: 600 042, Tamil Nadu, India Ph: 9600105739	Yes	Yes	
	Dr CP Thajudheen	Balakrishnan Building, 100 Feet Road, Coimbatore, Tamil Nadu, India Ph: 9362666789	Yes	Yes	
	Dr Maya Vedamurthy	RSV Skin and Laser Center, 9/5, Mahalingam, 2nd Cross Street, Mahalingam, Chennai: 600034, Tamil Nadu, India Ph: 9790943345	Yes	Yes	Whole body phototherapy chamber with UVA and UVB available, Excimer light, Hand and foot unit available
	Dr Anuradha Priyadarshini, SRMC	Dermatology Department, Sri Ramachandra Medical College, Porur, Chennai, Tamil Nadu, India Ph: 9843119213	Yes	No	Whole body NBUVB and UVA chamber
	Dr AV Kaleeswaran	AVM Skin, Hair Care and Laser Centre, 28/3, Veppanthoppu Street, Palani Road, Dindigul: 624001, Tamil Nadu, India Ph: 9442569301	Yes	No	Lumera targeted phototherapy available instead of Eximer. Daavlin full body NBUVB, UVA available
Telangana	Dr Ch Vijay Bhasker Reddy	Department of DVL,Sreepuram, KIMS, Narketpally, Telangana, India Ph: 9032445447	Yes	No	Whole body UVA
	Dr Pragathi Sankineni	Pragathi Skin and Cosmetology Clinic, Kaleelwadi, Nizamabad, Telangana, India Ph: 9908630783	Yes	No	
	Dr Vani Veggalam	Cleo Skin Clinic, MIG-549, 2nd floor, Ravi Hospital, KPHB Colony, Road Number 1, Hyderabad, Telangana, India Ph: 9550005777, 9032603777	Yes	Yes	Vitiligo surgeries

Continued

Continued

State	Name	Complete clinic address	Narrow-band full body UVB chamber	Excimer laser	Comments, if any
Telangana	Dr Purna Chandra Badabagni	ESIC Medical College and Hospital, Sanathnagar, Hyderabad, Telangana, India Ph: 1800 11 2526	Yes	No	Multiutility NBUVB phototherapy unit is also available
	Dr Sitara GL	4th floor, Above Reliance Trends Showroom, Madhinaguda, Hyderabad: 500049, Telangana, India Ph: 9392177173	No	No	NBUVB hand and foot unit available
	Dr Harshita Reddy	Apollo Hospital, Room No: 9063, Basement-1, International Block, Jubilee Hills, Hyderabad, Telangana: 500033, India Ph: 8008800123	Yes	Yes	Excimer lamp available
Uttar Pradesh	Dr Tarang Goyal	HOD, Department of DVL, Muzaffarnagar Medical College, Uttar Pradesh, India Ph: 7618230082	Yes	Yes	UVA and UVB both available, UVB hand foot unit also available, Excimer available
	Dr DK Omer	Dr Omer's Skin and VD Clinics, Jhansi, Uttar Pradesh, India Ph: 9621031298, 7991969669	Yes	No	NBUVB whole body
	Dr Meenal Mittal	Mittal Skin and Aesthetic Clinic, 1st floor, Mittal Diagnostic Centre, Opp. Eden Garden, Ramghat Road, Aligarh: 202001, Uttar Pradesh, India Ph: 8630327620	No	No	Vitiligo surgery available
	Dr Shashank Rastogi	38/2, Lowther Road, Opp. Bhola Hospital, Prayagraj, Uttar Pradesh, India Ph: 9554478567	Yes	Yes	Hand and foot NBUVB
	Dr Devesh Singh	B-1296, Indira Nagar, Lucknow: 16, Uttar Pradesh, India Ph: 8127180786	Yes	No	Whole body NBUVB
	Dr Shiwangi Rana	Department of Dermatology and Venereology, AIIMS, Gorakhpur, Uttar Pradesh, India Ph: 8860565443	Yes	Yes	UVA chamber

Continued

Continued

State	Name	Complete clinic address	Narrow-band full body UVB chamber	Excimer laser	Comments, if any
Uttar Pradesh	Dr Vibhor Kaushal	33/100, Namner, Agra: 282001, Uttar Pradesh, India Ph: 9926992693	No	Yes	
	Talwar Skin Centre	C-1113, Church Road, Indira Nagar, Lucknow: 226016, Uttar Pradesh, India Ph: 9621683219	Yes	Yes	Hand foot Unit also available
	Dr Pratik Shivhare	Nirvana Skin Clinic, Near Medical College, Jhansi, Uttar Pradesh, India Ph: 9580255710	Yes	Yes	
	Dr Gaurav Makhija	P & G SKIN CLINIC, H NO-56-SFS, Near Hanuman Mandir, Betiahata East, Gorakhpur, Uttar Pradesh: 273001, India Ph: 0551 2347093, 9554220700	Yes	Yes	Phototherapy UVA, UVB Excimer
	Dr Geeta Sharma	D' Skin N Laser Clinic, Kanpur, Uttar Pradesh, India Ph: 6393689466	No	Yes	Excimer available
	Dr Priyam Bhaskar Rai	Savitri Hospital, Near ITI College, Landmark: Sonda, Road: Barhaj Road, City: Deoria, Uttar Pradesh: 274001, India Ph: 8445218884	Yes	Yes	Phototherapy NBUVB, UVA
	Dr Nawed Khan	Rabia Skin Clinic, Campbell Road, Balaganj, Lucknow, Uttar Pradesh, India Ph: 9918595209	No	Yes	Excimer facilities available
	Dr Gagan Goyal	Dr Goyal's Skin Clinic, Patel Nagar, Ghaziabad, Uttar Pradesh, India Ph: 9818272622	Yes	No	
	Dr Himani Tandon	T. S. Misra Medical College and Hospital, opp. Railway Station, Amausi, Anora, Lucknow, Uttar Pradesh 226009, India Ph: 9369110563	Yes	No	Phototherapy chambers are available at both centers

Continued

Continued

State	Name	Complete clinic address	Narrow-band full body UVB chamber	Excimer laser	Comments, if any
Uttar Pradesh	Dr Shubhshree Misra	TSM Super Speciality Hospital, Lucknow, Uttar Pradesh, India Ph: 7800001204	Yes	No	
	Dr Rajeev Sharma	Bishen Skin Centre, M-69, Janakpuri Water Tank Ln, Janakpuri, Bank Colony, Aligarh, Uttar Pradesh 202001, India Ph: 9917018889, 0571-2409940	Yes	No	NBUVB full body chamber hand and foot unit
Uttarakhand	Dr Deepti Dhingra	Skin Station, 1st Floor, Bindal Tower, Chakrata Road, Bindal Bridge, Dehradun, Uttarakhand 248001, India Ph: 7617610000	No	Yes	Excimer available
	Dr Tarun Mittal	Ashrey Skin and Laser Clinic, 136/12, Mohit Nagar, Dehradun, Uttarakhand, India Ph: 9759344200	Yes	No	
	Himalayan Institute of Medical Sciences	Himalayan Institute of Medical Sciences, SRHU, Swami Ram Nagar, Jolly Grant, Dehradun, Uttarakhand: 248016, India Ph: 0135-2471158	Yes	No	
	Dr Kopal Maheshwari	Futela Hospital, Rudrapur, Uttarakhand, India Ph: 7500909919	Yes	No	NBUVB full body chamber and hand and foot unit
West Bengal	Dr Souvik Sardar	Eleganz Skin and Hair Clinic, Dhakuria, Kolkata, West Bengal, India Ph: 9830450415	No	Yes	
	Dr Souvik Sardar	Eleganz Skin and Hair Clinic, 118/A Selimpore Road, Kolkata: 700031, West Bengal, India Ph: 9433418181	No	Yes	Excimer phototherapy, vitiligo surgery
	Dr Dinesh Hawelia	Dr. Hawelia's Skin Clinic, 245A, Chittaranjan Avenue, Kolkata: 700064, West Bengal, India Ph: 9830274689	Yes	Yes	PUVA, NBUVB, Excimer lamp
	Dr Aniruddha Ghosh	Ghosh Clinic, Parnashree, Behala, Kolkata: 700060, West Bengal, India Ph: 8697354467	Yes	No	Full body NBUVB chamber

CHAPTER 15

Remembering Dr Sanjeev Mulekar

Madhulika Mhatre, Deepti Ghia, Iltefat H Hamzavi, Munish Paul

Section 1: Madhulika Mhatre

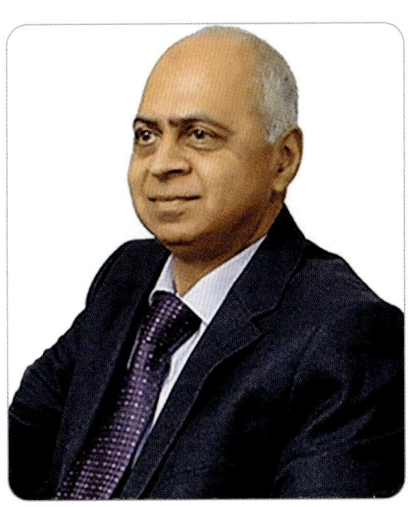

FIG. 1: Dr Sanjeev Mulekar Sir.

Dr *Sanjeev Mulekar* **(Fig. 1)** was not just a pioneer in vitiligo surgery, he was a visionary, a teacher, and a constant source of inspiration. For me, he was much more than a mentor—he was a guide who shaped my understanding of vitiligo and the art of compassionate care. His innovative approaches revolutionized vitiligo treatment, instilling hope where despair once prevailed.

I will always cherish the countless moments spent learning from him—his precise surgical techniques, his meticulous attention to detail, and above all, his unwavering empathy for patients. He taught me that medicine is not just about curing diseases but about restoring confidence and dignity to those we serve.

Dr Mulekar's passing away in March 2024 was a profound loss, not only to me but also to the entire medical community. Yet, his legacy lives on in every patient who regains their smile, in every doctor he inspired, and in every step forward the field of vitiligo research and surgery takes.

This book is a heartfelt tribute to a man whose life's work changed the course of vitiligo treatment forever. To me, he was, and will always be, "Mulekar Sir"—an extraordinary mentor and a compassionate human being **(Figs. 2 and 3)**.

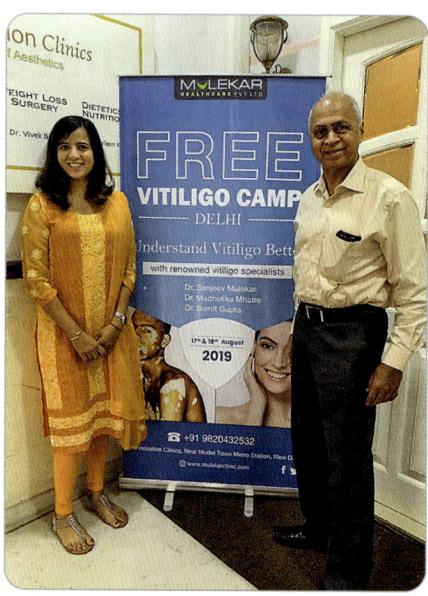

FIG. 2: Dr Sanjeev Mulekar and Dr Madhulika Mhatre.

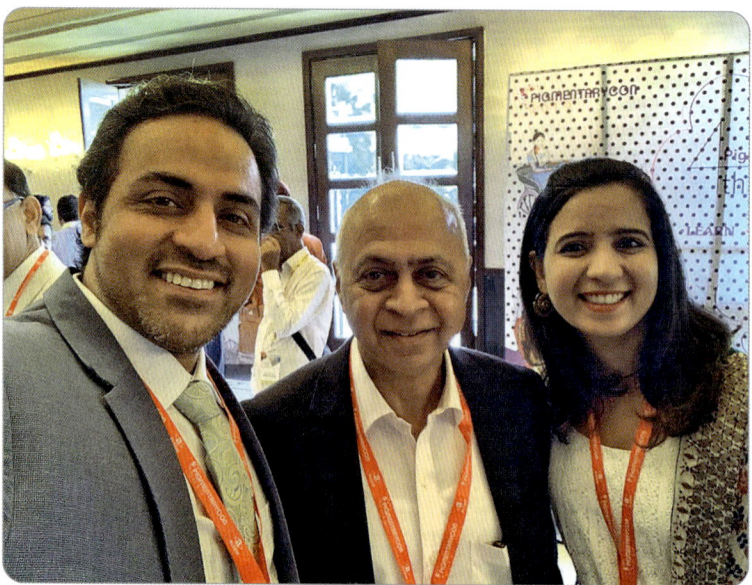

FIG. 3: Dr Sanjeev Mulekar, Dr Madhulika Mhatre, and Dr Aseem Sharma.

Section 2: Deepti Ghia

I was a first-year "Dermatology Resident" and was given a thesis topic on "Noncultured Epidermal Cell Suspension (NCES)" comparing it to the smash grafting modification—Jodhpur technique. Even today, vitiligo surgery remains a challenge, and as a resident, I was anxious about the mammoth task ahead of me. NCES, being the standard technique, required mastery before I could compare it to a new technique. I started searching for doctors who performed this highly specialized surgery. My teachers provided names of doctors in India; however, some were too busy with private practice to guide me, and others were too established to consider helping a first-year resident. I felt lost. When I reviewed publications on this technique, one name came up repeatedly: Sanjeev Mulekar.

When I read about him, I discovered he had completed his graduation and postgraduation from Topiwala National Medical College, which coincidentally was my alma mater as well. I felt an immediate connection and decided to email him, even though he was based in Riyadh, Saudi Arabia. He responded to my email and was initially skeptical about a resident undertaking this comparative study, especially when so few were performing the surgery. However, after I shared images of trypan blue staining used to prepare suspension from extra split-thickness skin sourced from the plastic surgery department, he agreed to meet me during his visit to Mumbai. He addressed all my queries about the surgery and allowed me to observe a few cases during his operations in Mumbai. He guided me through my thesis and played a crucial role in securing an observer position for me at Henry Ford Hospital in Detroit, USA, where he was a visiting faculty member.

When I presented my research work at the International Pigment Cell Conference in Bordeaux, France—my first solo international trip—Dr Mulekar and his wife, Mrs Smita Mulekar, were kind enough to care for me as guardians. His contributions to shaping my career, advancing my research, and connecting

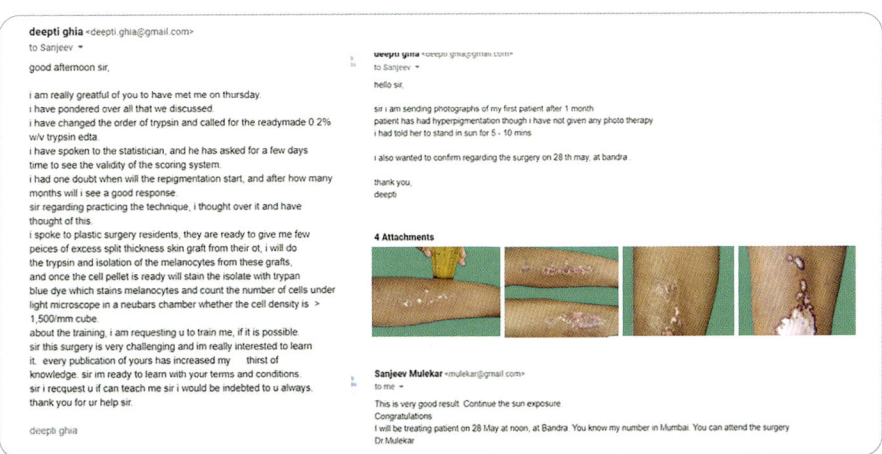

E-mails with Dr Sanjeev Mulekar

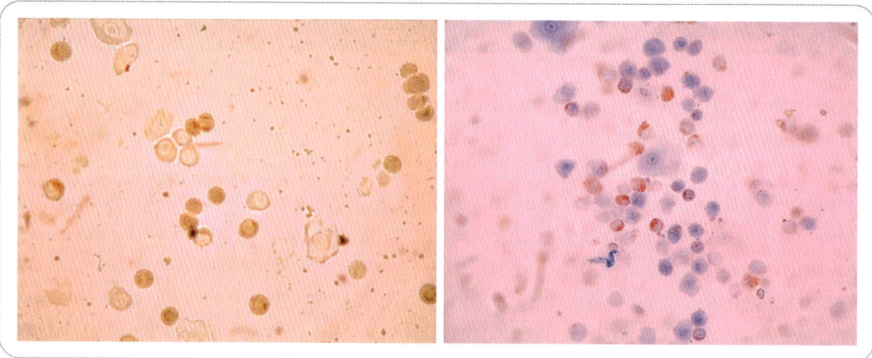

Trypan Blue Staining of Cell Suspension.

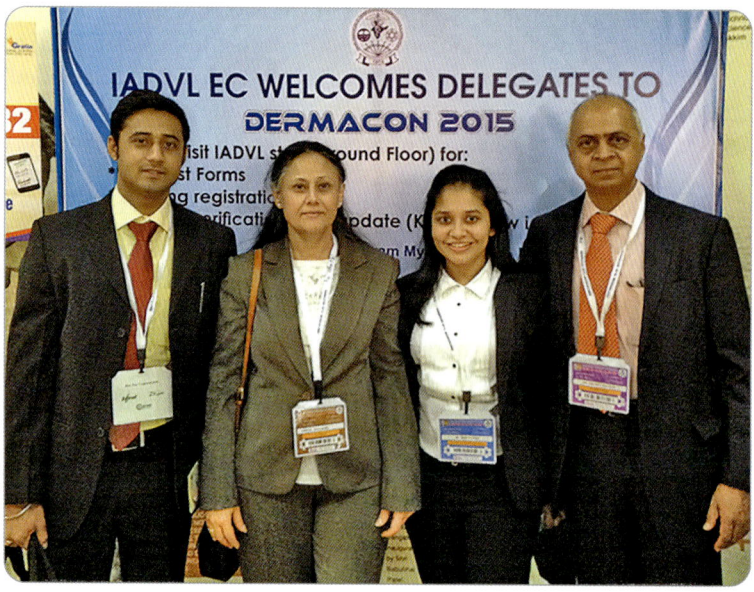

With Swapnil Mulekar, Smita Mulekar, and Dr Sanjeev Mulekar at Dermacon 2015.

me with the international vitiligo research community are invaluable. I had the privilege of working with him and spending quality time during the peak of his career.

Dr Mulekar's mentorship was not just pivotal for my thesis but became a cornerstone of my entire professional journey. His unwavering support, expert guidance, and generous encouragement left an indelible mark on my approach to research and patient's care. Through his teachings, he inspired me to strive for excellence, remain humble, and give back to the community. He was not merely a mentor but a role model whose influence continues to shape my career. I am deeply grateful for his belief in me and for being a guiding light in my journey through vitiligo.

Section 3: Iltefat H Hamzavi

It was so much joy, sadness, and longing as I have written these reflections on Dr Sanjeev Mulekar. When someone passes away you often think about their legacy and how he made you feel. You remember them because you miss them, but you also want to pass on their teachings to the next generation of leaders. Here is a list of points, I hope, that will endear their readers to Dr Mulekar.
1. Be confident in your work. He started working at a time when the Western countries were waking up to contributions from the East. He knew that he had something special to share with his work on vitiligo surgery. He worked so hard in submitting so many articles which were rejected by many journals till he found success.
2. Give credit to others. Dr Mulekar would often credit people like Mats Olsson, Yvon Gauthier, Somesh Gupta, Davinder Parsad, and many others for their work on vitiligo surgery. But, he also described his modifications in harvesting, processing, and skin preparation that made his protocols the one we followed in the United States of America.
3. Take joy in your work. Dr Mulekar was a man full of joy. Whether it was playing in the snow with our children in Detroit or caring for his patients with his wonderful wife Smita, there was joy. He was curious and confident at the same time.
4. Be patient with people and learn to work with others you disagree with. Dr Mulekar struggled to find long-term partners, but he worked with everyone across the globe. He would meet them where they were at. His results for patients with vitiligo were so dramatic that everyone wanted to give him a chance.
5. Be curious. Medicine is a vast field and there is so much we do not know. But, when we find our small area of comfort we often stop branching out. Dr Mulekar always worked to find new ways to do vitiligo surgery. Whether it was lasers, new cell processing kits or new dressings he was always willing to learn and team. He also wanted to keep the techniques of vitiligo surgery affordable. One innovation was to use an egg incubator to replace the expensive cell incubators we used in the United States. For a man, who was one of the first Indians to have front page, first author article in the Journal of the American Medical Association (JAMA) Dermatology, it was a testament to the range of his intellect and personality.

My father was born in India and never forgot the impact of its beautiful languages. He would recite a couplet in Urdu that I cannot trace the source for, but I believe that it is appropriate. *"We do not grieve your loss since we will all die. We grieve the loss of the key to the treasure of knowledge that was your life's work. That is irreplaceable."*

Dr Mulekar Academic Accomplishments:
- MBBS, Topiwala National Medical College and BYL Nair Charitable Hospital, Mumbai, 1977

- MD (Dermatology), Topiwala National Medical College and BYL Nair Charitable Hospital, Mumbai, 1993
- DVD, Topiwala National Medical College and BYL Nair Charitable Hospital, Mumbai, 1980
- Cover of JAMA*
- Over 20 groundbreaking papers
- One of the founders of Indian, Saudi Arabian, and American Vitiligo Surgery

Dr Mulekar and the Henry Ford Team **(Figs. 1 to 3)**

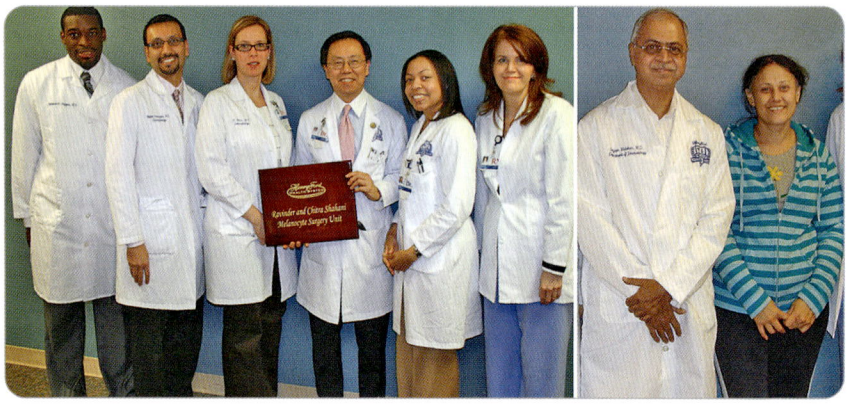

FIG. 1: Dr Mulekar and the Henry Ford team.

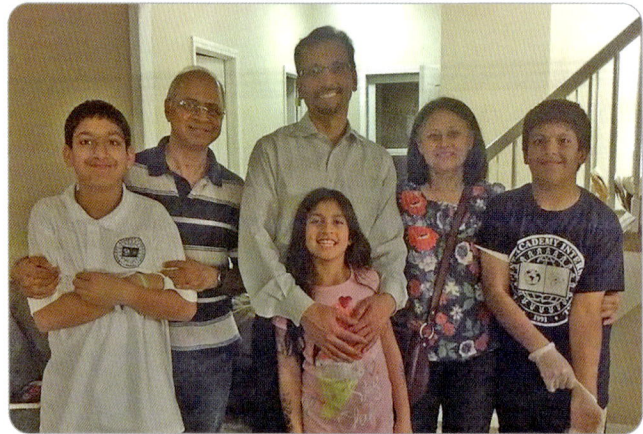

FIG. 2: Dr Mulekar, Smita Mulekar with the Hamzavi family in Detroit Michigan.

---

*Mulekar SV. Long-term follow-up study of segmental and focal vitiligo treated by autologous, noncultured melanocyte-keratinocyte cell transplantation. Arch Dermatol. 2004;140(10):1211-5. Now known as JAMA Dermatology.

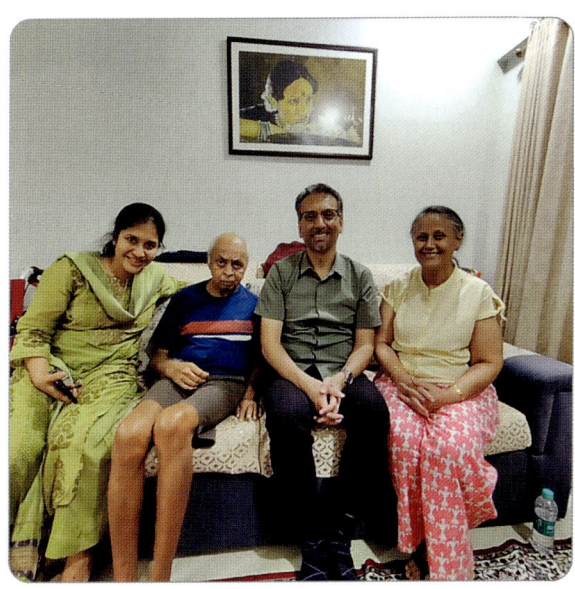

FIG. 3: Dr Mulekar, Smita Mulekar, Dr Deepti Ghia, and Dr Iltefat Hamzavi in Mumbai 2023.

Section 4: Munish Paul

It is said that sometimes you choose a path and sometimes the path chooses you.

I joined MD Dermatology in the year 1995 and was given my thesis "Topic as Oral Mini Pulse Therapy in Vitiligo" under Dr CR Srinivas. Little did I know that vitiligo would over the years become my specialty, my core branch, and my main focus of work literally for the rest of my life.

At Manipal, we got trained in "Phototherapy, punch grafting, and blister grafting" and I applied that in my practice at New Delhi to a huge number of vitiligo patients.

Even though we were repigmenting patients medically and surgically the results were far from perfect. And then a patient of mine got operated by Dr Sajeev Mulekar (I think in 2004) and I was literally blown away by the beautiful results, the excellent color, and texture matching.

Dr Mulekar used to operate with Dr Mukesh at that time, so I approached him, and he very graciously agreed to train me.

That was the start of a beautiful relationship way back in 2005 that is almost 20 years ago.

He literally handheld and trained me in cell transfer from taking grafts, dermabrading, cell separation, etc. Ma'am (Mrs Mulekar) used to accompany him when he used to operate in our center. We used to see the patients together, operate together followed by long discussions on patient's management, the need to publish, the need to present work, and share knowledge. Also, we used to discuss so much about life, family, etc.

Around that time, he joined Saudi and was operating in many more countries worldwide, but we were in touch, catching up in various conferences we were co-panelists sometimes or speakers in the same session and we used to always sit down after the lectures for our catching up and discussions.

I always remember him as a very simple, honest, and straightforward person, guess he was so straight in his thoughts that some people mistook it as arrogance; but, he was a simple man who meant no harm to anyone he was a physician and a surgeon and lived very modestly he did not understand business which is sad but good in a way.

It is amazing how one person can make such a big change and an impact on so many people's life; he was one of the pioneers to introduce cell transfer in vitiligo in India and he shared his work for me, Dr Mukesh, Dr Deepti, and so many. And through all of us so many more received trainings and so on. If we were to trace back the number of vitiligo patients who were benefited over the last 20 years, it would touch thousands. Is not it amazing how one person can make such a difference!

During one of the conferences, I felt him a bit slowed down and having a stretched skin on the face and I asked him if he was well and I told him to go and meet a neurologist as I suspected parkinsonism, he was taken aback but when he went to Mumbai the neurologist confirmed that. Unfortunately, he had a severe parkinsonism and his health deteriorated during the coronavirus disease (COVID) times.

We met him at his flat in Mumbai with Dr Deepti and it was so sad to see him in that situation and even though ma'am and his son tried their best we eventually lost him.

But, thanks to efforts made by Dr Deepti and others, an oration was started in his name recognizing his contribution to the subject of vitiligo.

We started "Vitiligo Foundation of India" with the blessings of so many senior dermatologists of India and held its first workshop/conference in Delhi which was a grand success with more than 250 delegates focused only on one subject, i.e., vitiligo. A full-day conference, Mrs Mulekar was gracious enough to join us and share her knowledge.

Since 1995, my main focus of work has been vitiligo that is almost 30 years. Patients of vitiligo have to go through so much pain, frustration, rejections, and discrimination in life that it literally snatches away their happiness, their souls, and their zest for life. We still do not have all the answers, but we are on the journey, the path to help so many people; every little development is like a stepping stone toward the bigger goal and I think that is the purpose of our life to make a difference in other people's life.

I feel so blessed that Dr Mulekar was my teacher, mentor, friend, philosopher, and guide and I feel that he still guides me and pushes me to do more.

Some call it coincidence I call it magic and destiny. Even a small pebble thrown in a still pond, it can create ripples and waves which may extend into infinity; that is what he did and that is what we should all strive to.

Love and Joy to everyone. Keep learning keep teaching ......

INDEX

Page numbers followed by *b* refer to box, *f* refer to figure, *fc* refer to flowchart, and *t* refer to table.

A

Activated T cells, nuclear factor of 57
Adenosine triphosphate 16
Adhesion 154
Adipose tissue extracellular fraction 171
Adjunct therapy 128
Adrenal corticotropic hormone 147
Aerobic incubator 96*f*
Afamelanotide 8, 59, 171
Afzelin 168
Airbrush technique 159
Alopecia areata 48
Alpha melanocyte-stimulating hormone 171
Alpha-lipoic acid 59, 166
Alpha-melanocyte-stimulating hormone 59
Ammi majus 116
Ammi majus linnaeus 3
Angelica dahurica 12
Animal studies 167
Antiatherogenesis 167
Antibacterial 168
Antibiotics 59
Anticancer 167, 168
Anti-CXCL10 antibodies 67
Antigen-presenting cells 5
    activation of 20
Anti-inflammatory 166
Anti-interferon-gamma 67
Antioxidant 59, 60, 166, 167
    defenses 16
    therapies 16
Antiviral 167, 168
Apigenin 168
Apoptosis 22
    inhibition of 167
Apremilast 8, 58, 60
Atopic dermatitis 48

Autoimmune
    cytotoxicity aggravates intrinsic defects 21
    diseases 14
    disorders 135
    hypothesis 14
    pathways 15
    response 20
    T cells, role of 63
Autoimmunity, evidence of 14
Azathioprine 5, 56, 60, 137

B

Baicalin 168
Baricitinib 47, 66
Basal cell cancer 121
Basal melanocytes 92*f*
Beta-fibroblast growth factor 46
Bimatoprost 8
Biochemical markers 32
Body dysmorphic disorder 147
Body surface area 58, 176, 177
Bone morphogenic protein 145
Broadband ultraviolet B 116
Broad-spectrum formulations 128
Butin 168

C

Calcineurin inhibitors 4, 43-45, 63
Calcipotriol 45
Calcitonin gene-related peptide 17
Calcium dysregulation 19
Camouflage
    application of 161
        techniques of 157
    cream 157
    preparation, ingredients of 155*t*
    removal of 159
    techniques 156

Index

Cannabidiol 168
Capsaicin 167
Catalase 32, 46
Catecholamines 32
Cell
   death debris 19*f*
   suspension, preparation of 95
Cellular grafting 100*f*
   principle of 92
   techniques, indications for 93
Cellular stability, concept of 38
Centipeda cunninghamii 172
Chemical triggers 16
Chemokines 15, 48
Circulating autoantibodies 51
Cobblestoning after mini-punch grafting 77*f*
Cognitive-behavioral therapy 147
Combination therapies 68
Complex disease 133
Consumables 94
Coronavirus disease 212
Corticosteroid 43, 44, 60, 177, 178
Cosmetic camouflage 153
   application of 161*f*
   impact of 160
   indications of 158*t*
   limitations of 162
Cryotherapy 106
Cultured epidermal suspension transplantation 170
Cultured epidermis 103
Cultured melanocytes 103
Cultured pure melanocyte transplantation 40
CXC motif chemokine 10 58
Cyanoacrylate gel 140*f*
Cyclic adenosine monophosphate 58
Cyclosporine 5, 51, 57, 58, 60
Cytokine 15
   dysregulation 64
Cytopenias 57
Cytotoxic
   CD8+ T cells 63
   T cells 15, 19*f*, 20

D

Danger-associated molecular patterns 20
Decapeptide 8
Delgocitinib 66
Dendritic cells 6, 47
Deoxyribonucleic acid 116
   methylation of 166
Depigmentation 112*f*, 115, 176
Dermatological life quality index 176
Dermatological treatments 150
Dermatology life quality index 127, 160
Dermatology resident 207
Dermatoscope, role of 38
Dermis 92*f*
Dermoepidermal junction with basal melanocytes 92*f*
Dermoscopy 31
Dicaffeoylquinic acid 168
Diet 166
   role of 165
Diphencyprone diphenylcyclopropenone 106
Disease chronicity 68
Dismutase superoxide 46
Donor site, preparation of 75
Donor skin, harvesting of 95
Dulbecco's modified eagle's medium 95, 97*f*
Dupilumab 67

E

Ebers papyrus 12
Egulatory T-cells 15
Electrolyte imbalances 58
Endoplasmic reticulum 21
Environmental triggers 12, 16
Epidermis 92*f*
Epigallocatechin-3-gallate 167, 168
Epigenetic factors 22
Epigenetic modifications 14
Epigmenting laser therapy 7*t*
Epitope spreading 21
Ethylenediaminetetraacetic acid 95, 96*f*
Excimer laser therapy, administration of 123
Extracellular exosomes 19*f*
Extracellular vesicles 22
Extracted hair follicles 99*f*
Eyebrow 141
Eyelids 139

F

Family history and heritability 13
Fatty-acid peroxyl 59
Filgotinib 66

First-degree relatives, incidence in 13
Fisetin 168
Flavonoids 168
Flip-top pigment transplantation 88*t*
   technique 86
Fluorouracil 170
Folic acid 166
Follicular and epidermal suspension 99*f*
Follicular unit transplantation 170
Fractional CO_2 laser 89, 170
   therapy, combination drugs of 170
Free radical scavenger 166
Full concealment 154
Full-body units 120

G

Galangin 168
Gastric intolerance 57, 58
Genetic factors 13, 22
Genetic predispositions 12
Genetic susceptibility loci 14
Genome-wide association studies 13
Giant congenital melanocytic nevus 173
Gingival hyperplasia 58
Ginkgo biloba 167
   extracts 59
Glutathione peroxidase 32
Grafting techniques 74*b*
   developments in 73
   types of 74
Grafts
   harvesting of 75, 78
   procedure and transfer of 75, 78
Green tea 167
Growth retardation 56

H

Hair
   follicle cell suspension 91, 99, 99*f*
   follicle grafting 84, 87*t*
   melanin extraction from 157
Handheld excimer lamp 123
Handheld narrowband ultraviolet B 121*f*
Handheld units 120
Handling sweat and friction 162
Harvesting donor skin 96*f*
Harvesting split thickness skin 96*f*
Heat shock proteins 20
Heliotherapy 116
Hepatocellular carcinoma 172

Hepatotoxicity 57
Herbal supplements 167
Hesperetin 168
Heterogeneous response 68
Home phototherapy 124
   reduction for 125
Hormone analogues 59
Human leukocyte antigen 14
Humoral immunity 39
Hydrogen peroxide 46
Hydroxyindoleacetic acid 146
Hydroxyl radicals 59
Hyperglycemia 58
Hyperoside 168
Hypertrichosis 56
Hypothalamic–pituitary–adrenal 17, 56, 147

I

Ibuprofen, role of 127
Imiquimod 106
Immune
   modulation 167
   modulators 21
   privilege in skin, loss of 21
   suppression 56
   tolerance 22
Immunomodulating agent 167
Immunomodulatory 166
Immunosuppressants 56, 60
Inflammatory cytokines 17
Infliximab 7
Ingle-cell RNA sequencing 15
Inhibits lipoxygenase 59
Inhibits platelet coagulation 166
Inhibits T-cell activation 166
Instruments 94
Intercellular adhesion molecule-1 5
Interferon gamma induced chemokine 165
Interleukin 17, 20, 22, 39, 68, 146, 173
   inhibitors 67
Intracellular redox status 165
Intrinsic defects 21
Issue-resident memory T cells 68

J

Janus kinase 4, 6, 13, 22, 47, 58, 63, 171
   inhibitors 47, 48, 58, 170
      representation of 65*f*
Jodhpur technique 170

K

Kaempferia galanga 168
Kaempferol 168
Keratinocyte 92*f*
  corticotropin-releasing hormone 146
  separated 92*f*
Khellin 167
Koebner phenomenon 2, 17, 37

L

Laser
  in depigmentation 108
  irradiation, immediate frosting after 110*f*
  role of 105
Laser-assisted grafting 86
Latanoprost 8
Lesions, classification of 177
Leukotrichia 31
Light amplification 45
Lip 138
  vitiligo 140*f*
Liposomes 49
Lip-tip involvement 28
Liquiritigenin 168
Liquiritin 168
Local innate immunity 21

M

Maintenance therapy 48
Matrix metalloproteinase 49
Melanin-concentrating hormone receptor 15
Melanin-loaded solid lipid nanoparticles 157
Melanocyte 16, 146
  death 146
    chemical mediators of 147
  detachment mechanisms 165
  development 149*f*
  and function 145
  ectodermal origin of 145
  functional 19
  improvement of 151*f*
  intrinsic defects 19
  promotion of 171
  replication 167
  stem cell
    activation 171
    therapies 22
  stress 22

Melanocyte-specific
  autoantibodies 15
  cytotoxic CD8 cells 38
Melanocytorrhagy 64
  theory 51
Melanogenesis, increases 166
Menstrual irregularities 56
Mesenchymal stem cells 22, 171
Mesh grafting 84, 88*t*
Methotrexate 51, 57, 60, 137
Methoxsalen 43
Microneedling 46
Microphthalmia-associated transcription factor 145
Microskintm skin camouflage kit 156
Miniature-punch grafting 76*f*
Minigraft testing 31
Minimal erythema dose 172
Mini-punch grafting 74, 74*b*, 87*t*, 142*f*
Minocycline 6, 59, 60
Mitochondrial dysfunction 16, 19
Mitogen-activated protein kinase 146
Modified silver's knife 96*f*
Mometasone 46
Monobenzyl ether of hydroquinone 16, 105
  reaction to 107
Monoclonal antibodies against CD-20 68
Morphological forms of vitiligo 30
Mosaic genetic skin disorder 29*t*
Mucosal vitiligo 28
Mycophenolate mofetil 60

N

Nanodrug delivery system 49, 169*f*
  mechanisms 49*f*
  principles of 170
Nanohydrogel 49
Nanoparticles 49
Nanostructural lipid carriers 157
Naringenin 168
Narrowband ultraviolet B 6, 7, 13, 37, 46, 66, 75, 116, 119, 135, 177, 178, 186
  adverse effects of 121
  chamber 120*f*
  therapy, administration of 121
  units, types of 120
Neoantigens 20
Neodymium-doped yttrium aluminum garnet 105
Neural theory 51
Neurogenic factors 16, 19

Index

Neurokinin-1 receptor 17
Neuropeptides 17
Neurotransmitters 17
Newer repigmenting agent 8*t*
Nigella sativa seed oil 167
Niosomes 49
Nitric oxide 147
Nivolumab 7
Noncoding RNAs 14
Noncultured epidermal cell suspension 207
  transplantation 170
Noncultured epidermal suspension 91, 94, 95*f*, 100*f*, 101*f*
  advantages of 102*b*
  comparison of 102*t*
  disadvantages of 102*b*
  equipment for 94*b*
  principle of 92*f*
Noncultured hair follicle cell suspension
  transplantation 170
Nonsteroidal anti-inflammatory drugs 109
Novel therapeutic targets 22
Numerous monoclonal antibodies 7

O

Oil-based foundations 155
Oil-free foundations 156
Opacity 154
Oral medications 134
Oral minipulse 5, 51
Oral steroids 5
Oral supplements 166
Oral therapy 137
Outer root sheath 92
Oxidative damage 16
Oxidative stress 12, 16, 19, 19*f*, 20, 64
  enhances autoimmunity 21
  increasing 17
  induced cellular damage 20
  theory 51
Oxygen species, reactive 16, 20, 64, 146

P

Panel narrowband ultraviolet B 121*f*
Panel units 120
Pentachrome 30
Pharmacological treatment 44
Phenol 106
Phenolic compounds 16

Phenylalanine 166
Phosphatase 173
Phosphodiesterase 58
Photochemotherapy 118
Phototherapy 86, 137, 211
  mechanism of 116
  non-responders to 127
  sessions, integration with 128
Phyllanthus emblica 167
Pigment blending 154
Piperine 167
Plant-derived compounds 168
Plaque psoriasis 48
Platelet-activating factor antagonist 167
Pluripotent stem cells 171
Plurisegmental 177
Plus ultraviolet A 57
Polyphenol 168
Polypodium leucotomos 167
Post-psoralen 118
Pre-camouflage counseling 159
Pregnancy, phototherapy in 135
Programmed cell death 15
  ligand 15
Proinflammatory cytokines 20, 21
  decreases 167
Promising advanced therapy medicinal products 171
Promotes glutathione synthesis 59
Prostaglandin 46
  E2 46
Protein tyrosine phosphatase non-receptor 14
Pseudocatalase cream 46
Psoralea corylifolia 3, 116
Psoralen 118
  and ultraviolet A therapy 3, 6
  types of 119*t*
  plus ultraviolet A 46
Psychological distress 147
  level of 176
Puerarin 168
Pulse therapy 56
Punch grafting 170

Q

Q-switched ND:YAG laser
  immediate reaction 111*f*
  induced depigmentation 114*f*
  induced full depigmentation of arms 112*f*

sequelae-frost-edema-crust-exfoliation-lightening 113
Quadrichrome 30
Quality of life 147, 176
 health-related 126

R

Radiation, stimulated emission of 45
Reactive oxygen species, generation of 165
Regulates gene expression 166
Regulatory T cells, role of 20
Renal toxicity 58
Renewcell 173
Repigmentation 176
 drugs for 6
Ringer's lactate 81
Ritlecitinib 171
Rituximab 68
Robotic-assisted skin grafting 86
Ruxolitinib 47, 65
 targets janus kinase 6

S

Secukinumab 67
Skin
 camouflage techniques, classification of 154*fc*
 crust 110*f*
 disorders, immune-mediated 48
 graft
  split-thickness 38, 80
  thin 170
  types of split-thickness 80
 microbiome, role of 22
 phototype 176
 repigmentation 22
 tone variations 161
Small molecules 58
Smash graft technique 85
Smash grafting 88*t*
 in beard area 85*f*
Smudging and wear-off 163
Spotted repigmentation after sun exposure 115*f*
Stem cells 22
Stress 146
 enduring cells, multilineage differentiating 171
 hormones, role of 146

Substance P 17
Subtle coverage 155
Suction blister epidermal grafting 74*b*, 78
Suction blister grafting 87*t*, 170
Sun protection 154
Sunlight therapy 13
Sunscreens
 chemical 128
 physical 128
 role of 128
Superoxide dismutase 16, 32
 cofactor for 166
Surgical and adjunctive therapies 91
Surgical modalities 138
Sweat resistance 154
Systemic corticosteroids 56, 63
Systemic drugs, patients treated with 134
Systemic janus kinase inhibitors 63, 65
 safety profile of 67

T

T helper cells 19*f*
Targeting interleukin 22
T-cell
 clones 39
 dysregulation 51
Tensin homolog 173
Test graft, validity of 35, 37
Therapeutic agents, penetrate capacity of 170
Thyroid disease 135
Tissue grafting 73
 history of 72
 techniques 72, 74*b*
Tissue-resident memory 48*t*
 T cells 64, 68
Tofacitinib 47, 48, 60, 66
Tofacitinib cream 48
Toll-like receptors 20
Topical calcineurin inhibitors 4, 135, 137, 138*f*, 177
Topical corticosteroids 4, 63, 135, 136, 177, 178
Topical janus kinase inhibitors 137
Topical psoralen ultraviolet A 137
Topical therapies, types of 43*t*
Topical treatments 43, 44*t*
Transcription pathway, activator of 22
Transcription proteins inhibitors 6
Transcutaneous drug delivery 170

Treatment protocols 59
T-regulatory cells 22
Trichrome 30
Trimester of pregnancy 134
Trioxsalen 43
Tumor necrosis factor alpha 15, 20, 67, 146, 173
Twin studies 13
Typical ingredients 155
Tyrosinase 14, 20
  related proteins 22
Tyrosine kinase 172

U

Ultrathin skin grafting 74b, 80, 81f, 82f
  on leg 83f
Ultrathin split skin grafting 87t
Ultraviolet
  A 116, 118
    instructions 118
    therapy 118
  B 59, 116
  exposure, enhanced sensitivity to 128
  light therapy 37
  radiation 16, 137
  therapy 167
Upadacitinib 66

V

Vasoactive intestinal peptide 17
Vitamin
  B12 166
  C 166
  D 166
  D3 analogs 4
  E 166
Vitexin 168
Vitiliginous patches on face 138f
Vitiligo 1, 65, 72, 73, 84-86, 124, 133, 146
  acrofacial 27
  activity, assessment of 30
  area scoring index 47, 59
  area severity index 31
  biologicals in 7
  blue 30
  camouflaging techniques for 153
  cellular grafting in 91
  childhood 135
  classification of 3, 26, 27t
  contact 29
  cycle of stress and 146
  depigmentation in 105
  disease activity 31, 37, 73
  drugs for stability of 4
  effect of pregnancy on 133
  emerging biologics in 67
  etiology of 13
  focal 28
  Foundation of India 212
  future trends and diet 165
  global issues consensus conference 26, 28
  historical aspects of 2
  impact patient scale 176
  in child 135, 136f
  in pregnancy 133
  International Patient Organizations Committee 183
  light-based therapy in 116
  management of 128, 176
  medical management of 3
  mixed 3, 28
  newer therapy in 7
  nonsegmental 1, 3, 26, 27, 27t, 29t, 177
  occupational 29
  on pregnancy, effect of 134
  over feet 161f
  over hands 161f
  patch on fingertip, micropigmentation over 141f
  patch on medial canthus region 140f
  pathogenesis of 19, 63
  pathogenic mechanisms implicated in 64f
  patient support group board members 182f
  psychosocial
    aspects of 145
    impact of 134, 147
  quality of life with 126, 160
  research, historical context of 12
  segmental 1, 3, 22, 26, 27t, 28, 29t, 82f, 100, 139f, 177
  stability of 35
  surgical management of 133
  systemic treatments in 51, 63
  therapeutic algorithm for 177fc
  therapy 170
    of localized 50
  treatment 43, 47, 169f
    guideline for nonsegmental 178fc

guideline for segmental 178*f*c
modalities for 179*t*
type of 93, 134
unclassified 3
universal 28
vulgaris, patient of 123*f*
Vitiligoid conditions, generalized 29
Vitilinex 172
Vogt–Koyanagi–Harada syndrome 28
Vulvar quality of life index 184

W

Water-based foundations 155
Waterproof 154
Wood's lamp examination 176

Z

Zinc 166